Social Aspects of Health, Illness and Healthcare

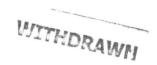

Social Aspects of Health, Illness and Healthcare

Mary Larkin

Open University Press

Open University Press
McGraw-Hill Education
McGraw-Hill House
Shoppenhangers Road
Maidenhead
Berkshire
England
SL6 2QL

email: enquiries@openup.co.uk
world wide web: www.openup.co.uk

and Two Penn Plaza, New York, NY 10121-2289, USA

First published 2011

A catalogue record of this book is available from the British Library

ISBN-13: 978-0-33-523662-6 (pb)   978-0-33-523661-9 (hb)
ISBN-10: 0-33-523662-6 (pb)   0-33-523661-8 (hb)

Library of Congress Cataloging-in-Publication Data
CIP data applied for

Typeset by RefineCatch Limited, Bungay, Suffolk
Printed in the UK by Bell & Bain Ltd, Glasgow

Fictitious names of companies, products, people, characters and/or data that may be used herein (in case studies or in examples) are not intended to represent any real individual, company, product or event.

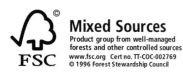

Mixed Sources
Product group from well-managed
forests and other controlled sources
www.fsc.org Cert no. TT-COC-002769
© 1996 Forest Stewardship Council

FSC

The *McGraw-Hill* Companies

Contents

This book is dedicated to my late grandmother – Alice Rebecca Mayhew (1908–2007) – for being such a source of inspiration to me.

Praise for this book

"This is an easy-to-read introductory text exploring the social aspects of health, illness and healthcare. Key concepts are introduced carefully and there is a helpful glossary of key terms. Activities and discussion points enable students to pace their learning and illustrative case studies bring the text to life. In short, this is a gentle yet comprehensive introduction which will no doubt become popular with lecturers and students alike."

Dr Sarah Earle, Associate Dean Research, The Open University, UK

"Larkin's book provides an excellent and accessible read for students studying health related disciplines . . . a useful resource for those new to the subject area of social aspects of health, health care and illness and a good refresher for those that may not have studied the subject for some time or those returning to study. The reader will be left feeling informed around the key issues and theories."

Sabina Sattar, Senior Lecturer, University of Central Lancashire, UK

"I wish to congratulate Mary Larkin for creating such a useful resource. The structure of this book and the writing style employed makes light work of complex subjects. The overview at the beginning of each chapter is useful to signpost the student to the topics covered. Because the book is well explained throughout it would be a useful core text for level 4 5 & 6 modules in pre- and post registration nursing in the UK. Each chapter of this book directs the students reading and the interactive design fosters independent learning. This is a well written comprehensive text and is a 'must' for students in the pursuit of understanding the social aspects of health."

Peggy Murphy, Senior Lecturer (Nursing), Glyndwr University, UK

"Mary Larkin's textbook offers the nursing student a lively insight into many applied aspects of the social aspects of health and illness. It uses a variety of theoretical perspectives, and all concepts are clearly extrapolated. A variety of devices are then utilised to facilitate knowledge and understanding. This is an excellent resource, which I would highly recommend."

Siobhan McCullough, School of Nursing and Midwifery, Queen's University Belfast, UK

"Mary Larkin has written a comprehensive survey of contemporary health issues well suited to the needs of students of social aspects of health. Written in an accessible and lively style, the book covers an impressive range of theoretical approaches and substantive material, complemented by summaries, discussion questions and learning activities, to prompt students to reflect on their reading and to engage with the text."

Hannah Bradby, University of Warwick, UK

"I find this to be one of the most intuitive texts I have read to date as a student. Mary Larkin has an obvious passion for and belief in what she has written, making this all the more enjoyable and interesting to read."

Roisin Kiernan, Student nurse, Queen's University Belfast, UK

List of figures and tables

Figures

Tables

List of figures and tables

Acknowledgements

The publishers would like to thank the copyright holders of the following material for permission to reproduce material in this book:

Before I Say Goodbye by Ruth Picardie, 1998, London, p. 38. Copyright © Ruth Picardie, 1997; and Justine Picardie, 1997. Foreword and Afterwords copyright © Matt Seaton, 1998. Reproduced by permission of Penguin Books Ltd.

"Observer Life, 22 June 1997" from *Before I Say Goodbye* by Ruth Picardie.
Copyright © 2000 by the Estate of Ruth Picardie and Justine Picardie.
Reprinted by arrangement with Henry Holt and Company, LLC.

Every effort has been made to trace and acknowledge ownership of copyright and to clear permission for material reproduced in this book. The publishers will be pleased to make suitable arrangements to clear permission with any copyright holders whom it has not been possible to contact.

Introduction: understanding the social aspects of health

Health is a physiological and psychological state but it is also, fundamentally a social state.

(Jones 1994: 1)

Aims and rationale of the book

This is an introductory text to a wide range of topics within the broad subject area of the social aspects of health. It simultaneously addresses the social aspects of illness and healthcare because health, illness and healthcare are intrinsically intertwined. Without assuming prior knowledge, the book will draw on several academic disciplines and theoretical perspectives in order to provide clear explanations of basic concepts and issues within each topic. A further aim is to help students feel more confident with this subject area and increase their chances of greater success in their courses of study.

The nature and scope of the book mean that it meets many learning and teaching needs. For instance, it can be used by first- and second-year students on undergraduate courses related to health, social care, youth and community work and social work, as a core/supplementary text, and for reference purposes. It is also for use by students taking pre- and post-registration courses in nursing and midwifery. In addition, lecturers can use relevant chapters as a teaching resource to support and reinforce student learning.

This chapter introduces you to the subject of the book, its structure and the topics it covers. Hence careful reading of it will ensure that you know how to maximize its potential benefits for both your current and future study of the 'social aspects of health'. The introduction to the social aspects of health is twofold. First of all, there is a brief historical contextualization to show how western society's views of health evolved and the how realization dawned that there are many social aspects to health. This involves a discussion of the biomedical approach to health, the ways in which it was challenged and the ensuing changes that led to multidimensional views of health more generally, and a greater awareness of the social aspects of health more specifically. The second part of the introduction to the social of aspects health comprises an outline of the way that subsequent changes in the study of health have raised the profile of the social aspects of health across many different levels. These include the fact that the increase in research into the social aspects of health has led to the acknowledgement of an extensive number of social influences on health and the development of theoretical perspectives. The main group of social factors that are now recognized as being central to the study of social aspects of health are then outlined. How these are addressed in the book is explained in the final section of the chapter, in which details of the content, organization and features of the book together with summaries of each chapter are also set out.

Activity 1.1

List all the factors that you think affect your health. Now compare them with those that are discussed below.

Contextualizing the 'social aspects of health'

The rise of biomedicine

Until the middle of the nineteenth century, healthcare was mainly carried out by women within the **private domain**. If medical problems could not be solved, the services of a variety of health practitioners (with or without medical training!) could be called upon in exchange for payment. Examples of these health practitioners include apothecaries (who offered and produced a range of medicines), barber-surgeons (who carried out limited surgical procedures), village herbalists, bone-setters and midwives. There were few hospitals and it was only the rich who could afford to consult learned physicians. In part, the multiple sources of provision were the consequence of minimal knowledge of illness and disease, due to a lack of understanding of anatomy and physiology and the causes of disease. The reality was that most practitioners offered the same treatment based on the same assumptions and relied on ancient theories without exploring or developing them (Pelling and Harrison 2001; Porter 2002).

From the beginning of the sixteenth century onwards, several significant developments laid the foundations for changes in medicine. Amongst these was the Enlightenment, during which geographical exploration and scientific discoveries flourished. For instance, Columbus made his famous voyage to the Americas in 1492 and Copernicus disturbed the received view of the universe in 1507 with his discovery that the Earth revolved around the Sun. In addition, the new 'art' of artists such as Leonardo da Vinci (1452–1519) and Michelangelo (1475–1564) reflected a desire to reach a greater understanding of man and nature by using more accurate representations in paintings and sculpture. One of the consequences of these developments was that the laws of nature had to be reinterpreted and applied in a variety of situations. This involved scientific hypothesizing and empirical testing. Another was that people's knowledge of the human body changed and, more importantly, there was the realization that the only way to find out more about human anatomy and diseases was through the dissection and study of human bodies. These consequences in turn led to new ways of thinking – referred to as **discourses** – in medicine which emphasized the need to 'study' not one sick person, but a group of sick people displaying particular symptoms in order to gain a scientific understanding of disease. As hospitals ensured a plentiful supply of patients for clinical observation and studying anatomy and physiology, these discourses, in combination with the continued growth in 'scientific' theories throughout the eighteenth century, resulted in an expansion in the number of hospitals. Simultaneously, medical practice and education began to develop and change significantly, with an increasing requirement to study organized courses in anatomy, surgery and the administration of medicines as well as undertaking hospital and surgical practice. The number of medical schools in London rose from 3 to 12 between 1820 and 1858. With theoretical and practical education and training, medicine not only developed as a powerful profession in its own right (see Chapter 12) but gradually expanded to encompass a growing number of specialisms as well (Loudon 1997; Naidoo and Wills 2008).

As the impetus to develop medical theory supported by research through the bringing together of clinical observation and pathological research gained momentum, progress in medical science and technology also accelerated rapidly. Among the most notable were the:

- development of new academic and professional subject areas such as bacteriology, germ theory and microbiology;

- introduction of aseptic techniques;

- introduction of anaesthesia;

- technological developments, such as stethoscopes, thermometers, microscopes and X-rays (Wear 1992; Jones 1994; Loudon 1997).

All these developments contributed to the development of **biomedicine**. This draws heavily on scientific knowledge in general and emphasizes scientific method and objectivity (the hypothecodeductive method). It sees health in terms of biology, attaching supreme importance to learning about anatomy and physiology. Consequently the biomedical approach rests on the assumption that all causes of disease – mental disorders as well as physical conditions – can be understood in biological terms. Disease and sickness are therefore explained in terms of their specific or multiple causes, tracking the cause and the course of disease as it affects particular parts of the human body. In addition, disease and sickness are viewed as deviations from normal functioning.

The adoption of biomedicine shaped approaches to health and healthcare until the 1970s. It meant that health was seen largely in mechanical terms, as a state where all parts of the body function 'normally' and there is an 'absence of disease'. Within the biomedical approach, health services are mainly geared to treating sick and disabled people, and their function is remedial or curative. Biomedicine's pathogenic focus, emphasis on risk factors and establishing abnormality also promoted an interest in the health of the population and influenced the growth of the **public health** movement in the nineteenth century (see Chapter 6) (Wear 1992; Jones 1994; Loudon 1997; Pelling *et al.* 2001).

Challenges to biomedicine

Questions were raised about the effects of medical progress inherent in the biomedical approach from the beginning of the twentieth century, and in the 1960s the level of questioning escalated with the result that direct challenges were made to biomedicine. A main protagonist was Illich (1976) who argued that biomedicine did more harm than good and highlighted its damaging effects. He put forward the theory of **iatrogenesis** which he used to refer to the harmful and detrimental effects of medical interventions, such as hospital-induced infections and adverse reactions to medical treatment. Such harm does not occur in the absence of medicine and medical practice and hence is medically caused. There are different types of iatrogenesis within Illich's theory and these are discussed in depth in Chapter 6 (Jones 1994; Naidoo and Wills 2008).

There were also those who challenged biomedicine's view of mental illness as being biologically caused. They disagreed with the way that its focus on normal bodily functioning led biomedicine to see mental illness as being due to biochemical changes in the brain. One of the outcomes of this dissension was the formation of the **anti-psychiatry movement** which was particularly active in the 1960s and 1970s. This movement criticized traditional theory and practice in psychiatry, arguing that this was incorrect and that mental illness was not a deviation from normal bodily functioning but created by social processes, such as labelling (see Chapter 7) (Szasz 1974; Rogers and Pilgrim 2005).

The move to a multidimensional view of health

In response to such challenges to 'scientific' techniques and drug treatments, the many factors that influence health started to be identified. For instance:

- **psychological factors:** the rise of psychology highlighted the role of psychological factors, such as the link between emotional stress and illness, on our health;

- **social divisions:** the role of social divisions such as class, income, race, gender and age in shaping health emerged from several reports about health inequalities, such as the *Black Report* (Black *et al.* 1980) and *The Health Divide* (Whitehead 1987);

- **economic and social differences:** the World Health Organization (WHO) drew attention to the poorer health experienced by those living in developing countries compared to those living in the developed world, due to economic and social differences;

- **environmental factors:** the effects of environmental factors, such as work environments and housing and air quality, were acknowledged from the 1960s, and this was reflected in the public health acts, slum clearance programmes and pollution controls introduced at that time;

- **healthcare delivery systems:** research demonstrated the varying impacts of the different healthcare delivery systems nationally and internationally.

As a result of the recognition of the multitude of factors that need to be taken into consideration when talking about health, there has been a move towards a more holistic approach to defining health in the last 50 years. This was encapsulated in the World Health Organization's definition in 1946: 'Health is a state of complete physical, mental and social well being, not merely the absence of disease or infirmity'. This definition was significant as it highlighted the importance of a multidimensional view of health for the first time. Subsequent definitions have promoted even broader conceptions of health which also go beyond the narrow focus on 'scientific' biological conceptions of health in the biomedical discourse, and emphasize its social and environmental dimensions. For example:

> to reach a state of complete physical, mental and social well-being, an individual or group must be able to identify and realise aspirations, to satisfy needs, and to change or cope with the environment. Health is therefore seen as a resource for everyday life, not the objective of living. Health is a positive concept, emphasising social and personal resources, as well as physical capacities.
>
> (World Health Organization 1986: 100)

Although there is evidence that western 'scientific' biological conceptions of health still dominate, as these definitions testify, there has been a move away from a purely clinical focus. In addition, there has been professional and public acceptance that there are a wide range of influences on health. Furthermore, as indicated in the reference to health as a 'positive concept' in the last sentence of the second definition of health above, there are now a variety of conceptualizations of health. Currently there are four main concepts in current use: *negative, positive* and *social* health, and *quality of life*. As demonstrated in the outline of each concept below, their understandings of health range in breadth from narrow to very wide.

- **Negative health:** this concept emphasizes the absence of symptoms and regards being healthy as *not* feeling unwell, and/or *not* having a diagnosed illness or disease. However, only 15 per cent of the general population in a western society will have chronic physical limitations and only some 10–20 per cent will have a substantive psychiatric impairment. Therefore, using the negative concept of health where the focus is on departure from health means there is no information about the remaining 80–90 per cent of the population.

- **Positive health:** the concept of positive health is more than the mere absence of disease or disability and is therefore a broader concept than the narrower disease-based concept of negative health. It refers to a positive state of well-being, 'equilibrium' or fitness and energy, all of which are required to function effectively from day to day (often referred to as *functional ability*). This concept of health has many distinct components which focus on both mental and physical health – it can be described as embracing the ability to cope with stressful situations, the maintenance of a strong social support system, integration into the community, high morale and life satisfaction, psychological well-being and high levels of physical fitness as well as physical health.

- **Social health:** the third concept of social health presents a broader view of health again, in that it goes beyond the reporting of symptoms, illness and the ability to meet the demands of everyday life. It focuses on the extent of a person's **social support** systems (e.g. the extent of their social interaction and social participation) and argues that these influence mental and physical health.

Although social health incorporates physical and mental health, it is measured apart from physical and mental health.

- **Quality of life:** this multidimensional concept is the broadest of the four. While it lacks definitional consensus, it generally refers to a range of components relating to satisfaction with life, general levels of physical and mental health, satisfaction with economic and social status, sense of self-worth, social health and functional ability (Currer and Stacey 1986; Blaxter 1990).

The focus on the social aspects of health

As indicated above, the adoption of a multidimensional view of health from the 1980s meant a general acknowledgment of the fact that there were social aspects to health. Since then, interest in and research into these has burgeoned. The social dimensions of health have been the subject of major government reports, and in 1980 the *Black Report* (mentioned above) highlighted the persistence of correlations between social class and infant mortality rates, life expectancy and inequalities in the use of medical services. In 1998 the *Independent Inquiry into Inequalities in Health Report*, headed by Donald Acheson, came to similar conclusions as the *Black Report* as it also found health inequalities in the UK and that poverty was a significant determinant of health. During the first decade of this century, the number and range of social influences on health that feature in policy documents that address health and health inequalities has increased. Examples are housing, communities, education, level and type of early years support for children and families, access to public services and unemployment (Department of Health 1999, 2003).

Moreoever, there has been a growing emphasis on the **social determinants of health** at local, national and global levels. These are the economic, political and social conditions under which people live and which determine their health. The term 'social determinants of health' grew out of the search to identify the specific factors which lead to members of different socioeconomic groups experiencing varying degrees of health and illness. This search gathered momentum and in 2005 the World Health Organization established the Commission on Social Determinants of Health (CSDH) to support countries in addressing the social factors that lead to health inequalities. As part of its remit, the CSDH draws attention to those social determinants of health that are known to be among the worst causes of poor health and inequalities between and within countries. These determinants include unemployment, unsafe workplaces, urban slums, **globalization** and lack of access to health systems. Indeed, the Commission's recent report embodied principles of action aimed at addressing these in its recommendations (Commission on Social Determinants of Health 2008). Simultaneously, there has also been an emphasis on the social determinants of **global health** such as pollution, climate change, environmental degradation, conflict between countries, domestic and foreign policies, international trade and the role of international health organizations and development agencies (Marmot and Wilkinson 2006; Department of Health 2008a).

One of the consequences of the surge of activity around the social aspects of health is that their identified number and range has increased dramatically. They now include several groups of factors. One is the effect of income, employment, unemployment, social class, gender, race, age, education and culture on health. A second is the impact of social environmental factors such as housing, neighbourhoods and communities, support systems and conditions at work. A third group comprises particular features of a **society**, such as the distribution of power, money, resources, goods, the strength of its public sector and the accountability of its private sector, and its social and economic policies, which are now regarded as key influences on health. The provision and delivery of healthcare, access to healthcare, and the systems put in place for health protection, health improvement and to deal with illness, have also received much attention. Last but not least, as mentioned above, global factors (e.g. globalization and the impact of climate change on health) have more recently featured in research and reports into the social aspects of health.

A further consequence is the steady growth of a body of theoretical approaches that acknowledge there are a broad range of social factors that can influence health, and that health is the result of the complex interactions that occur between such factors. Indeed, the concept of the 'social model of health' is now used within the field of health (Lupton 1996; Earle 2005).

Content and structure

Organization of the content

This book provides a comprehensive and contemporary exploration of the factors mentioned above which are now recognized as being key social aspects of health. The material has been organized in terms of the following three broad themes:

■ The relationship between social categories and health.

■ The experience of health and illness.

■ The delivery of healthcare.

These themes will be adopted as headings for the three main sections of the book. The first chapter will furnish the reader with an understanding of the academic and theoretical underpinnings of the social aspects of health required to study this subject area. In order to reinforce and develop students' understanding further, the theoretical perspectives introduced in Chapter 1 will be revisited during the course of the book and applied to the issues addressed. Although the intention is that the chapters can be read independently, it is strongly suggested that readers familiarize themselves with the material presented in Chapter 1 in order to gain a fundamental intellectual and theoretical knowledge of the social aspects of health before starting any of the other chapters.

The chapters within each section of the book present a detailed exploration of a specific topic, drawing on a wide range of literature and documents from many different sources as well as recent statistical data. While the emphasis will be on the contemporary UK, material will also be drawn from historical, European and wider international contexts as the need arises. The nature and extent of the discussions of theoretical perspectives in each chapter will vary according to the topic addressed and be supplemented with other perspectives relevant to specific issues as appropriate. In addition, these theoretical discussions will either be integrated into the individual sections of the chapters or addressed in separate sections. This variation in approach is designed to ensure that the material is organized in a way that makes the presentation of each topic as accessible as possible to the reader.

Reference has already been made to the interactions that occur between factors within the social aspects of health. Although the chapters appear as discrete entities, this form of organization is to enable you to gain a comprehensive overview of each topic. Any interactions between the factors addressed in each chapter will be acknowledged where appropriate.

Chapter features

Every effort has been made to ensure that the text is as readable and interactive as possible. Features include the following.

- An overview of each chapter.

- An outline of the content and structure of each chapter. This will include details of the way in which the relevant theoretical perspectives will be addressed.

- Key concepts will be highlighted in the text the first time they are used and are clearly defined in the glossary at the end of the book. The glossary provides relevant understandings for those with differing levels of social science knowledge. Its comprehensive nature means that it can also be used independently for reference purposes across a range of other modules and/or courses.

- Activities based on extracts from primary sources (e.g. case studies, historical documents, news-paper articles, policy documents and statistical data). In the 'Activity feedback' chapter that precedes the glossary, some suggestions and comments are made to help the reader reflect on their work on the activities and relate issues to relevant theoretical perspectives. Some of the activities can also be used and/or adopted by lecturers and tutors for workshops and class-room discussions. The presentation of these activities is designed to reinforce and support students' learning as opposed to being essential to the main text in each chapter. They are easily identified as they are presented in boxes and can be omitted by those students who do not require them.

- Links with other chapters are highlighted.

- Figures and tables to illustrate key concepts and data.

- Discussion points for either individual study or teaching purposes.

- Suggestions for further study and reading, plus web resources.

Chapter outlines
Section 1: The relationship between social categories and health
Chapter 1: Studying the social aspects of health
This chapter begins with outlines of the main academic disciplines that inform the study of the social aspects of health. The theoretical perspectives that will be used and referred to in the book are then addressed. Several key concepts and issues that will be frequently discussed are also intro-duced in this first chapter.

Chapter 2: Gender and health
The concept of 'gender' is defined at the beginning of this chapter. This is followed by an explora-tion of the differences in men and women's physical and mental health and the types of factors that shape these differences. The final section of the chapter discusses the theoretical explanations that have been developed about the relationship between gender and health.

Chapter 3: Social class and health
At the beginning of this chapter is an exploration of the concept of class. This includes class as a form of social stratification and the different conceptualizations of class used in theoretical approaches and social research. The relationship between social class and health is then explored by

examining relevant data on morbidity and mortality rates, the influences on this relationship and the insights provided by key theoretical explanations.

Chapter 4: Ethnicity and health
The concepts of ethnicity and race are distinguished before defining ethnicity and outlining the main minority ethnic groups in the UK. An overview of current findings about the different types of physical and mental illnesses experienced by members of these minority ethnic groups follows. The role of income and poverty levels, housing and healthcare in the health inequalities identified are considered before evaluating the explanations of the relationship between ethnicity and health that have been developed.

Chapter 5: Ageing and health
This chapter starts by examining the concept of age itself before moving on to discuss the relationship between the life course and our physical and mental health. Given the strength of the relationship between ill health and old age, there is then an in-depth exploration of this phase of the life course. This includes a discussion of the life course perspective and relevant research findings.

Section 2: The experience of health and illness
Chapter 6: Experiencing illness
The emphasis in this chapter is on the experience of illness in general. It starts by explaining the differences between acute and chronic illness, and then examines the theoretical insights into the experience of both these types of illness that have been developed. The last section explores how our experience of illness is shaped by changing definitions of illness and disease, and refers specifically to the medicalization thesis and the rise of health surveillance.

Chapter 7: Experiencing mental illness
This chapter starts with an overview of mental illness and its incidence. It then outlines the two main types of explanation of mental illness within the study of the social aspects of health. These outlines include discussions of models that have been developed to explain mental illness. This is followed by an in-depth exploration of the experiences of those who live with a mental illness, and how these and the interrelationships between them can lead to their exclusion from many aspects of life in our society.

Chapter 8: Experiencing disability
As the experience of disability is very much shaped by societal approaches to it, this chapter looks at the changes in definitions and models of disability that have occurred over time. Examples of disabled people's life experiences in contemporary society are then discussed. These examples illustrate the way that disability still leads to discrimination and inequality, despite the improvements in our approach to those who are disabled in our society.

Chapter 9: Dying, death and grieving
This chapter considers the contribution that the study of the social aspects of health has made to understandings of dying, death and grieving. In so doing, it explores the evidence and arguments that these experiences are strongly influenced by both the personal and social contexts in which they take place. The social context is the main focus as this is the specific area to which the study

of the social aspects of health has made the most contributions. The chapter ends with a discussion of possible theoretical interpretations of the material presented.

Section 3: The delivery of healthcare

Chapter 10: Families, communities and healthcare

In order to address the policy initiatives that have moved the care of both the acutely and chronically ill out of formal healthcare organizations and into the community, this chapter explores the two concepts which are central to the changes involved: the 'family' and 'community'. It then discusses these policy trends and, more specifically, the increases in informal healthcare they necessitate. The implications for family members providing the additional care and for those receiving it, as well as the issue of the 'community' as a source of the informal support required, are also explored.

Chapter 11: Healthcare organizations

The focus of this chapter is the organization and delivery of formal healthcare. It is divided into three sections. This first explains what the terms 'organization' and 'healthcare organizations' mean, the second examines examples of theoretical approaches to healthcare organizations and the third evaluates the main changes that have been made to healthcare organization in recent decades.

Chapter 12: Health professions

This final chapter explores the meaning, the extent and some of the implications of the power of those professionals who deliver healthcare. In order to do this, it explores the concepts of 'profession', 'professional socialization' and 'professionalization' in relation to both the medical profession and other health professions. It then considers the different ways that professional power has been found to operate in healthcare by examining changes in the power of health professions and the challenges to the autonomy of the medical profession.

Key points

- The evolution of western society's views of health has led to multidimensional views of health.

- There is now a greater awareness of the social aspects of health and it is widely acknowledged that there is an extensive number of social influences on our health.

- The range of social influences on our health and theoretical perspectives within the study of the social aspects is constantly changing as further research is undertaken.

Discussion points

- What are the advantages and disadvantages of the biomedical approach to health?

- What recent examples of iatrogenesis can you think of?

- To what extent are varying concepts of health useful?

Suggestions for further study

- Webster (2001) provides a highly readable account of the historical development of health-care systems if you wish to explore this further.

- More detailed explanations of the different concepts and models of health can be found in Chapter 1 in Taylor and Hawley (2010).

- A visit to the World Health Organization website will provide a wealth of information about definitions of health and the factors that influence health.

Studying the social aspects of health

1

Theories are lenses through which we investigate the social world.

(de Maio 2010: 28)

Overview

Introduction

The main aim of this chapter is to provide you with the understandings you require before embarking on your study of the social aspects of health. These understandings will also help you to apply your knowledge of this subject area in any professional roles you undertake. Comprehensive outlines of relevant academic disciplines and theoretical perspectives are provided. These can be used for reference purposes when reading specific chapters in the book and during any future study of the social aspects of health you may undertake. To further assist you with your current and future explorations of the social aspects of health, towards the end of the chapter there is an explanation about how health data are used and a summary of the established influences on health.

Academic underpinnings

Although several disciplines inform the study of the social aspects of health, it is the sociology of health and illness and the sociology of the body which are most frequently drawn upon. As the discipline of sociology underpins the sociology of health and illness, this section starts with an overview of this subject. The nature and scope of both the sociology of health and illness and the sociology of the body will then be explored, together with their contributions to knowledge about the social aspects of health.

Sociology

Activity 1.1

Which do you think is the most accurate description of sociology?

- Social work

- The study of individuals

- The study of society

- The study of the human social world

- The study of individuals and society

Sociology is the systematic study of the human social world or human society, in that it studies human beings in the social world. Although it sees individuals as highly significant, sociology is different from psychology in that it rejects any explanation which just focuses on 'individuals', or argues that individuals are autonomous, and challenges the assumption that social behaviour can be reduced to the study of the individual alone. While sociology looks at both individuals and society, it does more than this in that it looks at individuals operating in the social world and their relationship with that world. It maintains there is a two-way relationship between the individual and society, in that individuals are influenced by society and in turn can influence their social environment. This is represented diagrammatically in Figure 1.1.

Figure 1.1 The relationship between the individual and society in sociology

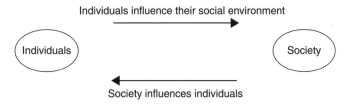

The development of sociology is relatively recent as it originated in the early nineteenth century during **industrialization**. The rapid industrial change that occurred at this time led to questions being asked about the sources of social change, social order, the relationship between the individual and society, and how the society into which people are born shapes their behaviour as individuals (Earle and Letherby 2008; Naidoo and Wills 2008). Sociology augments and supplements knowledge through a range of perspectives in three ways.

- **By giving us new understandings of society.** Sociology tries to understand how the social world 'works' – what's going on in society and the changes in society. It also investigates how the two-way relationship between social structures and individuals shapes the actions of each over time. In order to do this, sociology unravels and interprets the structure of society as well as the actions of individuals in a unique way. Consequently, it helps us to see what is going on in society in a new light. The well-known sociologist C. Wright Mills captured this perfectly when he said that 'doing' sociology requires thinking in a particular way. He describes this as thinking beyond our own essentially limited experiences and observations of the human social world, and challenging what appear to be the accepted explanations of social phenomena. The ability to adopt such a critical and questioning approach involves what C. Wright Mills describes as a **sociological imagination** which is seeing 'personal troubles [as] public issues of social structure' (Mills 1959: 8).

- **By providing us with evidence and explanations of an extensive range of facets of our human social world.** For instance, how society works in terms of what the different institutions do and how they function together. Sociology can also explain the actions of individuals and groups, and patterns of similarity and difference between people within a single society and between societies. Furthermore, it helps us to understand the distribution of social, political and economic resources and power within society. Consequently, sociology can account for why some groups are more powerful than others.

- **By offering explanations that are distinctive from other subjects.** Sociological explanations always look beyond the individual to take into account the wider social causes of individual behaviour. For example, when explaining why someone is unemployed, psychological explanations would perhaps look at personality traits such as lack of self-esteem, motivation or particular abilities. A sociological explanation would look at a number of crucial factors that are 'beyond' the individual and out there in society and how they affect individuals. As there is a social class gradient in unemployment, with those from the lower social classes experiencing much higher rates of unemployment than those in the higher social classes, one such factor would be social class. A sociological account would also consider the way that some occupational groups are more able to protect themselves from unemployment: higher occupational groups have more contacts and family ties in business which means they can use these to keep and find employment. In contrast, those in lower occupational groups are often less skilled and less well trained and are consequently more vulnerable to unemployment. Therefore, sociology does not only consider personal characteristics but all those factors in society that could affect an individual's lack of employment.

The sociology of health and illness

Early sociologists did not discuss health and illness directly. It was not until the 1950s that the value of sociological analysis in this field achieved recognition and even then it did not become established as a sub-discipline until the 1960s and 1970s (Earle and Letherby 2008). Initially it focused on criticizing traditional medical views as being value-laden and highlighted the social control exerted by health professionals through the practice of medicine. During the 1980s, those working within the sociology of health and illness extended its boundaries further and added its voice to the questions that were being raised about the biomedical model's physiological focus. In doing so, because of its sociological underpinnings, the sociology of health and illness emphasized both the roles of different aspects of our social world beyond the individual and the role of the individual in determining health. The former include social categories, social conditions and social processes. The latter include patients' own perceptions and knowledge of health.

The sociology of health and illness has now achieved professional and academic recognition. As a result of its further development and sociological underpinnings, it is concerned with *all* aspects of contemporary life that impinge on well-being throughout the life course. Examples of the wide range of issues that the sociology of health and illness currently addresses are:

- patterns of health and illness in relation to the wider social structure;

- lay perceptions of health and illness;

- the experience of health and illness;

- how certain conditions come to be viewed as illnesses or diseases;

- globalization and health;

- the social organization of formal and informal healthcare;

- the analysis of medical knowledge and professional power;

- lay-professional interactions in healthcare;

- the social and cultural aspects of the body.

In exploring these issues, the sociology of health and illness adopts an eclectic approach in that it embraces other disciplines, such as epidemiology, public health, social policy and psychology. It also employs many well-established sociological perspectives in its explanations.

While the diversity of the content of the sociology of health and illness has been criticized, it has significantly expanded awareness and knowledge of the breadth of social influences on health as well as its social context. In addition, it provides a recognized and dynamic academic base from which to explore, interpret and analyse many social aspects of health.

The sociology of the body

By challenging conventional assumptions about the body and disease, and studying people's own knowledge of their bodies and perceptions of their bodily experiences, the sociology of health and illness has generated a plethora of studies concerned with the body from a sociological viewpoint. These have been carried out not only within the sociology of health and illness but also in other areas, such as ageing and disability studies. Furthermore, many social changes have increased sociological interest in the body as a social product. For example, the cult of the body in consumer culture means that much modern consumption, such as in the areas of beauty, fashion and leisure, now focuses on goods for body maintenance. Hence the body has become a carrier of commodities which signify particular lifestyles, and create both identity and social status. Medical advances in transplants and cosmetic surgery mean that the concept of a 'natural body' is no longer tenable and are further indications of how the body is socially shaped. Demographic changes also mean that there is now a much higher proportion of older people in western societies (see Chapter 5), which has drawn more attention to the physical changes arising from the ageing process and the consequences of living with an ageing body (Shilling 2003; Twigg 2006).

As a result, over the past two decades, much sociological attention has turned to the previously neglected study of the body as both a natural phenomenon and a product of factors 'beyond' the individual within the social environment. The body now forms an important dimension of the sociological debate. This in turn has led to the development of the sub-discipline of the sociology of the body, which uses sociological perspectives to provide theoretical insights into key social aspects of the body (Williams 2003; Twigg 2006). These include:

- the impact of environmental, social, political and cultural influences on the body;

- the way the body is shaped by dominant discourses;

- lived experiences of health and illness.

The sociology of the body therefore adds academic rigour to the analysis of many issues about the social aspects of health addressed in this book, and will be used to add depth and understanding to the explorations of chronic illness and disability in particular.

Theoretical underpinnings

The discussion of academic disciplines in the first section makes reference to different theoretical perspectives. When social scientists talk about a **theory** they mean the set of ideas used to explain aspects of the social world in a systematic and consistent way. These explanations are also supported by evidence and extrapolate from this to develop understandings of social phenomena and predict future occurrences. The set of ideas within each theory are referred to as concepts (see Figure 1.2) which can be single words or a phrase.

The world view of the proponent(s) of a theory influences their interpretation of the evidence, the nature of their explanation and the concepts they develop. The variation in viewpoints is reflected in the differing theoretical perspectives about our social world. In addition, the sets of

Figure 1.2 Theoretical approaches

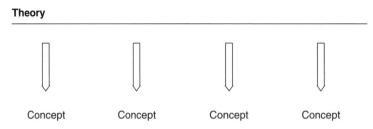

concepts within each theory are distinctive. For instance, a key concept within Marxist theory is 'capitalism' whereas feminist theory uses the phrase 'inequalities between the sexes' as one of its main concepts. As many of these theoretical perspectives have both informed, and continue to inform, the study of the social aspects of health, it is therefore essential that the reader is familiar with the main theoretical perspectives. Outlines of the theoretical perspectives that will be used in this book, together with an indication as to which areas of the social aspects of health they will be applied, are set out below.

Marxist theory

The emphasis in this theory is on the larger, structural elements of society such as the social, economic, legal and political systems. These are known as the **macro** elements of social structure. However, Marxist theory places most emphasis on the economic structure, as it maintains that the way the economy of a society is run determines the social relationships in that society. More specifically, it argues that the organization of the ownership of the predominant **means of production** within an economy leads to specific patterns of class relationships which inevitably entail power differentials and lead to social inequalities. For example, when feudalism was the dominant means of production, there were lords and serfs whose relationships were based on unequal rights and obligations, some of which were established in law. According to Marxist theory, such social relationships only change when the economic relationships change within a society.

Although Marx himself wrote about different historical epochs he concentrated on modern, western economies. He said that these are based on **capitalism**; within capitalist societies the means of production is profit-making and produces goods for sale using waged labour. There are those who privately own the means of production and those who have to sell their labour power to make a living. The former are called the **bourgeoisie**. They are the minority and their livelihood is based on the ownership of capital (hence they are also referred to as capitalists), and on producing and trading in commodities by employing waged or salaried labour. Those who have to sell their labour for wages are called the **proletariat**. They form the majority of the population in capitalist societies and they neither own capital nor do they have any choice about being workers. The bourgeoisie and the proletariat are the two main classes in capitalist societies. The relationship between them is unequal as the bourgeoisie exploit the proletariat in the pursuit of profit. This is described in the following extract from Marx's work about how capitalists make a profit from the labour of their workers.

In a certain period of time the worker will have performed as much labour as was presented by his weekly wages. Supposing that the weekly wage of a worker represents three workdays, then if the worker begins on Monday, he has by Wednesday evening replaced to the capitalist the full value of the wage paid. But does he then stop working? Not at all. The capitalist has bought his weeks' labour and the worker must go on working also during the last three week days. This surplus labour of the worker, over and above the time necessary to replace his wages, is the source of surplus value, of profit, of the [capitalist's] steadily growing increase in capital.

(Marx 1867: 58)

Hence, capitalism produces social divisions based on the ownership and non-ownership of the means of production. According to Marx, another consequence of the exploitation of the proletariat by the bourgeoisie was that the former would experience increasing **alienation**. He predicted that this would lead to social conflict which would result in the eventual overthrow of capitalism and the emergence of socialism (Marx 1867; Giddens 2009).

Marxist theory has been criticized on several counts. One is that it overemphasizes the economic determinants of social relationships and hence class is given primacy in any social analysis using this approach. In addition, Marx's predictions about such social changes have not been realized and Marxist social analysis has lost some of its pertinence and popularity. Nonetheless, aspects of this theory are frequently referred to in explanations of health and illness. For instance, the sort of inequalities that arise within capitalism, as identified by Marx, have been used to help explain class inequalities in health. Therefore Marxist theory will be returned to in Chapter 3. As it addresses inequalities in power, it is also useful in analyses of experiences of health and illness and the medical profession, and will inform discussions in Sections 2 and 3 of this book.

The emphasis in Marxist theory on the structure of society and the way that it constrains and shapes people means that it provides what is referred to as a structuralist view of society. Structural sociologists, conforming to **structuralism**, focus on how people's social behaviour, values and attitudes are largely determined by the organization and structure of the society in which they live, and more particularly, the social groups to which they belong in their society.

As there is coercion by one class and subordination of another within capitalist society, Marxist theory maintains that there is a fundamental conflict between the two classes. It has therefore been argued that it also offers a **conflict theory** of society. Conflict theorists argue that conflict is inherent in society and question the possibility of ever achieving social stability and equilibrium. This is because they see the unequal distribution of power and resources between groups in society as inevitably leading to some groups being more dominant than others. As a result, interests clash and there is conflict between dominant and subordinate social groups. The assumption in conflict theory that social order can only be maintained by the dominant social groups coercing the subordinate groups strengthens its assertion that consensus cannot exist in society, particularly as this coercion may involve physical force. However, the operation of informal and formal mechanisms of social control engineered by the dominant social groups is more likely to be used for such purposes in western societies (Dahrendorf 1959; Giddens 1984; Steel and Kidd 2001).

Another conflict theory is feminism. This argues that gender conflict is intrinsic to social life and it is to this sociological theory that we now turn.

Feminism

Feminism is a body of thought and a social movement which sees the equality of the sexes as essential and therefore argues for this equality in all areas of life. It explains the inequalities that exist between the sexes, and links this to the way that women have been historically oppressed and excluded from economic power and politics, and have had restrictions placed on them by society.

The impossibility of developing 'a holistic feminist account that speaks for all women' (Ramazanoglu and Holland 2002: 5) has been a constant theme within feminism. Although there are indeed striking differences between feminists in their values and perspectives (as discussed below), a central theme running through them is that it is men who have oppressed and excluded women because our social system is based on **patriarchy**. As a result, it is assumed that men can and should dominate and have most of the power because they are superior and that women should be subordinate to them. Feminists argue that patriarchy and the power it gives to men results in men being in control of the key institutions that shape our society, such as the judiciary. Our patriarchal social system is also embedded in and reinforced by social institutions. Commonly cited examples of these are the family and the education system. With regards to the former, feminists point to the way that girls, unlike boys, are socialized within the family into thinking that their primary responsibilities are to the home and family. They blame the education system for the **gender** stereotyping in the careers that girls and boys are trained for and encouraged to pursue (Barker 1997).

Therefore, the main thrust of feminist argument is that the inequalities between men and women are due to the way that patriarchy works in our society, as this means that female inequality and subordination to men is seen as 'natural'. The most well-known feminist theories are Marxist, radical and liberal feminism. These are discussed in Box 1.1 below.

Box 1.1 Well-known feminist theories

Marxist feminism
This feminist theory says capitalism is the cause of the unequal distribution of power between men and women. It focuses on women's position within the family in capitalist societies and argues that although women play an important role in the production of capital, they are exploited both in the private domain of the home and family, and the **public domain/sphere** of paid work within the economy.

In terms of the private domain, Marxist feminism sees women as slaves within the family who provide what is called 'free labour' which reproduces the workforce that capitalism requires at no cost. The word 'reproduce' is used in two senses here. One is in terms of the way that women literally 'reproduce' because they produce children who will be future workers. The other relates to the Marxist feminist argument that women also 'reproduce' the workforce because the caring work they undertake within the family enables their children and their husbands to function effectively as workers under capitalism. This caring work is not only unpaid but unnoticed and undervalued. In the public sphere, women are exploited in several ways. For instance, they are overrepresented in caring occupations and the aforementioned undervaluing of caring work is reflected in the occupational structure of capitalist societies. They are also viewed as a **reserve army of labour** to be used in the economy to increase the labour supply when required and therefore reduce wages.

Thus, Marxist feminists conclude that within capitalism women are exploited as reproducers **and** producers. It is this emphasis on capitalism within Marxist feminism that has led to criticisms of its analyses for prioritizing capitalism over patriarchy and not attributing relevant significance to the latter (Barker 1997; Steel and Kidd 2001).

Radical feminism
Radical feminists emphasize that men, as opposed to the economic system, are the primary exploiters of women. For them, patriarchy is based on the fundamental biological differences

between men and women and hence women's oppression by men is inherent in patriarchal socie-ties. Patriarchy is 'transhistorical' and 'transcultural' in that whatever the historical period or culture, men systematically dominate and shape society to meet their needs rather than the needs of both males and females. Such domination is both physical and sexual (Firestone 1979). According to radical feminists, women can achieve freedom by wresting control of their bodies and fertility from men. They also argue that new technology can help eliminate some of the obstacles to achieving this freedom.

Criticisms of this feminist theory include its lack of recognition of the variations in the interpreta-tion of biological differences between men and women across time and between cultures. For instance, during the First and Second World Wars, women's biological inferiorities were over-looked in the need to fill gaps in the workforce created by the absence of men from traditional 'masculine' jobs (Oakley 1972, 1984). Another flaw in radical feminism that has been highlighted is that not all gender relationships are characterized by oppression and exploitation. Furthermore, despite all the changes in women's position in society over the past 50 years, there is no evidence to suggest that a matriarchal society would be preferable.

Liberal feminism
In line with the thinking of **liberalism** – that individuals should be treated in accordance with their efforts as opposed to their birth or heredity – liberal feminists argue that men and women should have equal rights. Such gender equality should be achieved through the existing legal structures in society. Hence, rather than advocating a radical transformation of gender relationships, liberal feminists believe in campaigning to remove all social, political, economic and legal obstacles that prevent women having the same rights and opportunities as their male counterparts.

While many liberal feminists maintain that there have been moves to greater equality between the sexes as a result of campaigning, the extent to which this has occurred in both the public and private spheres is much debated. Critics of liberal feminism also point to the evidence that although the gender pay gap is decreasing, women are still primarily responsible for the day-to-day running of the home (Sullivan 2000; Abbott 2006; National Statistics 2007; Gatrell 2008).

The development of these different strands has led to feminism in general being accused of lacking internal coherence as a social theory. However, it has had substantial impacts both intellectually and as a social movement. It challenged earlier sociological theories because of the way they focused on a narrow range of topics and ignored gender. Indeed, feminism's greatest contribution is probably its attack on the 'malestream' tradition of mainstream sociology which renders women invisible. Hence it not only forced an intellectual reconsideration of established thinking and theories but also stimulated research into gender issues nationally and internation-ally. As a social movement it has helped women to achieve greater economic, political, legal and social equality and still strives for improvements in women's lives. In relation to the study of the social aspects of health specifically, it has drawn attention to many important, yet previously unrec-ognized, issues about women's health. These include the social causes of women's illness which were ignored because women were defined within medicine soley by their biology and reproduc-tive capacity. By offering varying analyses, the broad tendencies within feminist theory enhance understanding and help to shape effective action aimed at addressing such issues (Barker 1997; Abbott *et al.* 2005).

Activity 1.2

The different types of feminism can be confusing when you first come across them. Read through them once again and complete the following table. This activity will help to consolidate your understanding. Some suggestions about what you could have included in each box can be found in the 'Activity feedback' chapter on page 223.

FEMINIST THEORY	CAUSE(S) OF INEQUALITIES BETWEEN MEN AND WOMEN	SOLUTIONS	CRITICISMS
Marxist feminism			
Radical feminism			
Liberal feminism			

Functionalism

In contrast to the preceding theories, functionalism focuses on those factors that bind society together to make it stable. This theory sees society as a biological organism (such as the body), made up of different integrated social structures which have to work together (as the different parts of the body do) in order for society to function properly and for social order to be maintained. These social structures comprise sub-systems and social institutions. Within these, individuals are allocated to **social roles**. Correct performance of social roles is essential for the maintenance of social stability. A central value system ensures that there are shared cultural and social expectations about the way each role should be carried out and the way others should respond. These social expectations are called role relationships, each of which carries with it a specific set of rights and obligations. For instance, in a classroom, a teacher has the right to control the class and is expected to teach the class effectively. The children in that classroom have a right to the education being provided and are expected to behave in a responsive manner. Social institutions themselves also have to perform specific functions that are necessary to maintain social order and for the continuation of social life. Using the family as an example, this social institution uses the process of **socialization** to ensure that the next generation continues to perform social roles.

Returning to the analogy of the body, according to functionalism, malfunction occurs when individuals within their sub-systems and social institutions solely pursue their own interests and do not adhere to the central value system in fulfilling their roles and relationships. Such malfunction can cause damage across the whole social system in the same way that disease does when it affects a part of the human body. Similarly, if the malfunction is not addressed, society cannot operate effectively and loses its order and solidarity (Parsons 1964; Jones 1994).

Functionalism presents an essentially 'consensual' representation of society; the consensus is based on an agreement to sustain society and shared norms and beliefs. When change occurs, a state of equilibrium is restored through the establishment and acceptance of new consensual agreements. Some everyday activities can also have a latent consensual function in maintaining the system as a whole. For example, in addition to the nutritional function of food, this perspective would also point to the way it reinforces social groupings and cultural practices within a society (Lupton 1996).

Therefore, functionalism is viewed as a **consensus theory**. Such theories use organic analogies and argue that society survives and remains stable because of the broad acceptance by the majority of its citizens of consensual beliefs. They also assert that the natural state of society is one of dynamic equilibrium which copes with change by restoring balance and harmony. However, functionalism has been criticized for assuming that all those within the sub-systems do actually share the same understandings about situations to such an extent. In addition, criticisms have been levied at its prescribed and static notions about social roles and the way that individuals passively carry out those roles. Nonetheless, this perspective has made significant contributions to the understanding of key areas of the social aspects of health, such as the experience of illness and health-care systems. One of the most influential theorists within functionalism is Parsons, and we will be referring to his work when these issues are discussed in Chapters 6 and 11 respectively.

Symbolic interactionism

As indicated above, functionalism is concerned with how individual motivations and actions are in alignment with the central value system of society rather than an individual's own aims, beliefs and consciousness. Symbolic interactionism puts forward a different view of the role of the individual in social life. This theory is interested in people as active social actors; it focuses on how they make and define their own reality through their perceptions and interpretations of the social world that arise from their interactions with each other. Furthermore, social roles and norms are learned through these interactions. Indeed, symbolic interactionism developed as a reaction against perspectives such as functionalism which presented individuals as passively responding in a puppet-like way to the social system. Another point of distinction between functionalism and symbolic interactionism is the views they adopt about the nature of the social world. We have seen how functionalism makes use of analogies associated with the natural world, such as the human body. This means that it sees the social world as objective and observable. In contrast, symbolic interactionism sees the social world as being made up of its individual participants motivated by human consciousness. Consequently, symbolic interactionism argues that the meaning of human action is not observable but is subjective and has to be interpreted by studying the meanings that people attach to their behaviour.

Hence, this theoretical perspective focuses on **micro** elements of society which are the small-scale aspects of human behaviour such as the face-to-face interactions between individuals and between individuals and groups. Research adopting a symbolic interactionist approach begins with the individual and focuses on explaining the social world from the point of view of the subjective individual as a social actor. Criticisms of symbolic interactionism have centred around the way it ignores structural factors, does not place individuals and groups within a wider social context and offers depth at the expense of breadth. Despite these criticisms, this perspective has generated invaluable understandings of meanings and their fluidity. It has also produced many insights into the social aspects of health, and work carried out within a symbolic interactionist theoretical framework will be referred to in Section 2 of this book when discussing experiences of health and illness (Hochschild 1983; Cuff *et al.* 2006).

Postmodernism

The term postmodernism itself is broad and is used in a range of academic disciplines when describing the profound social changes that occurred at the end of the twentieth century in what sociologists refer to as the move from **industrial** to **post-industrial society**. These changes not only include the transformation of industrial organization but also of class structure, religious allegiances and political life. As a result, contemporary life is less certain, identities are more fluid and society has become more diverse, pluralistic and fragmented. Stuart Hall, a leading sociologist, summarized this phenomenon in the following quotation from an article written in the 1980s:

> *Our world is being remade. Mass production, the mass consumer, the big city, big brother state, the sprawling housing estate, and the nation state are in decline: flexibility, diversity, differentiation, and mobility, communication, decentralization and internationalization are in the ascendant. In the process our own identities, our sense of self, our own subjectivities are being transformed. We are in transition to a new era.*

(Hall 1988: 24)

As this book will demonstrate, many existing sociological theories, such as Marxism and functionalism, have become unsustainable in their original form and have required adaptation because they are historically and culturally relative. Postmodernism is the most recent sociological theory and challenges the all-embracing nature and expressions of certainty about the social world of its theoretical predecessors. It searches for new ways of explaining our changed social world with its decline in absolutes and the collapse of meaning. In doing so, it emphasizes that we can never uncover the truth, be objective or have a theory about the social world. This is because social life is continually constructed and reconstructed through our everyday interpretations and actions, and therefore knowledge about the social world is constantly changing. Indeed, postmodernism argues that we are 'agents' who can make an increasing number of choices about how we shape our lives and identity, rather than having our behaviour and roles prescribed by the society in which we live. This focus on human subjects and human action has also led sociologists to direct their attentions to *agency* as opposed to *structure*.

Postmodernism has several strands. One of these is **social constructionism**, which refers to how social reality is actively viewed or 'constructed' in a particular way by individuals and groups as a result of social relations and human agency rather than being 'natural' or biological in origin. Social constructions of different aspects of society or behaviour vary historically, socially and culturally. Thus, there is no obdurate reality because we make our own and social reality is essentially contestable (Giddens 1992; Cuff *et al.* 2006).

Postmodernism has been accused of not being a unified theory and overemphasizing choice in its conceptualization of human beings as 'agents'. Nonetheless, this theory has been credited with extending the boundaries of sociological enquiry and challenging analyses proffered across a range of theoretical bases. Using feminism as an example, postmodernism has questioned whether patriarchy is so pervasive throughout society and in women's lives, and consequently has raised awareness of the variations in the experiences of womanhood. It has also contributed to the study of the social aspects of health. An example is the way it shows how medical knowledge is a product of those engaged in its practice in particular societies and historical periods. This has in turn highlighted the fluid and dynamic nature of medicine and the extent to which it lacks neutrality. Therefore, postmodernism has challenged the 'truth' of medical knowledge, and we will draw on this work throughout the book. Furthermore, many of the societal changes it refers to have been used in the exploration of new areas in the study of health. For instance, the growth in individualization and reflexivity that postmodernists assert are features of post-industrial society has been used in relation to lifestyles and risks to health (Giddens 1992).

Activity 1.3

The following concepts are all referred to in the discussions of the theoretical perspectives above. Using the table below, place them under the correct perspective. When you have finished, compare them with the list of key concepts within each perspective that are set out in the answer to this activity in the 'Activity feedback' chapter on page 224.

Concepts

Active social actors
Agency
Alienation
Analysis should begin with
    the individual
Bourgeoisie
Capitalism
Central value system
Consensual representation
    of society
Cultural and social
    expectations
Women's subordination to
    men is 'natural'
Proletariat

Economy of a society
Education system
Equality of the sexes
Equilibrium
Exploitation
Human consciousness
Impossibility of
    uncovering the truth
Individuals make their own
    reality
Knowledge about the
    social world is
    constantly changing
Society is like a biological
    organism

Lack of objectivity
Means of production
Oppression and exclusion
    of women
Patriarchy
Post-industrial society
Social construction
Social order
Social roles
Socialization
Understand and interpret
    human action
Sub-systems
Focus on the individual
    rather than society

Marxist theory

Feminism

Functionalism

Symbolic interactionism

Postmodernism

Health data

An important issue in the study of the social aspects of health is the use of data about variations in health in our society. Differences in health between various groups in society are usually measured in terms of **morbidity** and **mortality rates**. The former refer to the numbers and patterns of physical and mental illnesses within a designated group at a given time, while the latter refer to numbers and causes of deaths within a designated group at a given time. Both are expressed as a rate per 100,000 of the population and reductions in either or both are equated with improved health. Mortality rates are also used to calculate the most widely used indicator of population health in general – life expectancy at birth. This provides an estimate of the average number of years a newborn baby can expect to live if patterns of mortality at the time of their birth were to stay the same throughout their life.

The measurement of health is controversial. One area of controversy has been the indicators used, which have been accused of lacking objectivity. Taking morbidity rates first, these are compiled using self-reported health, and yet such self-reports have been found to consistently underestimate disease which is clinically identified and people inevitability define their health in different ways. Service utilization rates (such as visits to GPs and number of inpatient hospital stays) have also been used as indicators of morbidity but these can be inaccurate because the extent of a patient's use of health services can be influenced by a variety of individual and social factors. These factors include changes in policies on service provision and length of utilization – for instance, policy initiatives over the past two decades have resulted in considerable increases in day surgery and reductions in the length of inpatient hospital stays.

With reference to mortality rates, a key indicator used is occupation. As we shall see in Chapter 3, the way occupations are classified is regularly revised and also varies between studies. Therefore, comparisons of findings can be questionable. Furthermore, important information has been omitted because married women have typically been classified according to their husband's occupation (Bowling 2005; Steel *et al.* 2008; Graham 2009). More generally, concern has been expressed about the way that the social processes involved in measuring health introduce varying degrees of bias and subjectivity.

Hence, refinements to the methods and models used for measuring health differences are continually being made. Although it is important to be aware of the problems associated with measuring morbidity and mortality rates, it is equally important to realize the full potential of such data in increasing knowledge about the social aspects of health. The patterns that emerge from careful analyses of morbidity and mortality data have been invaluable in showing how health and illness are produced by social relationships and inequalities, as opposed to random biological events. These insights are often further enhanced by the use of data from other indicators, such as smoking rates, obesity levels and data about specific illnesses. Therefore, in order to develop your understanding of the social aspects of health as much as possible, morbidity and mortality figures will feature in several chapters of this book, and, where necessary, they will be used in conjunction with other health indicators.

Influences on health

During the course of the discussions in this book, reference will also be made to many of the influences on health. Those that are most frequently discussed in the study of the social aspects of health, plus a summary of their specific impacts on health, are set out below. The reader will be referred back to this list as appropriate.

- **Smoking:** more deaths can be attributed to smoking than to any other single risk factor. It causes a third of all cancers: lung cancer, cancer of the mouth, larynx, oesophagus, bladder, kidney, stomach and pancreas. Other smoking-related causes of death are chronic obstructive lung disease (including bronchitis), heart disease, asthma and brittle bone disease (osteoporosis) (Department of Health 1998; Office for National Statistics 2006b, 2009).

- **Drinking:** consuming alcohol above the recommended guidelines leads to health problems both immediately and in later life. These problems include cirrhosis of the liver, heart disease, strokes and some cancers (Busfield 2000a; Office for National Statistics 2006a, 2009).

- **Exercise:** the beneficial effects of physical exercise are extensive and include the way it promotes mental well-being and musculoskeletal health. Lack of physical exercise contributes to many chronic diseases such as cardiovascular diseases, strokes, Type 2 diabetes, osteoporosis and some cancers (Department of Health 2004a; Graham 2009).

- **Weight:** being overweight, and particularly being obese, is linked to many health problems which range from poorer self-rated health and infertility to much more significant illnesses such as diabetes, cardiovascular disease, certain cancers, hypertension, respiratory problems and musculoskeletal diseases. It can also contribute to premature death (Simonsen *et al.* 2008; Weaver *et al.* 2008; Marmot 2009).

- **Substance misuse:** in addition to leading to death, substance misuse has many negative effects on health. These include anxiety, memory and cognitive loss, psychiatric disorder, HIV infection, accidental injury, hepatitis and coma. It may also result in an increased risk of sexually transmitted diseases (National Institute for Health and Clinical Excellence 2007; Bradby 2009).

- **Poor housing:** this often goes hand-in-hand with overcrowding, lack of central heating, and damp, rot, mould, lack of light and a poor state of decoration. Such living conditions can adversely affect mental and physical health. Examples of mental health problems identified are anxiety and depression. Physical health problems include increased vulnerability to respiratory illnesses (such as asthma) and enteric diseases (such as vomiting and diarrhoea) (Wilkinson 1999; Krieger 2002).

- **Deprived neighbourhoods:** living in a deprived area inevitably involves experiencing many disadvantages, for instance, higher crime rates, lack of amenities and low employment opportunities. These have been linked to higher anxiety and depression rates. Furthermore, such areas are less conducive to a healthy lifestyle – residents have higher smoking rates and lower rates of exercise (Wilkinson 1999).

Conclusions

This chapter has provided you with comprehensive explanations of issues that are central to the study of the social aspects of health in this book. Having developed your knowledge of these issues, you are now in a position to begin to explore the chapters in the rest of the book. Readers are advised to return to this chapter should they wish to refresh their understanding of any of the points discussed when they are referred to in later chapters. Enjoy and good luck!

Key points

- Several disciplines inform the study of the social aspects of health, however it is the sociology of health and illness and the sociology of the body which are most frequently drawn upon.

- Many theoretical perspectives about our social world have both informed, and continue to inform, the study of the social aspects of health.

- Although health measurement is problematic, data on health is essential to the study of the social aspect of health.

- The most frequently discussed influe nces on health within the study of the social aspects of health are smoking, drinking, exercise, weight, substance misuse, poor housing and deprived neighbourhoods.

Discussion points

- What do you think having a 'sociological imagination' requires?

- What are the main differences between conflict and consensus theories?

- In what ways do you think sociology can enhance the study of the social aspects of health, illness and healthcare?

Suggestions for further study

- Chapter 4 in Naidoo and Wills (2008) provides a good overview of the contribution of sociology to the study of health as well as addressing some of the central concerns and debates in the sociology of health.

- If you wish to explore the latter in more depth, Earle and Letherby's (2008) highly readable book, *The Sociology of Healthcare* comprises a collection of readings which cover a range of issues within the sociology of health and illness. While these encourage the reader to think sociologically, they do not assume prior knowledge of sociology.

- A quick look at the indexes to the journals *Sociology of Health and Illness* and *Social Science and Medicine* will give you a greater insight into the range of issues included in this subject area and furnish you with ideas for future sources of material.

- Should you wish to explore the theoretical perspectives in more detail, see Cuff *et al.* (2006). Chapter 1 in Barry and Yuill (2008) will also be useful.

The relationship between social categories and health

Introduction to Section 1

This section addresses the first of the three broad themes identified in the factors mentioned in the Introduction as now being recognized key social aspects of health. In the exploration of 'The relationship between social categories and health' that takes place in this section, four such social categories are discussed:

■ Gender and health

■ Social class and health

■ Ethnicity and health

■ Ageing and health

Each of these topics is dealt with in a separate chapter and hence there are four chapters. The chapters all include relevant key concepts and theoretical perspectives. Although the chapters in this section can be read independently, you are advised to refer to both the Glossary at the end of the book and to the outlines of the theoretical perspectives that inform the study of the social aspects of health in Chapter 1 to enhance your understanding of each topic.

Gender and health

2

Women are sicker but men die quicker.

(Quoted in Gatrell 2008: 2)

Overview

Introduction

The relationship between gender and health has been debated since the 1970s and was one of the first topics to be addressed within the sociology of health and illness. During this time, the many contradictory trends that have emerged, such as that in the quote above, have been extensively researched, contested and theoretically explored. As we shall see in the course of this chapter, gender is a major social division in our society and an appreciation of the impact of gender on health is central to the study of the social aspects of health. This chapter aims to capture the main themes in the literature about this important social aspect of health and starts by clarifying the concept of gender. It then looks at the differences in men and women's physical and mental health. This is followed by an exploration of a range of influences on men and women's health. The chapter ends with a discussion of theoretical explanations that have been developed about the connections and interactions between gender and health. The emphasis throughout is on both men and women's physical and mental health.

<table>
<tr><td colspan="2">

Activity 2.1

Using the boxes below, jot down some examples of what is 'typically' associated with being male and female in our society.

</td></tr>
<tr><td>**Males**</td><td></td></tr>
<tr><td>**Females**</td><td></td></tr>
<tr><td colspan="2">There are some ideas in the 'Activity feedback' chapter on page 225.</td></tr>
</table>

What is gender?

Gender means something different from **sex**; sex can be distinguished at birth and refers to being biologically male or female. In other words, sex refers to having male or female genitals and to the ways in which we develop anatomically in certain predictable ways. In contrast, gender means the social, as distinct from purely biological, characteristics associated with masculinity or femininity in a particular society (Janes 2002). For example, in the UK, wearing make-up, dresses and high heels, passivity, tenderness and caring roles are associated with being a female. In contrast, masculinity is associated with physical strength, undertaking physically demanding work, aggressiveness, toughness, and being emotionally unexpressive and adventurous. These associations often lead to unwarranted generalizations from sex differences, referred to as **gender stereotyping**. They also vary over time and between societies and cultures. For instance, Reynolds (1996: 66) describes how up until the late 1800s all young children, irrespective of whether they were boys or girls, were dressed in what would now be described as feminine clothes. Interestingly, their activities were simultaneously portrayed in literature and the arts as gender stereotypical: 'Well into the last century, infants and young children were effectively genderless. Boys and girls were both dressed in skirts and frocks . . . images of children tended to conform to gender stereotypes, with boys engaging in activities out of doors while girls busied themselves at home'. In relation to changes in adult gender stereotypes, during the Second World War women successfully undertook all forms of manual work which previously had not been associated with being female (Jones 1994; Abbott 2006).

Such changing gender stereotypes show that gender is not linked to biological necessity. Therefore, sociologists argue that gender is socially constructed because of the way it owes so much to social and cultural influences. The social process whereby biological differences are given social and cultural significance and used as a basis for the social classification of males and females is called **gender differentiation**. Another important concept about the social construction of gender in these arguments is **gender role**. This refers to the social and behavioural characteristics that a society assigns to masculine and feminine roles. These can form the principal categorization within social life and in some societies there are radical divisions between gender roles (O'Donnell 2002; Gatrell 2008).

Extreme social constructionists argue that gender differences have no biological or genetic basis (Oakley 1972). Those that refute this view point to a variety of evidence. This includes the fact that although societies do differ in terms of the exact characteristics they assign to males and females, there is evidence that these 'gendered roles' are relatively consistent across time and space. Moreover, there are very few societies where gender roles are completely reversed and females are expected to be 'masculine' and vice versa. Other evidence cited is that from studies which show preschool children prefer gender stereotyped toys despite being bought gender neutral toys from the age of 1 (Robinson and Morris 1986; Servin *et al.* 1999).

In defining gender, reference has already been made to the fact that gender differences can lead to radical divisions in social life between males and females. One of the main areas where this is most apparent is in health.

Activity 2.2

See how much you already know about gender differences in health by ticking whether the following statements are true or false! All of these points are covered in the text in Sections 2 and 3, but the answers can also be found in the 'Activity feedback' chapter on page 225.

Women have a lower number of inpatient hospital stays than men	**T/F**
Women are twice as likely to suffer from depression than men	**T/F**
Women live around four years longer than men	**T/F**
Heart disease and cerebrovascular disease are a major cause of death among women	**T/F**
Men tend to find their work more alienating and stressful than women	**T/F**
Smoking rates are higher for women	**T/F**
Women are more physically active in every age group	**T/F**
Men are more likely to be obese than women	**T/F**
There is a general reluctance among men to report ill health and access healthcare services	**T/F**

Gender differences in health

As mentioned in Chapter 1, morbidity and mortality rates are used to measure differences in health between various groups in society. Analyses based on these rates show that gender has a significant impact on physical and mental health. Let's look at some of these gender differences in health by analysing morbidity and mortality rates further.

Morbidity rates

Studies about gender differences in health traditionally use indicators of health service use, such as visits to GPs and number of inpatient stays in hospital. These indicators show that women get physically and mentally ill more often. Figure 2.1 illustrates this in relation to the frequency with which women visit their GPs.

However, such statistics have been questioned for several reasons. Women are more likely to have to visit their GP and experience inpatient stays because of certain biological conditions related to pregnancy and childbirth, contraception, menstruation and the menopause. In addition, as women live longer than men they are likely to use health services for a greater number of years. Indeed, when this fact is taken into account, women only have a slightly higher morbidity rate with the exception of mental health. This is supported by recent statistics that showed the overall difference between the sexes in self-reported rates of 'not good health' was just one percentage point (7 per cent and 8 per cent respectively), once the age distribution of the population was taken into account (Busfield 2000a; Office for National Statistics 2006a).

Irrespective of whether women do have higher morbidity rates than men or not, some common illnesses which are unrelated to physiological sex differences are gendered. For instance, women are more likely to suffer from cancer, arthritis and rheumatism than men, while men have higher rates of circulatory diseases including ischaemic heart disease (i.e. heart attack or angina) and strokes (Office for National Statistics 2006a, 2008a).

With reference to mental health specifically, while females have higher rates of mental ill health at most stages of their lives, men and women seem to be prone to particular types of mental illness. The following figures illustrate this:

Figure 2.1 Gender and morbidity rates – percentage of males and females consulting an NHS GP in the 14 days prior to interview, Great Britain, 1971–2002

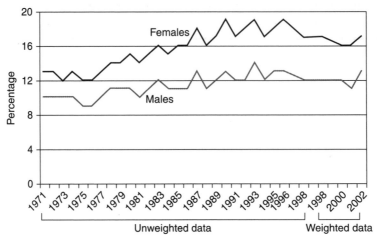

Source: National Statistics (2004a)

- women are twice as likely to suffer from depression;

- women are 10 times more likely to suffer from bulimia nervosa and anorexia nervosa;

- men are more likely to receive a diagnosis of schizophrenia and other serious psychoses;

- men are three times more likely to commit suicide;

- more men than women are treated for problems with drug and alcohol abuse (Doyal 1995; Allen 2008; McCrone *et al.* 2008).

Although such findings do clearly show there are gender differences in physical and mental illnesses, evidence is starting to emerge of reductions in some of the observed differences. Among the most interesting developments are the increases in numbers of young men with anorexia nervosa and young women with drinking problems (Drummond 2010; Plant *et al.* 2010). These changes will inevitability impact on illness rates for males and females and will therefore need to be taken into consideration in future discussions of gender and health.

Mortality rates
Figure 2.2 shows that while there have been improvements in life expectancy at birth in the UK since 1981, there is still a four-year difference in life expectancy between males and females, and this looks set to continue. When considering this difference, it is important to note that not all the years females gain through increased life expectancy are lived in relatively good health and free from a disability or limiting long-term illness. Healthy life expectancy at birth for females in 2004

Figure 2.2 Male and female life expectancy at birth, UK, 1981–2056

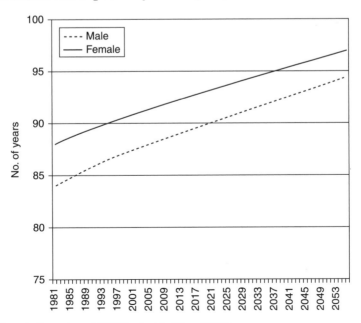

Source: Government Actuary's Department (2006), cited in Allen (2008)

was 70.3 years compared with 67.9 years for males. Disability-free life expectancy for females born in 2004 was 63.9 years and for males 62.3 years. Consequently, while women live longer than men, they are also more likely to spend more years in poor health or with a disability (Office for National Statistics 2006a, 2008a; Allen 2008; Department of Health, 2009a).

As with morbidity, causes of death are gendered, with heart disease and cerebrovascular disease being major causes of death among men. Although these diseases also result in the deaths of a substantial number of women, they manifest themselves in lower mortality rates than for men. The most common causes of death among women are breast cancer and cancers of the genito-urinary system (Hayes and Prior 2003).

Influences on men and women's health

So what factors lead to these gender differences in health? Much research has been carried out into several aspects of men and women's lives which shows that there are a variety of influences. Examples of these are illustrated in the case study below and then discussed in the rest of the section. Where details of their specific impacts on health are required, these will either be given or the reader will be referred to the list of 'Influences on health' on page 27 of Chapter 1, as appropriate.

Case example: Peggy and Stuart

This middle-aged couple had just celebrated their twenty-fifth wedding anniversary. Since the last of their three children had reached school age, Peggy had a part-time office job to fit in with caring for the family and to supplement the family income. Stuart was a warden in their local country park.

Peggy had always been careful of the family's health, paying great attention to the quality of their diet and encouraging the children to take part in sports activities at school. She applied the same care to her own health, swimming twice a week and accessing health screening programmes when invited to do so.

Stuart enjoyed his food but because of the nature of his job did not gain weight until his mid-forties. When the pounds started to pile on, he refused to reduce the amount he ate or undertake any exercise outside work. In his early fifties he started to have headaches that lasted several days and found that his increasing girth was slowing him down at work. He initially refused to attend a 'well-man' clinic at the local GP surgery but did give in to Peggy's 'nagging' when the headaches increased in intensity. He was diagnosed with high blood pressure and was also found to have considerably raised cholesterol levels. Despite medical advice to reduce his salt and fat intake, plus lose two stones in weight, he strongly resisted changing his lifestyle.

Work and gender

In order to explore the relationship between gender and work, it is necessary to explain how the sociological concept of work is different from the everyday meaning of work. Work for sociologists has two meanings.

- An activity which brings in money. This is therefore called **paid work** and is done outside the home in the public domain.

■ An activity which contributes to the reproduction of society. This means that the activity is necessary for a society to run but it is **unpaid work**. These activities enable people to go on living and indeed to undertake paid work. They include all forms of domestic labour such as producing the next generation, caring for children, shopping and cooking for a household, washing clothes, and providing a clean and warm place to relax and sleep. Unpaid work is done in the private domain of the home, does not have as much status as paid work and does not receive the public recognition of money.

Sociological research has shown that there are differences between the type of 'work' that men and women do in both the public and private sphere. Let's take the public sphere first.

Public sphere
Women now make up 45 per cent of the workforce in the UK. Even though there is legislation protecting women's position in the labour market and more women are educated to degree level than in the past, there are considerable differences in the type of work that men and women do. This means that women do not have the same pay, status and power as men because they are more likely to:

■ be concentrated in certain types and areas of employment such as care work, personal service, shop work, cleaning and clerical work;

■ work part-time and/or in temporary jobs;

■ be in the less well-paid and less powerful posts.

For instance, only 10 per cent of women in the UK are judges, 8 per cent are in top management positions and 5 per cent are MPs. A trend of lower pay and less power also applies in those occupations where the number of men and women is equal, such as teaching and health. With reference to health occupations, although the fact that the number of women entering medicine now exceeds the number of men (the ratio is 60 women to 40 men) only 5 per cent of surgeons are female and women typically end up in part-time GP work with smaller caseloads and smaller salaries than their male counterparts (Janes 2002; Gatrell 2008).

   Despite these inequities, the gender pay gap between men and women has been decreasing since the late 1990s. As Table 2.1 shows, the pay gap (as measured by the median hourly pay excluding overtime of full-time employees) narrowed between 2006 and 2007 to its lowest value since records began. However, this trend can be adversely affected by changes in the economy, particularly

Table 2.1 Gender pay gap

Employees on adult rates, whose pay was unaffected by absence (%)	Median	Mean
Full-time/full-time	12.8	17.1
Part-time/part-time	–3.5	13.2
All employees/all employees	22.5	20.9

Note: The data represent the gender pay gap for hourly earnings excluding overtime

Source: Hicks and Thomas (2009)

economic downturns and realignments of different employment sectors. An example of the latter is the continuing decline of the manufacturing sector. One of the outcomes of this decline is that men are predicted to take a bigger share of the part-time jobs in the service sector that have to date been mainly undertaken by women (Sunderland 2009; UK Commission for Employment and Skills 2009).

There are proven health advantages related to pay, status and power. These include enhanced quality of life and higher rates of self-esteem. It is clear from the preceding discussions that these health advantages are not equally shared between men and women and that this situation may also worsen. Furthermore, there is some evidence that the types of jobs women undertake are hectic with little control over their hours or conditions of employment. As such characteristics have been linked to increased stress levels, it has been argued that women are much more likely to suffer from stress from their employment outside the home. On the other hand, women are less likely to be in dangerous and/or polluting occupations such as the armed forces, agriculture, construction and mining. Men also tend to find their work more alienating and stressful than women because they see their jobs as their key role in life, have higher aspirations and are less likely to be motivated by a desire for sociability and social interaction than women. In fact, being in paid employment has been found to be beneficial to women's health in terms of enhancing their self-esteem and extending their **social networks** (Doyal 1995; Annandale and Hunt 2000; Busfield 2000a).

Private sphere
Regardless of whether they or their partners/husbands are employed, women are *primarily* responsible for the day-to-day running of the home and carry out the bulk of all domestic and caring work. This includes cooking, cleaning, the washing and ironing, shopping, and caring for both children and elderly/frail relatives. Although men provide some help with such activities, the only area of domestic life where they are likely to make a significant contribution is repairs around the house (Sullivan 2000; Abbott 2006; National Statistics 2007; Gatrell 2008).

Thus, even though women are now recognized as being a crucial part of the workforce, and their wages are essential to the economic well-being of the family, they continue to bear substantial domestic responsibilities. The way that working women tend to combine their paid work in the public sphere with their unpaid work in the private domain of the home has led to the development of the concept of the **dual role**. Fulfilling a dual role has implications for women's health. With respect to domestic tasks specifically, these have many of the characteristics that occupational psychologists have shown to be most stressful for waged workers. This is because they are of service to others, monotonous, boring and repetitive, and they are not done through choice. The fact that there is also no recognition for this work because housework is rarely noticed unless it is *not* done can lower self-esteem and promote feelings of worthlessness. The emotional and mental strain of meeting the demands of their roles in the private and public spheres has been shown to lead to exhaustion and depression in women (Oakley 1974; Doyal 1995).

These sorts of findings about the different activities and roles that men and women undertake in the private sphere of the home and the public sphere of paid employment are referred to as the **sexual division of labour**. It is important to note that both men and women are constrained by this sexual division: just as it is difficult for a woman to advance in her career in a way she might wish, so it is also difficult for a man to participate fully in family life. Each is constrained by the gender expectations of their respective roles and there are financial as well as social penalties for those who do not conform (Janes 2002; Abbott 2006). This is illustrated in the following quotation from Abbott (2006: 67): 'structural constraints continue to limit the opportunities available to women in a masculine culture. At the same time, although men benefit from this relationship, the same masculine culture also imposes constraints on men'.

Poverty and gender

As we saw in Chapter 1, poverty is an important determinant of physical and mental health. The different positions of men and women in the public and private domains is one of the reasons why women are more vulnerable to poverty than men throughout their lives. Indeed, 20 per cent of women compared to 18 per cent of men in the UK belong to households in poverty (Palmer *et al.* 2007). Particular groups of women are more vulnerable to poverty than others, such as those who are lone parents (especially teenage lone parents) and older pensioners (see Chapter 5) (Gardiner and Millar 2006; Levitas *et al.* 2006; Patsios 2006).

Women are also more likely to experience poverty at particular stages of their lives – for example, when caring for children and following divorce. With reference to the latter, it has recently been established that women suffer more financially than men after a divorce: men's incomes rise by a third and women's incomes (regardless of whether they have children or not) fall by more than a fifth and remains low for many years. This has important implications for women because almost half of marriages in England and Wales will end in divorce. When they live in poor households, women often bear the brunt of poverty and they are the ones who 'do without'. Studies have shown that they make sacrifices in terms of going without food, clothes and entertainment to provide for their children, in order to manage with scarce resources (Abbott 2006; Jenkins 2008).

Women's increased risk of, and greater vulnerability to, poverty in their lives means that they are therefore at risk of the adverse effects of poverty on their health, as discussed in Chapter 1 (see page 27).

Health-related behaviour and gender

Men and women's health-related behaviour varies and while there are some exceptions, men tend to engage in more risky behaviour that is a threat to their health. Some examples are set out below.

Smoking

Figure 2.3 shows that although smoking prevalence has declined dramatically during the past four decades, men are still more likely to smoke than women across all ages. In 1974, 51 per cent of men and 41 per cent of women smoked whereas in 2007 these figures had dropped to 22 per cent and 20 per cent respectively. The gap between men and women therefore fell from 10 per cent to 2 per cent (Office for National Statistics 2006a, 2009).

Although the consistently higher smoking rates among men have been attributed to conformity to ideas of masculinity, some of the complexities of the relationship between women and smoking have also been unravelled. For instance, studies have found that certain groups of women, such as young mothers on low incomes, are more likely to smoke than others despite the fact that they acknowledge smoking is irrational from a health and financial point of view (see Chapter 1, page 27). They say they smoke because they feel that it creates space and time out for them from their daily routines of caring for their families and helps them cope (Graham 1993; Graham and Blackburn 1998).

Drinking

More men than women exceed the recommended daily alcohol intake benchmarks (40 per cent of men compared to 23 per cent of women). Men are also more likely to drink more heavily than women (23 per cent compared to 9 per cent). Death rates for men from alcohol-related causes, including accidents, alcohol-related illnesses and accidental poisoning with alcohol are over double those for women (Busfield 2000a; Office for National Statistics 2006a, 2008a).

Figure 2.3 Prevalence of cigarette smoking, Great Britain, 1974–2007

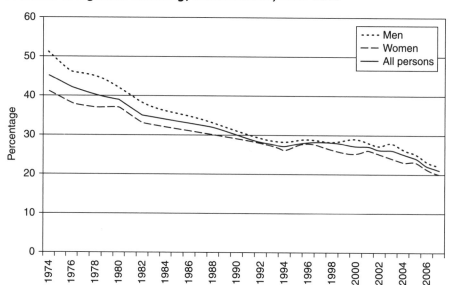

Source: Office for National Statistics (2009)

Diet

Although both men and women generally have a good knowledge of what constitutes a 'healthy diet' and the ways in which such a diet benefits their health, men report greater difficulties acting upon their knowledge for various reasons. These difficulties include increasing responsibilities at home and at work. Hence, women have healthier diets and are more likely than men to eat whole-meal bread, fruit and vegetables once a day, drink semi-skimmed milk and eat less 'unhealthy foods' like cakes and chips (Office for National Statistics 2006a; Weaver *et al.* 2008).

Exercise

Although the percentage of adults who meet the recommended levels of physical activity has declined since 2003, men are more active in every age group (Office for National Statistics 2006a; Weaver *et al.* 2008). The general reduction in adults taking the recommended levels of exercise is a risk factor in the health of both men and women (see Chapter 1, page 27). The fact that women are less active indicates that they are at greater risk than men.

Weight

Men are more likely to be **overweight** but less likely to be obese than women. **Body mass index** (BMI) is the indicator of healthy and unhealthy weight that is now used and is a measurement of a person's weight in kilograms divided by their height in metres squared. A BMI of more than 25 is regarded as being overweight and about 65 per cent of men currently have a body mass index of more than 25 compared to 55 per cent of women. Being **obese** is defined as having a BMI of 30 or more. Although the gap between the sexes in terms of obesity has been closing during the past two decades, overall obesity rates have increased and women are still more likely to be obese. As Figure 2.4 shows, in 1993 the obesity rates were 13 per cent and 16 per cent for men and women respectively. In 2005, the equivalent figures were 23 per cent and 25 per cent (Office for National Statistics 2006a, 2008a).

Figure 2.4 Prevalence of obesity in adults: by gender, 1993–2005

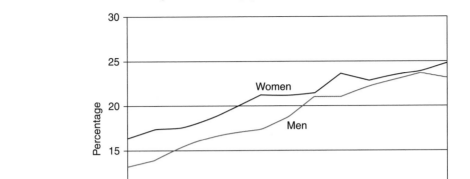

Source: Office for National Statistics (2008a)

Therefore, significant numbers of men and women are at risk of the many health problems associated with being an unhealthy weight, and women in particular are more likely to develop the more severe health problems that obesity brings (see Chapter 1, page 27).

Substance misuse
Both the number of, and the gender difference in, those reporting use of illicit drugs has decreased since 1998. Nonetheless, 9 per cent of men and 7 per cent of women still report such usage which indicates that men are still more likely to experience the negative effects of substance misuse on their health than women (see Chapter 1, page 27) (Office for National Statistics 2008a).

Healthcare and gender
The ways in which men and women's experiences as recipients and providers of healthcare vary are yet another set of influences on gender differences in health. Although some aspects of the examples discussed in this section are addressed in more detail in other parts of the book, the following overview of the gendering involved in receiving and providing healthcare will give you an appreciation of the relationship between gender and healthcare.

Recipients of healthcare
We saw earlier in this chapter that medicine plays a greater role in women's lives because they visit their GPs more frequently than men and have a higher number of inpatient stays in hospital. Feminists have argued that as the senior levels of the medical profession are male dominated, research and therapies are shaped by male interests. As a result, women are subject to control by men within the healthcare system and their medical diagnoses and treatment are adversely affected (Oakley 1993; Doyal 1995, 1998).

On the other hand, men's medical needs are not always met through healthcare services. This is partly because of a general reluctance among men to report ill health and access services that are available and partly because of inadequate levels of healthcare provision for men, such as less than comprehensive screening for testicular and prostate cancer (Luck *et al.* 2000). The following quote illustrates this; it is about treatment available through the NHS and how this is 'more focused and holistic for female health needs but more fragmented for male health needs. The result is that the NHS generally provides health services for males only in indirect and implicit ways' (Luck *et al.* 2000: 145).

Providers of healthcare
Community care policies since the 1970s have led to an increasing reliance on family carers, most of whom are women. Women are also expected to make sure their children are healthy, take appropriate action if they are ill and provide **informal healthcare**. It is well established that informal caring negatively affects physical and psychological health (Lewis and Meredith 1988; McLaughlin and Ritchie 1994; Brown and Stetz 1999; Hirst 1999; Bond *et al.* 2003) (see also Chapters 5 and 10). Despite the increase in the number of male nurses, nursing is still a female-dominated profession. Although many find being a nurse a satisfying job, they face several health hazards in the course of their duties. In hospitals, risks include lifting heavy patients, allergic reactions to drugs they have to administer and violence from patients. Nursing, particularly mental health nursing, can be psychologically stressful because of the responsibility involved, workplace culture, understaffing and lack of resources (Doyal 1995, 1998; Hayes and Prior 2003; Gabe *et al.* 2004).

Activity 2.3

Now that you have read through the above account of the influences on men and women's health, what do you think are the problems of studying gender differences in health? You may wish to compare your ideas with those presented in the 'Activity feedback' chapter on page 225.

Theoretical approaches to gender differences in health

The nature and the extent of the sort of differences in men and women's lives that have featured in the discussions of the influences on gender and health in this chapter are examples of the evidence used to argue that gender is a major social division. As we have seen, gender structures and organizes our public and private lives and opportunities, leading to inequalities between men and women.

There are several theoretical approaches which specifically address gender inequalities in health. Although biological factors (such as the way women's experiences of health are shaped by menstruation, pregnancy and childbirth) are acknowledged, within the study of social aspects of health explanations tend to emphasize socially constructed gender differences. For instance, cultural and behavioural explanations have focused on the extent to which women suffer from ill health because they take on too much responsibility if they accept the role of housewife as well as undertake paid employment and/or do not take regular physical exercise. Another important approach has adopted the concept of **hegemonic masculinity**. This concept is used to explain how particular versions of masculinity come to be idealized and embedded in culture and in institutions in society. Characteristics of such ideals of masculinity typically include stoicism and invincibility, which in turn are seen as demonstrating manliness. Hegemonic masculinities lead to alternate forms of masculinity being regarded as less legitimate. Explanations which apply the concept of hegemonic masculinity to gender differences in health highlight the ways in which men's poorer health in general is due to their health-related behaviour. They link this behaviour to the construction of masculinity in our society which inhibits self-care and healthy lifestyles. These approaches therefore argue that in order to change men's attitudes to their health and health behaviour, hegemonic masculinity needs to be challenged (Connell 1995; Gough and Robertson 2010).

Although the above theoretical approaches are very useful, it is feminism that has had the most impact on the development of theoretical explanations of gender differences in health. Hence the rest of this section will look at these in more detail

Feminist explanations of gender differences in health

Some of the work of leading feminists in the field of gender and health (most notably Oakley and Doyal) has been mentioned in this chapter already. Despite their differences, feminist perspectives have certain commonalties. For instance, they all acknowledge that differences in patterns between male and female health and illness stem in part from obvious biological differences. In addition, they assume that patriarchy is an important consideration in health and point to the way that women have been excluded from the medical profession because of male domination, and how men have taken over aspects of women's lives, such as childbirth, and imposed their views about what is regarded as abnormal physical and mental symptoms in women patients. Nonetheless, feminist views on gender and health do vary and the interpretations put forward by Marxist, radical and liberal feminists are outlined below to illustrate some of these variations.

- **Marxist feminism:** according to Marxist feminists, women are exploited as reproducers and producers. When analysing gender differences in health, the emphasis in this perspective has been twofold. The first is on the way women's fertility is exploited because of the need to produce the next generation of workers required by capitalism. The second is women's exploitation in their role as providers of free childcare and increasingly as informal carers of old and/or disabled family members.

- **Radical feminism:** as radical feminists argue that it is men, as opposed to the economic system, that dominate and shape society to meet their own needs rather than the needs of both males and females, they maintain that it is men who control and benefit from healthcare.

- **Liberal feminism:** the emphasis within liberal feminism is on gender equality through campaigning for equal rights. This has led liberal feminists to focus on the inequalities in women's participation in medicine as a profession.

With reference specifically to mental health, some feminist writers have argued that the gender differences in mental health are constructed by psychiatry and psychiatrists. The categories and concepts used in psychiatry mean that women and their behaviour are more likely to be defined as pathological and hence there is more chance of them being wrongly diagnosed as mentally ill than there is for men. There is also a greater likelihood of discourses from criminology being used to construct men's behaviour and this is yet another reason why men do not receive psychiatric diagnoses as often as women. With regards to psychiatrists, these feminist writers have focused on the way that gender shapes the encounter in consultations between male professional psychiatrists and female patients; as the psychiatric profession is male dominated, patriarchal power is exercised during consultations. Within patriarchal power, women's behaviour is typically devalued and pathologized and they are, by definition, viewed as being psychiatrically impaired. Thus during consultations between male psychiatrists and women, women tend to be labelled as mentally ill (Showalter 1987; Ussher 1991).

There is evidence to support such views from studies on the diagnosis of mental illness. One such study is that by Floyd (1997) who found that the diagnosis of depression in women is inaccurate with a misdiagnosis in 30–50 per cent of female patients. This study identified some of the causes of misdiagnosis by psychiatrists, such as a woman's age, sexual orientation, menstrual, occupational and/parental status. These are therefore potential areas for discrimination against women used within the psychiatric diagnostic process which can lead to them being wrongly diagnosed as depressed.

Criticism of feminist approaches to gender differences

Critics of the aforementioned feminist approaches highlight how they ignore the way in which healthcare can also harm men – for example, because of lack of screening programmes for men's diseases (Abbott *et al.* 2005). They also argue that there is a need to look at the changing social constructions of gender and illness. This can be illustrated by another reference to mental illness: Payne (1998) described how young men have come to be constructed as being more likely to be highly mentally disordered than women. She attributes this to several highly publicized incidents involving mentally disordered young men in the 1990s which led to the construct of the 'highly disordered male' being created. This coincided with other representations of young men that were emerging at the same time, such as their increased levels of involvement with the criminal justice system, dramatic increases in suicide and higher rates of youth employment. Thus, fears about the danger of the mentally disordered came to focus on young men and madness was consequently reconstructed in gendered terms as being associated with this group.

Conclusions

The powerful influence of gender on our physical and mental health is clear from the material and information presented in this chapter. Both sociology and the sociology of health and illness have made and continue to make valuable contributions to understandings of gender differences in health. Among the most significant of these is the acknowledgement that the health of men and women is shaped by a multitude of social factors that interact in a variety of ways and change over time. This leads to the conclusion that the study of gender differences in health is dynamic and, furthermore, cannot be studied without due consideration of the other social divisions that impact on our health during our lives (Seale and Charteris-Black 2008). Therefore, the next three chapters will assess the effect of social class, ethnicity and age on health.

Key points

■ Gender differences can lead to radical divisions in social life between males and females.

■ In relation to health, gender significantly impacts on both physical and mental health.

■ Factors that lead to gender differences in health include the type of 'work' that men and women do in both the public and private spheres, women's greater vulnerability to poverty, men and women's health-related behaviour, and the ways in which men and women's experiences as recipients and providers of healthcare vary.

- Although there are several theoretical approaches which specifically address gender inequalities in health, it is feminism that has had the greatest impact on the development of theoretical explanations of gender differences in health.

Discussion points

- What are the main problems of using mortality and morbidity rates to measure gender differences in health?

- To what extent do you think current mortality and morbidity rates will continue? What changes do you think will influence them?

- How useful is the concept of gender when explaining differences in men and women's physical and mental health?

Suggestions for further study

- Useful statistics on gender and health can be found in the Office for National Statistics publications *Focus on Health* (2006a) and *Focus on Gender* (2008a).

- There are various books that can provide you with in-depth explorations of particular influences on the health of men and women. For example, Gatrell (2008) offers original insights into the gendered nature of paid and unpaid work, and Hayes and Prior (2003) can help with detailed analysis of the relationship between gender and healthcare.

- Different perspectives on key influences on health and causes of ill health can be found in Busfield (2000a), Chapter 3, and Part 3 of Graham (2009).

There are marked inequalities in health between the social classes in Britain . . . Mortality tends to rise inversely with falling occupational rank or status, for both sexes and at all ages . . . data on (self-reported) morbidity tend to reflect those on mortality.

(Black et al. 1980: 55)

Overview

Introduction

The above quote is taken from one of the most influential documents about the relationship between social class and health, the *Black Report* (Black *et al.* 1980). As indicated in the Introduction to this book, it is regarded as a milestone in health inequalities research in that it systematically demonstrated the highly significant impact of social class on physical and mental health. The impact of class continues to be of great social, political and economic concern and is also yet another cause of health inequalities fundamental to the study of the social aspects of health. This chapter therefore explores the relationship between social class and health. It starts by looking at class as a form of social stratification and in so doing outlines other forms of social stratification and the different conceptualizations of class used in theoretical approaches and social research. Data on social class and morbidity rates, and social class and mortality rates are then presented. This is followed by an analysis of the sorts of factors that influence this relationship. The chapter ends with a discussion of some of the key theoretical explanations of the relationship between social class and health.

Social stratification

Social class is a form of social stratification. So what does this mean? It refers to the way society is divided into groups which are organized into a hierachy in which the most favoured are at the top and the less privileged are at the bottom. These groups are often referred to as 'strata' and the structure of the strata is called 'social stratification'. Several systems of social stratification exist, as explained below.

Caste

In a society based on a caste system of social stratification, social position is ascribed at birth and is unchangeable. Hence, individuals remain in the same social position throughout their lives. There are usually four major castes with a fifth group whose members are regarded as being outside the caste structure because they are 'untouchable'. Although the castes correspond with occupational groups, they are simultaneously ranked in order of religious purity, with those in the higher castes being regarded as the most pure. Intimate contact with those who are not members of your caste should be avoided, and indeed, sexual relations or marriage with members of other social groups is forbidden.

Prior to industrialization, caste societies existed throughout the world but there are now only a few, mainly in rural India. The expansion of capitalism into India's economy has meant that adherence to the caste system has been weakened because of the contact with those in other castes demanded by capitalist economic relations. As India is increasingly influenced by globalization, it is predicted that the caste system will become less and less sustainable and will give way to the class-based system of industrial societies (Sharma 1999; Giddens 2009).

Slavery

This form of stratification was very common in the USA, South America and the West Indies in the eighteenth and nineteenth centuries. Slavery meant that some individuals were literally owned by others as their property. Although some slaves were treated reasonably well, those working on plantations or in mines were often treated very harshly and brutal methods of punishment were used to try to increase their productivity.

As slaves often rebelled and fought back against their subjection, social systems based on slave labour were unstable. Slavery was also inefficient economically and from the eighteenth century onwards its morality was increasingly challenged. Although slavery is now illegal, it still exists in different forms throughout the world. For instance, there are sex slaves in Thailand and in Pakistan, and millions of people are in bonded labour because they have been tricked into a loan that leads to generational enslavement (Anderson 1974; Matthewman *et al.* 2007; Giddens 2009).

Social class

This differs from the other two forms of social stratification not only because it is less rigid but also because there is usually social mobility due to the fact that social status is in part achieved rather than given at birth. Class differences also depend on economic inequalities between groups of individuals. A very general definition of class is a system of social stratification in which there are groupings or classifications of the population with broadly similar occupations, resources and lifestyles. There can be some shared perception of their collective condition too – for example, those in the middle class identify with their position and others in it (Braham and Janes 2002; Matthewman *et al.* 2007). However, the precise meaning of class varies considerably, and it is to these variations that we now turn.

Conceptualizing social class

Definitions of social class vary from the everyday through to theoretical and official definitions. In addition, there are variations within these categories which also vary over time. This section aims to introduce you to these variations by exploring theoretical approaches to class as well as classification systems used for research into social class and official data-gathering purposes.

Theories of social class

An exploration of the concept of class cannot take place without reference to the historical approaches to class within sociology – namely the work of Karl Marx and Max Weber. The discussion of their theories of social class illustrates how theoretical concepts of class vary.

Activity 3.1

Think back to the discussion of Marxist theory in Chapter 1. What did Marx have to say about social class? Now read the following and see how much you have remembered.

Marx's theory of class

As explained in Chapter 1, Marx saw the organization of the ownership of the predominant means of production within an economy as the basis of class relations. He maintained that there were two main classes in contemporary societies – the bourgeoisie and the proletariat. Thus for Marx, social class refers to 'a group of people who stand in a common relationship to the means of production – the means by which they gain a livelihood' (Giddens 2009: 439). Although he did not systematically analyse the concept of class itself, Marx provided further details about these two main classes in various parts of his work. The bourgeoisie comprised those who owned and controlled capital, such as landowners, industrialists, bankers and those who could live on unearned income from investments. The proletariat were characterized by their lack of ownership and their use of labour power in their employment. The types of jobs they did were skilled and unskilled manual work and office work.

Marx argued that movement between these two classes was severely restricted. This was because the bourgeoisie tended to intermarry and their children inherited accumulated capital, whereas the proletariat tended to move between similar jobs and unemployment and to marry other workers, and their children had no option but to do the same. Consequently, people in each class had 'shared experiences' and developed a 'class consciousness'.

Although the relationship between these two classes was interdependent, it was based on the exploitation of the proletariat by the bourgeoisie and was essentially unequal and conflict-ridden. Furthermore, the inequalities between the two classes were not just economic but also caused inequalities in life chances that were likely to be perpetuated. Marx predicted that the 'class consciousness' of the proletariat would be fuelled by such persistent inequalities and exploitation, the two classes would polarize, and the proletariat would rise up against the bourgeoisie and over-throw capitalism. The resultant demise of capitalism and the emergence of socialism would be the only way that social conflict could be resolved and inequalities eradicated.

Among the strengths of Marx's two-class model is the way it could help to explain class issues involving industrial conflicts between capitalists and workers. Its critics have focused on the fact that it is too simplistic and does not capture the complexities of the class system in capitalist socie-ties. In response to such criticisms, Marxists have modified the original theory to acknowledge that there are more lines of differentiation within the two main classes. Other modifications include the recognition of an intermediate social class, referred to as the 'petit bourgeoisie' and those who occupy what Marxists refer to as 'contradictory class positions'. The former is made up of those who own capital but do not employ labour, such as shopkeepers. The latter refers to those groups who play a role in controlling capital and others, such as managers who manage budgets and those who design work systems, but are still exploited by capitalists (Wright 1989; Scott 2006).

Weber's multiclass model
Other sociologists have built on Marx's ideas. One of these was the German sociologist, Max Weber. He accepted the validity of Marx's theory of social class but rejected his economic determinism and developed his own model to present a more complex view of class. Weber proposed that class is not based solely on the ownership or non-ownership of the means of production and adopted a multifactorial approach to social stratification, using several concepts to describe the various economic and non-economic factors that may combine or diverge in different ways, depending on particular circumstances, to determine class (Weber 1997). These are as follows.

- **Market situation:** according to Weber, class is not only determined by control or lack of control over the means of production but by many other economic resources. These include skills, qualifications and expertise which influence the type of work people can undertake to make them 'marketable' to a greater or lesser extent and which lead to varying earning opportunities. He referred to these as an individual's 'market situation'. In turn, as market situation determines level of income and working conditions, it influences life chances and inequalities in these areas between social groups.

- **Status:** this is the difference in honour or prestige accorded to different social groups. While it is often related to symbols of status in people's lifestyles (e.g. expensive clothes, houses, cars and holidays) it is not always determined by wealth, as evidenced by the social esteem enjoyed by the aristocracy despite the fact that their assets have been compromised over time.

- **Party:** Weber saw this as an important component of class because being part of a party organi-zation, be it employment-related (e.g. trade unions and employers' organizations) political or religious, gives individuals access to power.

Table 3.1 Weber's four main classes

I	Propertied class
II	White-collar workers
III	Petty bourgeoisie (shopkeepers and small proprietors)
IV	Working class

Weber developed a four-class model (see Table 3.1) based on these overlapping elements of stratification. Hence, according to his model, inequalities between classes are the product of unequal access to a range of social resources to which those in the higher social classes have the greatest access. Weber also maintained that groups within this structure try to preserve their prestige by monopolizing resources and restricting access to their ranks, and called this process **social closure**. Examples of social closure include the way doctors' and lawyers' professional associations determine who qualifies for entry into their respective professions and actively protect their members. Furthermore, Weber argued that an individual's class position is a result of the diversity of such sources of inequality in society and their responses to them. Therefore, although class position leads to inequalities in life chances, individuals can act to change their position in society and hence do have social mobility (Scott 2006; Giddens 2009).

Weber's multiclass model is very useful in explaining how subdivisions arise within society and how life chances vary between groups. Despite the fact that his theory has been criticized for ignoring the role of gender, because of these qualities it has influenced studies on social mobility and social inequality.

Activity 3.2

Many of the differences between Marx and Weber's theories of class have emerged from the above summaries. Some of the similarities have also been alluded to. In order to help you revisit the main tenets of their arguments and check your understanding of them, read through the theories again and have a go at completing the table below on their main similarities and differences. If you only find a few similarities, don't worry, that is to be expected given how different the two theories are! Some suggestions about what you could include are in the 'Activity feedback' chapter on page 226.

Similarities	
Differences	

Social class classification systems for research

A number of indicators of social class have been used in social research into issues such as health. Some have been devised by researchers themselves. Examples include the Cambridge Scale, Townsend's Deprivation Indices and the Goldthorpe Class Schema. The latter is shown in Table 3.2.

Table 3.2 The Goldthorpe Class Schema, nine-category version

Class label	Occupational group	Level
I/II/IVa	Professional and managerial salariat and employees	1
IIIa	Routine non-manual employees, higher grade	2
IVb	Self-employed workers (non-professional)	2
IVc	Farmers	2
V	Foremen and technicians	2
VI	Skilled manual workers	2
IIIb	Routine non-manual workers, lower grade	3
VIIa	Semi-skilled and unskilled manual workers	3
VIIb	Agricultural workers	3

Source: Goldthorpe (1980)

Table 3.3 Registrar General's Social Class categories

Class label	Occupational group
I	Professionals
II	Managerial and technical
IIIN	Skilled occupations (non-manual)
IIIM	Skilled occupations (manual)
IV	Partly-skilled manual occupations
V	Unskilled manual occupations

Source: Office of Population, Censuses and Statistics (1998)

In official statistics and surveys, official classification systems for social class are used. The current one is the National Statistics Socioeconomic Classification (NS-SEC). This was introduced in 2001 and for several decades prior to this the two most widely used official socioeconomic classifications were the Registrar General's Social Class (see Table 3.3) and Socio-economic Groups (SEG). The NS-SEC is an occupationally-based classification system and was developed from a sociological classification that had been widely used in pure and applied research. It has eight classes and is set out in Table 3.4. As you can see, occupations are classified into agreed subgroups within these major groups, an example being the way that managers can be classified into corporate, production, and quality and customer care managers (Office for National Statistics 2002; National Statistics 2005a).

The above discussions about theories of social class and classification systems used in research about social class clearly demonstrate not only historical variations but also inconsistencies in the conceptualization of class. Nonetheless, a constant theme throughout the discussions was the way that class causes divisions between social groups in society. More importantly, the theories in particular highlight the way that the relationships between classes (whatever definition is used) lead to inequalities in terms of material and economic resources and social power. One of the most significant ways in which these inequalities are reflected is in the differences in health between social classes and the persistent class gradient that exists in health.

Table 3.4 The National Statistics Socio-economic Classification (NS-SEC) system

Class label	Occupational group
1	Managers and senior officials
2	Professional occupations
3	Associate professional and technical occupations
4	Administrative and secretarial occupations
5	Skilled trades occupations
6	Personal service occupations
7	Sales and customer service occupations
8	Process, plant and machine operatives
9	Elementary occupations

Source: National Statistics (2005a)

The relationship between social class and health

The use of morbidity and mortality rates to measure health has already been established. However, questions have often been raised about the use of these data to explore the relationship between health and social class. The data on mortality in Britain is derived from death certificates, and studies have shown that the information on these varies across the classes, which means that accurate comparison of the causes of death between the classes can be problematic. For instance, middle-class death certificates have been found to have more than one description of cause. It has been suggested that this is because those in the middle classes request more detailed explanations of the cause of death. Despite such problems, certain patterns indicative of a relationship between class and health have been observed and documented by researchers and policy-makers since the mid-nineteenth century (Black *et al.* 1980; Taylor and Field 2007).

As mentioned in the introduction to this chapter, the first significant piece of research about the inverse relationship between health and social class was the *Black Report* (1980). Subsequent important research has included Margaret Whitehead's survey *The Health Divide* (1987) (also known as the *Whitehead Report*), the *Independent Inquiry into Inequalities in Health Report* (Acheson 1998) (also known as the *Acheson Report*) and *Fair Society, Healthy Lives: A Strategic Review of Health Inequalities in England Post-2010* (Marmot 2010) (also known as the *Marmot Review*). The findings in these reports demonstrate the consistency of the trends in health inequalities between the social classes. These trends are illustrated in the case study below and explained in more detail in the following discussions about recent mortality and morbidity figures.

Case example: Once upon a time there were two little boys . . .

One was called Sam and the other was called Shaun. They both attended the primary school in their village, although Shaun was frequently absent because he suffered from asthma. Sam's parents were both professionals; his father was a teacher and his mother was an accountant. Shaun's father was a self-employed builder and his mother did some part-time cleaning in various houses in the village. Both sets of Sam's grandparents were alive and well, and he also had two great-grandmothers. In contrast, Shaun's only living grandparent was his maternal grandmother. His maternal grandfather had died a year previously of untreated Addison's Disease (an endocrinal disease which results in the adrenal glands producing insufficient hormones) and his paternal grandparents had died in their sixties of lung cancer. Shaun's father had recently been diagnosed with a respiratory disease called chronic obstructive pulmonary disease (COPD).

Mortality rates

As we saw in Chapter 2, although average life expectancy has increased dramatically over the past 100 years, there are variations in life expectancy between males and females. There are also variations in life expectancy between social classes: Figure 3.1 shows that there is an inverse relationship between mortality rates and social class for both men and women. The nature of this

Figure 3.1 Life expectancy at birth by social class, a) males, b) females, England and Wales, 1972–2005

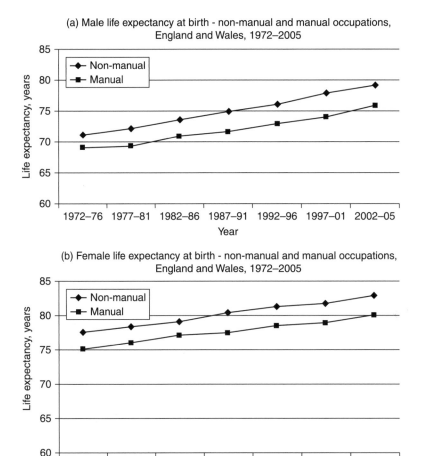

Source: Office for National Statistics (2007a)

relationship currently means that life expectancy at birth in England and Wales for males and females in the professional group is around 7.5 years more than that for those in the unskilled manual groups (Office for National Statistics 2006a, 2007a; Department of Health 2008b).

Cause of death varies with social class. For example those in semi-skilled and unskilled occupations are more likely than managerial, technical and professional workers to die from respiratory, endocrine, nutritional and metabolic diseases. Those in lower socioeconomic groups also have increased mortality rates for all cancers except breast cancer, which is most common among women with a higher social status. Furthermore, although there was a substantial fall in infant mortality rates during the twentieth century, infant mortality remains highest for babies with fathers in semi-routine and routine occupations. Moreover, decreases in the infant mortality rate for this group are usually smaller than those in the overall infant mortality rate (Office for National Statistics 2006a; Weires *et al.* 2008; Puigpinós *et al.* 2009).

Morbidity rates

Indicators of morbidity used in research into health differences between social groups are self-reported poor health and patterns of limiting long-term illness. While these indicators show that the health of the UK's population has improved steadily over the last century, they also show that there is still a strong relationship between social class and poorer health. Reporting of poor health is highest among those in the lower classes (including the unemployed) and lowest among those in the higher classes (i.e. those in professional and managerial occupations). Figure 3.2 is based on recent data and illustrates the extent of these variations between classes. For instance, it shows that the rates of 'not good health' for people in routine occupations are more than double those for people in higher managerial and professional occupations (8.6 per cent and 3.4 per cent respectively). The patterns for limiting long-term illness are similar to those of self-reported poor health

Figure 3.2 Self-reported general health (age standardized), UK, 2001

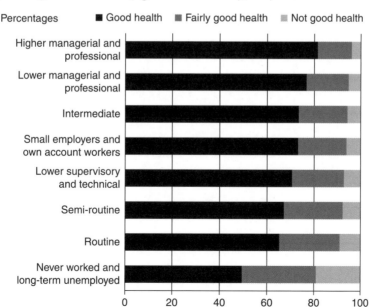

Source: Office for National Statistics (2006a)

Figure 3.3 Prevalence of neurotic disorders by social class

Social class	I	II	III Non-manual	III Manual	IV	V
Percentage	7	15	17	15	17	19.5

Source: adapted from Office for National Statistics (2006a)

(Office for National Statistics 2006a). This has led to conclusions such as 'those in the lower socio-economic groups experience a disproportionate burden of disease' (Naidoo and Wills 2008: 128).

Although there are some exceptions, as Figure 3.3 shows, mental illnesses are also generally greatest among the lower classes. However, one of the most notable exceptions is that eating and obsessive-compulsive personality disorders are more likely to occur in the higher social classes (National Statistics 2006a; Pilgrim 2007).

Activity 3.3

The following is an extract from the aforementioned *Marmot Report* (2010) into social inequalities in health. Read through it and note down any similarities with the information presented in this section of the chapter. There are some ideas to help you in the 'Activity feedback' chapter on page 226.

Not only are there dramatic differences between the best-off and worst-off in England, but the relationship between social circumstances and health is also a graded one: the higher a person's social position, the better his or her health is . . . In England, people living in the poorest neighbourhoods will, on average, die seven years earlier than people living in the richest . . . Even more disturbingly, there is a greater variation in the length of time people can expect to live in good health (their health expectancy). For example, the average difference in disability-free life expectancy is 17 years . . . In other words, people in poorer areas not only die sooner, but spend more of their shorter lives with a disability. To illustrate the importance of the gradient, even excluding the poorest five per cent and the richest five per cent, the gap in life expectancy between low and high income is six years, and in disability-free life expectancy 13 years.

(Marmot 2010: 37)

Influences on social class differences in health

Many influences on social class differences in health have been, and continue to be, identified, and the main ones have been selected for discussion in this section. As in Chapter 2, where specific details of the ways these influences affect health are required, these will either be given or the reader will be referred to Chapter 1.

Health-related behaviour

There is much evidence of class differences in health-related behaviour. This shows that those in the lower classes tend to take more risks in relation to their health (Lynch *et al.* 1997; Busfield 2000a; van Lenthe *et al.* 2009). Very recent studies have confirmed that *multiple* risk-taking behaviour in relation to health is more common among those in the lower socioeconomic groups (Drieskens *et al.* 2009). These patterns in health-related behaviour and lifestyle contribute substantially to class inequalities in health, and some examples are explored below.

Exercise

Although men in the lowest social classes are more physically active than other groups in society (mainly because they are less likely to have sedentary occupations), both men and women in non-manual occupations are much more likely to engage in leisure-time physical activity outside of the workplace. This is demonstrated in the following quotation: 'in men, age-adjusted rates of walking as a leisure-time activity are 38 per cent higher in social class 1 than in social class 5. For women, rates are 67 per cent higher in social class 1 than in social class 5. Similar trends are observed in sports participation' (Department of Health 2004a: 13).

Given the relationship between physical exercise and health (see Chapter 1, page 27), those in the lowest social classes who do not engage in work-related physical activity are at an increased risk of many chronic diseases because of their lower rates of physical exercise. Particular aspects of social disadvantage that can be associated with low socioeconomic status, such as low educational attainment, have been identified as contributing to the differences in non-work-related activity levels (Busfield 2000a; Department of Health 2004a; Graham 2009).

Diet

It has been recognized for some time that that there is a social gradient in diet quality, with those in the higher social classes having better diets than those in the lower classes. Darmon and Drewnowski (2008: 1107) found that: 'whole grains, lean meats, fish, low-fat dairy products and fresh vegetables are more likely to be consumed by groups of higher SES [socioeconomic status]. In contrast, the consumption of refined grains and added fats has been associated with lower SES'.

Alcohol consumption

Interestingly, the social gradient observed for diet quality is reversed for alcohol consumption. Those more likely to drink frequently are those in the highest income brackets, particularly those in the managerial and professional occupations (Busfield 2000a; Office for National Statistics 2004). Hence, higher socioeconomic groups face an increased risk of alcohol-related illnesses (both immediately and in later life) (see Chapter 1, page 27).

Obesity

Obesity is more common among those in the routine or semi-routine occupational groups than in the managerial and professional groups. Although women have higher obesity rates than men in general (see Chapter 2), statistics show that there is a strong link between social class and obesity for women, with those in the lower classes having the highest rates. For instance, the latest figures show that in 2001, 30 per cent of women in routine occupations were classified as obese compared with 16 per cent in higher managerial and professional occupations. Among those who had never worked and the long-term unemployed, 25 per cent of women were classified as obese, compared with 16 per cent of men (Office of Population, Censuses and Statistics 2002). As explained on page 27, obesity leads to a wide range of health problems which include serious illnesses such as diabetes, cardiovascular disease, certain cancers, hypertension, respiratory problems, and musculoskeletal diseases (Simonsen *et al.* 2008; Weaver *et al.* 2008; Marmot 2009).

Smoking rates
Although other factors such as gender and poverty are influential, there is a strong association between cigarette smoking and socioeconomic position. As discussed in Chapter 2, there has been a sharp fall in cigarette smoking over the past four decades. However, it is highest among manual social groups and lowest among higher managerial and professional classes. As Figure 3.4 shows, in 2006, almost twice as many adults aged 16 and over in routine and manual occupations smoked than in managerial and professional occupations (i.e. 29 per cent compared to 15 per cent). Such class differences have persisted since the 1990s, and recent data suggest no narrowing of the gap (Office for National Statistics 2008a; Gray and Leyland 2009). Consequently those in lower socioeconomic groups are, and will continue to be, more at risk of health problems caused by smoking (see Chapter 1, page 27).

Socioeconomic disadvantage has been identified as a cause of the continuing greater prevalence of cigarette smoking among lower socioeconomic groups (Graham and Blackburn 1998; Graham *et al.* 2006; Harman *et al.* 2006). This will be discussed in more depth in the next section of the chapter.

Figure 3.4 Cigarette smoking by socioeconomic classification, adults aged 16 and over, Great Britain, 2006

Socioeconomic classification	Percentage of cigarette smokers
Managerial and professional	**15%**
Large employers and higher managerial	14%
Higher professional	11%
Lower managerial and professional	18%
Intermediate	**21%**
Intermediate	20%
Small employers	22%
Routine and manual	**29%**
Lower supervisory and technical	25%
Semi-routine	31%
Routine	32%

Source: adapted from Office for National Statistics (2008b)

Breastfeeding
The benefits of breastfeeding are well established. It decreases the incidence and severity of many infections in infancy, including gastroenteritis and respiratory infections. It can also provide protection from later adverse health outcomes, such as diabetes. Furthermore, breastfeeding is beneficial to the mother's health; it increases the likelihood that mothers use up body fat deposited during pregnancy and can reduce the likelihood of developing epithelial ovarian cancer and premenopausal breast cancer.

Current recommendations are that, wherever possible, babies should be fed on breast milk exclusively from birth to 6 months. However, there are clear social class differences in both the initiation and duration of exclusive breastfeeding. With regards to the initiation of breastfeeding, mothers in higher managerial and professional occupations are four times as likely to initiate breastfeeding than mothers in routine jobs and those with the least favourable working conditions. In relation to the duration of exclusive breastfeeding, mothers in routine jobs are less likely to be breastfeeding their babies exclusively between 1 and 4 months than mothers in higher managerial and professional occupations (Acheson 1998; Kelly and Watt 2005; Dyson *et al.* 2007).

Living conditions

Higher proportions of those in the lower social classes live in social housing and poor housing in deprived areas than those in the higher social classes. As explained in Chapter 1, living in such conditions leads to poor health and is yet another influence on the social divide in health status (Office for National Statistics 2006a; Scott 2006).

Poverty and low income

Those in the lower social classes are more likely to live in poverty than those in the higher social classes because the nature of their work means they are more prone to unemployment and low income (Graham 2009). Several recent studies have attributed some of the poorer health outcomes and increased health risks experienced by those in lower socioeconomic groups to poverty and/or low income (Rose and Hatzenbuehler 2009). In terms of health outcomes, the low levels of income among these groups has been linked to higher incidences of mental health problems, cervical cancer, alcohol-related illnesses and lower survival rates after cardiac surgery (Currin *et al.* 2009; Dietze *et al.* 2009; Pagano *et al.* 2009; Tomlinson and Walker 2009). Examples from studies of the increased risk to their health include the way that their absence of adequate income means that the chances of reduced birth weight and pre-term birth are greater. Both of these lead to diseases in childhood and adulthood, such as cardiovascular disease, asthma and diabetes, and tooth, eye and ear problems. These poorer groups have also been shown to be more at risk of inadequate nutrition at all stages of life as well as obesity. As already established, these have short-term and long-term consequences on health (Nelson 2000; O'Donnell 2005; Law *et al.* 2007; DeFranco *et al.* 2008; Zeka *et al.* 2008).

Poverty and income inequality continue to rise (Brewer *et al.* 2008). The following extract from an article in *The Guardian* illustrates this point:

> Britain under Gordon Brown is a more unequal country than at any time since modern records began in the early 1960s, after the incomes of the poor fell and those of the rich rose in the three years after the 2005 election. Deprivation and inequality rose for a third successive year in 2007–8, according to data from the Department of Work and Pensions that prompted strong criticism from campaign groups for the government's backslidings on its antipoverty goals.
>
> (Elliot and Curtis 2009: 4)

Such inequalities seem to be firmly entrenched in our society, and for the immediate future at least are unlikely to reduce. Hence improvements in social class health differences associated with poverty and low income cannot be expected.

Healthcare

The inconsistent nature of data that has been produced about consultations with GPs has meant that it is difficult to come to any firm conclusions about variations between social groups in terms of their propensity to engage in such consultations. In contrast, data about the use of preventative services (e.g. screening and immunization services) show that there are social class differences in the use of these services. Preventative services contribute positively to health and are most frequently accessed by those in the higher social classes (Baggott 2004; Taylor and Field 2007).

In addition, those in the lower social classes are less likely to access outpatient and inpatient hospital care. Various reasons for this have been suggested. One is that more affluent groups may have enhanced access to specialist care through private health care insurance (Gulliford 2003). Others have identified a range of factors, as illustrated by Adamson *et al.* (2003: 18): 'There must be barriers at the referral, diagnosis or treatment stage of healthcare provisions. Such barriers may be due to differences in presentation of symptoms, communication problems between doctors and patients or systematic differences in the referral and treatment behaviours of practitioners'.

Some of the other factors that influence use of healthcare, such as age, gender and ethnicity, are discussed in other chapters. Although there have been and are several initiatives which aim to ensure greater equity in meeting healthcare needs across the social spectrum, it has been argued that policies need to focus on the source of inequalities, and make use of the sociological literature to identify the barriers to access experienced by different social groups (Dixon-Woods *et al.* 2005; Goddard 2009).

Activity 3.4

Here is an extract from a 2009 newspaper article entitled 'And you thought it was just the proles who ate all the pies'. It makes several points about social class and health-related behaviour. Read it through and then think about the questions that follow it.

> *Could doctors, lawyers and others of the professional persuasion put down their kebabs and pay attention? This obesity alert relates to you. A survey by Quorn has revealed that it is the middle classes who are the biggest buyers of takeaways, more so than plumbers, taxi drivers or others of the so-called lower order . . . The reason given for the middle class take-aways binge is the financial climate, the stress and fatigue of dealing with ongoing global upheaval causing their terrible diets . . . but when the working classes stuff down their greasy, calorific, life short-ening take-aways, the fault is all theirs . . . it is said that they are feckless morons, who need to take personal responsibility for their lardy lifestyles and don't deserve any help from the NHS. By contrast, [when] the middle classes are caught vacuuming up nightly tubs of sweet'n'sour, it is magically not their fault; they are merely hapless victims of global financial forces. Poor things. Talk about convenience food. Isn't the credit crunch just the most convenient excuse ever?*
>
> (Ellen 2009)

(1) In what ways do the findings from the survey by Quorn, as reported in this article, conflict with the points made in the section on social class and health-related behaviour?

(2)   What possible causes of differences in social class and health-related behaviour are suggested in the article?

There are some suggestions to help you in the 'Activity feedback' chapter on page 227.

Theoretical explanations of the relationship between social class and health

Several of the discussions in the above section referred to underlying factors that can be used to explain some influences on social class difference in health. Examples are socioeconomic disadvantage, the state of the economy and how these can shape health across the life course. In the light of the substantial body of evidence about social inequalities in health and their resistance to attempts at their equalization, those working within different theoretical perspectives have tried to unravel the contributing factors and develop explanations. The result is that there is now a range of theoretical approaches which are often challenged and renamed as new evidence and interpretations emerge. In order to give you a flavour of the differences in theoretical approach to the relationship between social class and health, three contrasting theories will now be discussed. The first two are based on two of the perspectives on the social aspects of health from Chapter 1: Marxist theory and postmodernism. These will be followed by a discussion of the life course perspective.

Marxist explanations

The mode of production within capitalism is inevitability the focus of Marxist explanations. Contemporary Marxist analyses of the social class gradient in health, illness and mortality rates acknowledge the development of both national and global capitalism. Several themes feature in these analyses. One is the role of the class system within capitalism which results in those in the lower social classes being forced to sell their labour to survive. Another is the way that the capitalist class exploit this fact in order to maximize profit. This exploitative relationship and pursuit of profit by the capitalist class means that they will cut the cost of labour in terms of increasing working hours, compromising work safety, increasing job insecurity and reducing autonomy, job satisfaction and wages. All of these impact on physical and mental health (Doyal and Pennell 1979; Busfield 2000a; Bradby 2009).

Marxist explanations also see diseases and their unequal distribution as the product in part of the social and economic conditions of industrial capitalism. This view is found in both early and more contemporary writing within the Marxist tradition. For instance, Fredrich Engels, Marx's fellow writer, maintained that the poverty and poor living conditions of the working classes led to higher incidences of disease, as demonstrated in the following quote from his work: 'That the dwellings of the workers in the worst portions of the cities, together with the other conditions of life of this class, engender numerous diseases is attested on all sides' (Engels 1969: 126).

More recent writers have revisited this earlier work and broadened its scope. They argue that the large-scale economic, social, technological and environmental changes that have occurred as a result of the development of capitalism at national, international and global levels impact negatively on health (Doyal 1995; Busfield 2000a). Although critics argue that Marxists use evidence selectively to support their arguments, their analyses do highlight the ways in which social structure can contribute to social class inequalities in health. As mentioned in Chapter 1, Marxist theory provides a structuralist view of society. This is because it emphasizes the structure of society and the way that it constrains and shapes people. Marxist analyses have inspired the development of many other structuralist explanations of the relationship between social class and health. These perspectives emphasize the effects of social structure on health and tend to focus on the impact on health of factors such as poverty, the distribution of income, type of employment, unemployment, housing conditions, pollution and working conditions in both the public and the domestic spheres. Structuralist explanations show that those in lower social classes are likely to suffer worse health because of the way factors such as poverty and housing conditions feature in their lives and have a more detrimental effect on them than those in the higher social classes. These perspectives are sometimes incorporated into a **social causation** approach to social issues and problems, because they see social factors as *causing* differences in health (Barry and Yuill 2008; Bradby 2009).

Postmodernist explanations

Can you remember the main points about postmodernism from Chapter 1? If not, they were that it challenges existing theoretical certainties about the social world and its structure. It also argues that human beings are 'agents' who make their own decisions about their lives and construct social life through their everyday interpretations and actions. Hence, the social world is in a constant state of flux.

Two main tenets of postmodernism are central to its explanation of social class differences in health. One is that any analysis in terms of social class is irrelevant. The other is its concept of agency in relation to human beings. Essentially, as people now have the opportunity to create their own lifestyles and identity, society is much more individualized and there are no distinctive subcultures, like those traditionally found in social classes. Furthermore, individuals' ability to shape their own lives through the decisions they make also extends to health. Hence, they can choose from a range of lifestyles and risks that affect their health. This was demonstrated in the previous section on the influences on class differences and health. A postmodernist explanation would recognize that such choices are obviously socially, culturally and historically relative, but would argue that individuals do have some choice, and that health differences are not soley the product of the structure of society, as in structuralist explanations (White 2009).

Activity 3.5

The discussions of Marxist and postmodernist explanations both referred to issues addressed in the section 'Influences on social class differences in health', such as the way that occupation and health-related behaviour can play a role in social class differences in health. Can you see any other such issues that have emerged and how these could form the basis of other explanations such as the life course perspective outlined below? To help you to evaluate your own attempts at theory development, its links with the aforementioned influences are highlighted.

The life course perspective

As indicated at the beginning of this section, there is a wide range of theoretical explanations about the relationship between social class and health. The above outlines of the approaches based on two of the perspectives from Chapter 1 made reference to evidence presented in the previous section about influences on social class differences in health that supported aspects of their arguments. Another explanation that is similarly linked to other themes that emerged from the discussions of these influences has been put forward within social constructionism – a strand of postmodernism. One of the most well-established social constructionist accounts is the life course perspective and this is the third and last theoretical approach to the relationship between social class and health to be discussed.

Among the influences on social class differences in health addressed so far, there were several examples of how some of the adverse health effects of social class can accumulate across the life course. One of these was the way that those in lower socioeconomic groups are less likely to breastfeed than higher socioeconomic groups and how this means that babies of mothers in lower social classes can consequently be more vulnerable to many infections in infancy and in later life. Another example was that the higher poverty experienced by those in the lower social classes increases their chances of having pre-term births and reduced birth weight babies, both of which lead to certain diseases in childhood and adulthood.

There is now a substantial body of research that shows how the poorer health outcomes of those in lower social classes are cumulative from conception, through to infancy, childhood, adolescence, adulthood and old age. Such findings have led to the development of a life course approach to social class differences in health (Field and Taylor 1998; O'Donnell 2005).

Some of those working within this approach have focused on how both advantages and disadvantages in relation to our health accumulate over time and used the concepts 'biographical time' and 'historical time' to do this. The former refers to the more personal events in our lives, such as relationships and employment. The latter refers to the particular social and economic events that occur in the course of a person's life, such as changing attitudes to sexuality or a severe global economic recession. 'Biographical' and 'historical' time are seen as relating to each other in that what happens in 'historical' time can influence 'biographical' time. The human body 'stores' both the beneficial and damaging experiences of 'biographical' and 'historical' time. Any damage accumulates over time and results in health problems later on in the life course (Bury 2000).

Let us take the example of a man in a low-paid job who is made redundant during a global economic recession to illustrate this approach. He is unable to find further employment for over two years and this takes its toll on his marriage and a divorce ensues. This results in a further drop in income. According to the life course approach, the combined effects of damaging events in his 'biographical' and 'historical' time will have negative impacts on his health in later life.

The life course perspective has contributed to the recognition in healthcare of the development of disease over the whole life course. This has simultaneously led to the acknowledgement that the whole person within the ongoing context of their life in its entirety needs to be taken into consideration when addressing health issues. In relation to social class health inequalities specifically, one of the strengths of this approach is that it integrates individual life trajectories with evolving social structures. Another is that as a model it has inspired a raft of preventative policies which, for instance, are aimed at preventing the development of health problems from the very beginning of life and eliminating child poverty (Lynch et al. 1997; O'Donnell 2005; Bradshaw et al. 2006).

Conclusions

The evidence presented in this chapter should leave you in no doubt that social class has a major and enduring impact on physical and mental health. While theoretical insights are plentiful, inequalities in health between social classes are proving extremely hard to eliminate despite numerous health interventions (Marmot 2010). This is partly because of the interrelationships between social class and other social divisions in creating these inequalities. We have already explored the influence of gender on health in Chapter 2. The next chapter will address the effects of ethnicity on health. Once again, the contributions made by the main disciplines that inform the study of the social aspects of health will be used to develop understandings of this topic.

Key points

■ Several systems of social stratification exist, of which class is just one example.

■ The most well-known historical approaches to class within sociology are those developed by Karl Marx and Max Weber.

■ There is a longstanding and strong relationship between class and health variations in life expectancy between socioeconomic groups, with poorer physical and mental health among those in the lower groups.

■ Many influences on social class differences in health have been, and continue to be, identified. These include health-related behaviour, living conditions, poverty, low income and use of healthcare.

■ There is now a range of theoretical approaches which are often challenged and renamed as new evidence and interpretations emerge.

Discussion points

■ What problems are associated with the use of classification systems for social class?

■ 'Although it has been well known for over a hundred years that occupation and social class are implicated in the aetiology of many diseases there are still no regular and reliable official statistics of provision of (let alone need for) medical treatment by the social or occupational class of the patient' (Black *et al.* 1980: 75). To what extent do you think that this statement is still true?

■ What role do you think individual behaviour plays in socioeconomic health inequalities?

Suggestions for further study

■ Chapter 7 in Gidden's book (2009) provides an excellent overview of different systems of social stratification, and theories of social class.

■ The Office for National Statistics publication *Focus on Health* (2006a) provides up-to-date figures and commentary on the relationship between social class and mortality and morbidity rates.

■ Useful discussions of socioeconomic health inequalities can be found in both Busfield's (2000a) *Health and Health Care in Modern Britain* and Graham's work *Understanding Health* and *Unequal Lives* (2000, 2009).

■ Chapter 6 in Barry and Yuill (2008) and Chapter 8 in Denny and Earle (2005) contain useful overviews of some of the contemporary theoretical explanations of the relationship between social class and health.

Ethnicity and health

4

Black and minority ethnic (BME) groups generally have worse health than the overall population, although some BME groups fare much worse than others, and patterns vary from one health condition to another.

(Parliamentary Office of Science and Technology 2007: 1)

Overview

Introduction

Research over the past 25 years has highlighted the **social inequalities** experienced by many of those from other countries who have settled in Britain. Migration into this country is not a new phenomenon. For instance, in the nineteenth century, rising populations and bad harvests led to a mass influx of Irish people. At the turn of the twentieth century, virulent anti-Semitism led to the movement of Jews from Eastern Europe. After the Second World War a significant number of people emigrated from Britain's old colonies (e.g. the New Commonwealth and Pakistan) to settle in Britain. Many were responding to the demand for labour in various sectors of the British economy as opportunities were often more limited in their own countries of origin. Among the most recent groups to make their homes here are those from Eastern European countries, such as Poland (Mason 2006). However, it is the immigration from Britain's old colonies since the Second World War that has had the most impact on our society. This is because of the extent to which it has increased the proportion of people of colour in Britain. They now make up just under 8 per cent of the population and their presence has made the country a more ethnically diverse society (Mason 2006).

Most of the aforementioned research has been about these non-white ethnic groups and, although studies have been carried out into the experiences of other groups, this area of research is, by comparison, in its infancy. Nor as yet does it allow the identification of trends in the same way as the now extensive body of research about non-white ethnic groups. The gathering of reliable data is further complicated by the fact that the more recent immigrants often do not spend long in this country. Indeed, a recent study found short-stay migration is a growing phenomenon – the number of immigrants spending less than four years in the UK doubled between 1996 and 2007 (Finch *et al.* 2009).

Research has shown the extensive nature of the inequalities between white and non-white ethnic groups and how these inequalities have led to the development of racial divisions which are now regarded, along with class and gender, as major social divisions in society. One of the main areas where this division is most apparent is in patterns of health and illness (Payne 2006; Ahmad and Bradby 2008). Hence the choice of the topic of ethnicity and health for this chapter.

As indicated in the quotation at the beginning of the chapter, the relationship between ethnicity and health is very complicated and a good understanding of it is required for an appreciation of the full extent of this social aspect of health. In order to provide you with a comprehensive understanding, this chapter will start by clarifying the definition of ethnicity to be used. In view of the considerable knowledge that exists about non-white ethnic groups and the lack of substantive research about more recent immigrant groups, the focus of the chapter is on non-white ethnic groups in relation to health. The main findings about the differences in health status of minority ethnic groups in the UK and the factors that contribute to these will then be explored. The final section evaluates some of the contemporary theoretical explanations of ethnic inequalities in health.

Defining ethnicity

Activity 4.1

What factors do you think need to be taken into consideration when defining ethnicity? Now read the paragraph below and see how your list of factors compares with those mentioned as being integral to this concept.

When defining ethnicity it is important to distinguish it from the term 'race'. Although the two concepts do overlap, 'race' is used to refer to physical or biological differences between people, whereas 'ethnicity' is 'socially constructed difference used to refer to people who see themselves as having a common ancestry, often linked to a geographical territory and perhaps sharing a language, religion and social customs' (Dyson 2005: 20). Such 'social customs' include dress, eating habits and literature. Notions of shared experiences, similarities and connections are therefore integral to ethnicity. This means that ethnic groups usually have a strong sense of identity as well as extensive and supportive networks, irrespective of any blood relationships that exist.

Despite the identification of the characteristics of ethnicity in this way, there is nonetheless an inherent fluidity in the concept in that it varies across situations and generations, and with time. Systems of classification are also continually being contested and revised. Another complication when studying ethnicity and health is that different terms are used in the research carried out. In the light of any consequent confusion and for the sake of clarity in this chapter, the term 'minority ethnic groups' will be used and these are defined as those non-white groups who are from, or are descended from, populations in Caribbean and African countries, the Indian subcontinent, Hong Kong and South China. While the dynamism of the concept of ethnicity and within-group heterogeneity is acknowledged, fixed categories for minority ethnic groups are used to reflect those applied in the literature under discussion. When comparisons are made between studies, every effort will be made to ensure that the categories in question share the same characteristics.

Three very broad categories tend to be used for people from the aforementioned countries: 'black', 'Asian' and 'Chinese'. The composition of the main groups within these categories, together with a brief outline of where they originate from, can be found in Table 4.1.

Ethnic inequalities in health

The way official statistics were compiled meant that the links between ethnicity and health were not established until the 1980s. Since then there has been much research into the health status of minority ethnic groups in the UK. Although this consistently shows that these groups are more vulnerable to ill health *in general* than the white British, there is considerable variation between and within groups. For example, Pakistani, Bangladeshi and black Caribbean people report the worst general health. In contrast, black African, Indian, East African and Asian groups report the same general health as white British. Chinese people tend to report the best general health of all white and non-white groups. There are also significant differences in the *types* of physical and mental illnesses experienced by members of minority ethnic groups. An overview of these is set out below.

Physical illnesses
As the following examples show, some clear trends in the prevalence of certain physical illnesses have emerged.

- **Cancer:** although overall cancer rates for those in minority ethnic groups are lower than for the majority population, 'there is not an across the board inequality of cancer incidence' for these groups (National Cancer Intelligence Network 2009: 5). For instance, Asian people have higher rates of liver and mouth cancer than white British people. Black males of all ages are more likely to be diagnosed with prostate cancer than white males. The incidence of breast cancer among minority ethnic women who were not born in the UK has been attributed to the fact that it takes

Table 4.1 The main non-white, black and minority ethnic groups in the UK

Indian	This Asian group has its ancestry in the Indian subcontinent and comprises both Indian Sikhs and Indian Gujeratis. The former are from the Punjab in northern India and follow the Sikh religion. Indian Gujeratis have migrated from Gujerat in western India and are either Hindus or Muslims.
Pakistani	These people are also classified as Asian. They come from all over Pakistan and although they are therefore from several different races, they usually follow the religion of Islam.
Bangladeshi	The predominant religion among this third Asian group is Islam. They mainly come from the coastal areas of Bangladesh and from Sylhet, which is located in the north-east of the country. However, geographical and political changes mean that a sense of national identity may be elusive for those in this group.
African Asian	These people are also Asian and originate from various East African countries, such as Kenya, Uganda and Tanzania. They include Hindus, Sikhs and Muslims.
Black Caribbean	This group is referred to as 'black'. They often have African ancestral origins but their more immediate forebears settled in the Caribbean West Indian islands (excluding Puerto Rico, Dominica and Cuba, as people from these countries are Latin American).
Black African	This is another 'black' group. They mainly come from West Africa but exclude those of other ancestry, such as European and South Asian, living in Africa.
Chinese	These are natives of China. Not only does 'Chinese' refer to ethnicity but also to race, as the Chinese race approximates to the group known as 'Mongolian' in terms of historical racial classifications.

time for the detrimental lifestyle and other risk factors associated with living in this country to impact on health.

- **Heart disease:** as explained in Chapter 2, men have higher rates of ischaemic heart disease (i.e. heart attack or angina) in general than women. Men in certain minority ethnic groups are 50 per cent more likely to have ischaemic heart disease than other men in the population. These are the Bangladeshi, Pakistani and Indian groups. Chinese men and women have the lowest rates of any group in the UK. Mortality rates from coronary heart disease (CHD) for those who have migrated from the Indian subcontinent are more than 50 per cent higher than those in the majority population

- **Strokes:** high blood pressure (hypertension) contributes significantly to the risk of having a stroke. Caribbean men and women have the highest rates of hypertension while Bangladeshi men, Chinese and Bangladeshi women have the lowest. Caribbean men are 50 per cent more likely to die of a stroke than the general population.

- **Diabetes:** the prevalence of diabetes is five times higher among African Caribbean and Asian communities than other groups in the UK. Although Chinese people have the lowest rate of diabetes among the minority groups, this is still higher than in the white population.

■ **Maternal morbidity:** experiencing a severe illness during pregnancy, labour and birth is more common among non-white women, and particularly those within the black African and black Caribbean minority groups. This pattern is reflected in reported differences in maternal death rates.

■ **Sickle cell disorders:** sickle cell anaemia and thalassaemia beta are the most common forms of sickle cell disorders. While they do occur in the white majority population, this is only infrequently and the risk of their occurrence is elevated for particular minority ethnic groups. The sickle cell trait is carried by as many as 1 in 4 West Africans and 1 in 10 African Caribbeans. Thalassaemia beta is carried by 1 in 10 Pakistanis and 1 in 30 Chinese (Culley and Dyson 2001; Dyson 2005; Bhopal 2007; Parliamentary Office of Science and Technology 2007; Taylor and Field 2007; Knight *et al.* 2009).

Mental illnesses

Research concerned with the incidence of mental ill health among minority ethnic groups is more controversial. Until recently, findings showed that these groups shared a similar rate of mental illness to that of the indigenous white population but a more complex picture is now emerging. Surveys based on treatment rates show that those in minority ethnic groups are *more likely* to be diagnosed as having a mental illness than white British. In addition, 1 in 5 mental health inpatients come from a minority ethnic background, compared to about 1 in 10 of the population as a whole. However, surveys that have looked at the prevalence of mental illness in the community show smaller ethnic differences. Nonetheless, there is evidence that some minority ethnic groups are particularly susceptible to certain types of mental illness (Melzer *et al.* 2004; Parliamentary Office of Science and Technology 2007; Allen 2008). These are as follows.

■ **Psychoses:** the diagnosis of psychosis in general is seven times higher for black Caribbean people than white British, while the Chinese have the lowest rates of diagnoses for psychoses. Psychotic illnesses also include schizophrenia. When the figures for psychosis are disaggregated to show the different types of illness, they reveal that the incidence of schizophrenia is substantially higher for those who fall into the broad category of 'black' (see Table 4.2). Furthermore, there is evidence in one of the latest studies that the black Caribbean population experiences the highest psychosis rates.

■ **Depression:** Figure 4.1 shows depression rates for both men and women by ethnic group. Taking women first, when compared with the white population, rates of depression are higher

Table 4.2 Incidence of schizophrenia by ethnic group

Group	Number of new cases per 100,000
White	14.4
Mixed	22.8
Asian	17.0
Black	87.6
Other	26.9

Source: Fearon *et al.* (2006)

Figure 4.1 Percentage of people with depression, by ethnic group and gender

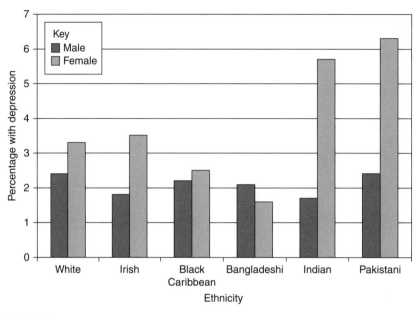

Source: McCrone *et al.* (2008)

among Indian and Pakistani women but lower for black Caribbean and Bangladeshi women. With reference to depression rates for men, although these are more uniform for men in black and minority ethnic groups, Pakistani men have the worst rates.

■ **Phobias:** these are more prevalent among Asian and Chinese people than in the indigenous British white population (Melzer *et al.* 2004; Fearon *et al.* 2006; Taylor and Field 2007; McCrone *et al.* 2008).

The evidence that has emerged about ethnic inequalities in health, as presented in this section, has led to conclusions such as 'the relationship between ethnicity and health is a very complex and changing one' (Taylor and Field 2007: 75). It also points to the fact that a range of influences shape the health of those in minority ethnic groups. For example, the statistics about diabetes and schizophrenia rates suggest that genetic factors are important. Heart disease and depression rates seem to be linked to gender. In addition, the findings about cancer and phobia rates indicate the role of cultural and environmental factors. Before considering the explanations that have been put forward about ethnic variations in health and illness, let us explore some of the main risk factors that have been identified.

Activity 4.2

Below is an extract from a Race Equality Foundation briefing paper on ethnicity and coronary heart disease. While it discusses the many influences on the link between high rates of coronary heart disease and people of South Asian origin specifically, it also illustrates the range of influences and explanations that need to be considered when addressing the complex relationship between ethnicity and health. Once you have read the rest of this chapter, try to identify any similarities with the points made in this extract.

> *Cardiovascular disease (CVD) is a progressive long-term condition in which the heart and/or circulatory system becomes 'diseased'. It includes a host of conditions, examples of which are coronary heart disease (CHD) and stroke. Living with one or more of these conditions has a significant impact on quality of life for both the individual concerned and those around them who provide care and support . . . South Asians living in the UK have a high rate of CVD compared to the majority population . . . the reasons for higher morbidity and excess death among South Asian populations remain unclear . . . conventional factors, such as high blood pressure and high blood cholesterol, undoubtedly contribute to this increase. On their own, however, they do not account for the full extent of increased risk . . . This has led to the proposition that there are differences, among ethnic groupings, in the role and potency of coronary risk factors . . . several risk factors might explain this. Diet and lack of exercise are perhaps generic problems for socially disadvantaged groups. People of South Asian origin living in the UK, for instance, tend to have low levels of physical activity and fitness compared to the general population . . . some biological factors linked with CVD are more common in people of South Asian origin than in other ethnic groups. Metabolic syndrome is one of these: a condition in which a group of risk factors (such as high blood pressure and large waistline) occur together, increasing the risk of CVD . . . other biological factors more common in South Asian people and linked to CVD are endothelial dysfunction (malfunctioning cells lining the inside of blood vessels) and high levels of other biological compounds such as homocysteine (a chemical building block used by the body to make protein) . . . Genetic factors also influence an individual's predisposition to CHD but should not be overestimated. Biological and behavioural factors cannot explain all ethnic variations either . . . socio-economic status, disadvantage and social exclusion, alongside inappropriate and inaccessible service support, are equally likely to be important. None of these factors, however, has been studied systematically and little is known about their actual impact.*
>
> (Astin and Atkin 2010: 1)

Influences on ethnic inequalities in health

As in Chapters 2 and 3, details of the ways these influences affect health are either provided or the reader will be referred to Chapter 1.

Income and poverty levels

These are adversely affected by the following factors.

- **Unemployment:** although unemployment rates for ethnic minority groups have decreased, they are twice those for the total working age population. There are considerable variations between groups and between males and females in certain groups. Figure 4.2 illustrates some of these: Indian men have a similar level of unemployment to other white men (7 per cent and 6 per cent respectively). However, the unemployment rates for black Caribbean, black African, Bangladeshi and mixed race men are around three times the rates for white British and white Irish men (between 13 and 14 per cent). Pakistani women have the lowest employment rates whereas the unemployment rate for Pakistani men is just over the average (National Statistics 2004b; Clark and Drinkwater 2007).

Figure 4.2 Unemployment by ethnic group and sex, Great Britain, 2004

Percentages

[Bar chart showing unemployment percentages by ethnic group, split by Males and Females, for: White British, White Irish, Other White, Mixed, Indian, Pakistani, Bangladeshi, Other Asian, Black Caribbean, Black African, Chinese, All ethnic groups. Horizontal axis: 0, 5, 10, 15, 20. Legend: Males, Females.]

Source: National Statistics (2006b)

■ **Type of employment:** research from the 1960s to the 1980s showed that those in minority ethnic groups were employed in particular industries and occupations and more likely to be in less skilled and lower paid jobs than other groups in the population. Current research indicates that the employment experiences of those in these groups are now more divergent – African Asian, Chinese and Indian men are just as likely to be in the top two occupational groups as those in the white population. While the proportion of those from all ethnic groups with managerial jobs is increasing, the biggest increases are for black Caribbean, black African and Indian men as well as Indian women. In contrast, Bangladeshi men remain concentrated in the lower skilled and lower paid jobs (Social Exclusion Unit 2004a; Department for Work and Pensions 2006; Mason 2006).

Improvements in occupational attainment have been most marked for those who have obtained higher qualifications. Nonetheless, there is statistical evidence that graduates from ethnic minority groups, particularly women, are less likely to be employed than white graduates and are increasingly experiencing more problems obtaining high status jobs. Such inequalities also have longer-term implications for retirement planning and pension entitlement (Clark and Drinkwater 2007; Platt 2007).

The persistence of such, albeit reduced and more variable, differences in occupational attainment are reflected in the way that the incomes of those in ethnic minority groups are generally lower than those of white people. Those who are most vulnerable to such income differentials are Bangladeshi men, who on average earn 27 per cent less than white men. There are also substantial earnings gaps within occupations, as illustrated by the fact that black Africans and Bangladeshis in professional and managerial occupations earn up to 25 per cent less than white men in similar positions.

Hence, minority ethnic groups experience higher unemployment levels and pervasive earnings disadvantages in the British labour market. These factors, in combination with their low uptake of some benefits, mean that income poverty rates among minority ethnic groups are, on average, twice as high as that of white British people. Moreover, this is despite a national reduction in income poverty over the last decade in this country. Some groups are particularly vulnerable – as Figure 4.3

Figure 4.3 Income poverty rates

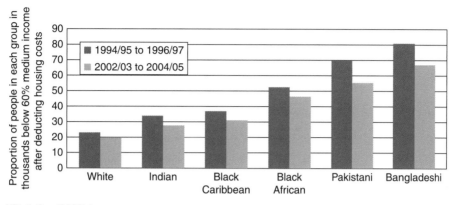

Source: National Statistics (2006b)

shows, income poverty rates are highest for Bangladeshis and Pakistanis (Clark and Drinkwater 2007; Palmer and Kenway 2007; Platt 2007).

Apart from the more general health problems associated with living in poverty (see Chapter 1, page 27), several specific effects of poverty on the health of poorer people in ethnic minorities have been identified. For instance, they are more likely to experience mental ill health and have higher rates of long-term illness (Culley and Dyson 2001; Melzer *et al.* 2004; Platt 2007).

Housing

Although both urban and rural areas are increasingly ethnically diverse, those in ethnic minority groups tend to be concentrated in certain parts of the most densely populated urban areas. Examples are London and the West Midlands. There are many reasons for this, such as the location of particular industries. Some studies have also shown that residential concentration of ethnic groups is driven by a preference for co-ethnic neighbours because of **discrimination** and hostility (Clark and Drinkwater 2007). Whatever the reasons, the outcome is that they live in some of the most deprived areas and experience the many disadvantages inevitably associated with this, which include poorer employment prospects and higher crime rates. They are also less likely to be homeowners and more likely to be living in social housing (Mason 2006; Platt 2007; Shelter 2007).

As discussed in Chapter 1 (see page 27), living in deprived neighbourhoods and poor housing have many adverse effects on physical and mental health and are not conducive to a healthy lifestyle.

Healthcare

There is relatively little research into the provision and use of healthcare in relation to those in minority ethnic groups. That which exists shows that their GP consultation rates tend to be the same or higher than those of the white population but this could be related to the higher incidence of illness that they experience. There is also some evidence that minority ethnic groups have lower utilization rates of hospital outpatient and inpatient services, as well as some preventative services such as cervical screening (Adamson *et al.* 2003; Gulliford and Morgan 2003; Taylor and Field 2007; Badger *et al.* 2009; Moser *et al.* 2009).

When the full range of healthcare services available are not being used by a particular group, they are obviously more at risk of adverse health outcomes than other groups. Several different types of barriers that exist for minority ethnic groups have been identified. These include language, lack of knowledge about which services to access, health beliefs, and attitudes towards health services. Some of these are highlighted in the case study below. Although lack of culturally sensitive services (particularly in mental health services) and discriminatory attitudes by staff have also been identified as barriers, very recent research has shown that there have been improvements in these areas (Culley and Dyson 2001; Adamson *et al.* 2003; Dixon-Woods 2005; Bhopal 2007; Badger *et al.* 2009).

Case example: Screening services

Priya was of South Asian origin and although she had lived in Britain for 25 years, she had not mixed much outside her own cultural group. She did not use any of the services at her GP surgery and her contact with the medical staff had been mainly limited to giving birth to her four children. The births had taken place at her local hospital where they were very good at meeting the needs of women from minority ethnic groups.

When she turned 50, she received an invitation to attend for breast screening. She had trouble understanding the letter but was encouraged by her daughter to access the relevant information in her own language and to attend.

She was extremely anxious about her appointment at the mobile breast screening unit that was set up in the car park of her local supermarket. When she got there, her daughter was not allowed to accompany her and she could not understand all the instructions that she was given, in English only, by the receptionist about undressing and the procedures that would be followed. Much to Priya's embarrassment the receptionist just repeated the instructions very loudly which made others in the waiting room look in their direction to see what was going on. The radiographer was pushed for time, somewhat abrupt with her and insensitive to her lack of English language skills. She came out of the breast screening unit in a very distressed state and refused to attend for further screening to check out an abnormality that had been identified.

In connection with the point made in the case study, minority ethnic groups are more likely to report negative experiences of healthcare and, more generally, health and social care. Asian and Chinese people are least likely to be positive (Lester and Glasby 2006; Healthcare Commission 2009).

Activity 4.3

Read the outline of postmodernism in Chapter 1. Think about the extent to which people from minority ethnic groups are 'agents' and have the sort of postmodernist choices described in relation to their health. Use the boxes below to jot down your thoughts. See the relevant section in the 'Activity feedback' chapter on page 227 for a detailed discussion.

Evidence of lack of 'agency' and choice	
Evidence of 'agency' and choice	

How can the relationship between ethnicity and health be explained?

The role of discrimination has been highlighted in several of the preceding discussions about ethnic inequalities in health. Discrimination is a dimension of **racism** which manifests itself when those groups who believe themselves to be inherently 'superior' discriminate in terms of their attitudes and behaviour against those who belong to ethnic groups because they are deemed to be 'inferior'. Such judgements are bound up with the idea that certain biological and racial characteristics make people different and less acceptable in terms of their social activities and abilities. There are different types of racism: **institutional racism** has been referred to as a 'corrosive disease' and is defined in the report on the enquiry into the death of Stephen Lawrence as:

> The collective failure of an organisation to provide an appropriate and professional service to people because of their colour, culture, or ethnic origin. It can be seen or detected in processes, attitudes and behaviour which amount to discrimination through unwitting prejudice, ignorance, thought-lessness and racist stereotyping which disadvantage minority ethnic people.
>
> (Macpherson 1999: 8)

Racism can also be **direct** and **indirect**. The former can take the form of physical and/or verbal abuse because of race, ethnicity and religion, whereas indirect racism is the fear of direct racism – it does not refer to the actual experience of being physically attacked or verbally abused but to the fear that that this *could* happen (Mason 2006; Barry and Yuill 2008).

Despite initiatives to address racism, it still exists in many areas of life and there is increasing acknowledgement that 'racism may be said to affect health adversely' (Dyson and Smaje 2001: 54). For instance, institutional racism subtly affects life chances and this leads to inequalities in standards of living which in turn can adversely affect the health of some minority ethnic groups. Where direct racism takes the form of physical assault there are obviously immediate health consequences. In addition, both direct and indirect racism have been shown to increase anxiety levels, inhibit social interaction and lead to social isolation. These effects in turn cause a range of psychological and physiological health problems such as increased depression levels, hypertension and cardio-vascular disease (Dyson and Smaje 2001; Harris *et al.* 2006).

While racism *per se* undermines health, there are many other factors that determine the health of minority ethnic groups. These are addressed in contemporary accounts of the relationship between ethnicity and health. As you will see in the outlines of selected examples below, the role of racism is nevertheless implicit in some of the explanations put forward.

Genetic explanations

The validity of explanations based on the role of genetics has been questioned because of incon-sistencies in the classification of minority ethnic groups over time and evidence of huge variations in risk within minority ethnic groups (Dyson and Smaje 2001; Iley and Nazroo 2001). Nonetheless it is important that genetic factors are not overlooked completely. This is because some specific genetic factors which contribute to certain illnesses – for example, inherited blood disorders – broadly correlate with some ethnic groups. However, in view of the strong influence of environ-mental and social factors on the incidence of certain diseases within minority groups the contributory nature of their role needs to be emphasized (Nazroo 2001; Denny and Earle 2005).

Cultural explanations

The role of minority ethnic **culture** in explaining the relationship between ethnicity and health has provided some useful insights in understanding concepts of health within ethnic groups and the impact of culture on health-related behaviour and lifestyle. An example of the latter comes from surveys in the UK on smoking rates which have shown that these vary dramatically between ethnic groups – for instance, smoking is much more common among Bangladeshi men (49 per cent) than among white British (29 per cent), Pakistani (28 per cent) or Indian men (19 per cent). The rate is particularly high (56 per cent) in Bangladeshi men aged 50–74 (Bush *et al.* 2003). On a more positive note, the extent of the cohesiveness of minority ethnic cultures is an important influence on health. As mentioned in the first section of the chapter, ethnicity can be a source of social networks. Studies have highlighted how involvement in such networks within minority ethnic cultures provides **social integration** and social support which have been found to have positive effects on physical and mental health.

The value of these insights is somewhat diminished by the fact that the overall evidence is that the role of culture in health is not very significant and criticisms have been voiced that its influence downplays key structural and environmental factors. Moreover, critics have warned against adopting a rigid and stereotypical view of minority ethnic culture, and of the need to acknowledge changes in cultures as well as variations within and across them (Berkman and Syme 1979; Berkman *et al.* 2000; Dyson and Smaje 2001; Karlsen and Nazroo 2001; Bradby 2009).

Materialist explanations

These focus on the ways in which material deprivation can cause variations in the health of minority ethnic groups. Materialist theories have been accused of not accounting for all significant variations, such as why the prevalence of diabetes is so much higher in most minority ethnic groups than among the white population, irrespective of social class. In the light of the association between depression and material deprivation, another example of the limitations of materialist explanations is the fact that Bangladeshi women, who are among the most economically disadvantaged in society, have low depression rates. Such criticisms have led to allegations that these explanations are imprecise about what mechanisms and mediating factors intervene in the relationship between material deprivation and the health of those in minority ethnic groups.

In defence of materialist explanations, it has been pointed out that they are plagued by the problems of measuring deprivation. Attempts have also been made to address some of the criticisms by developing more sophisticated approaches. These include identifying different dimensions of material deprivation (e.g. housing tenure, income and car ownership) and showing how each of these exerts a cumulative effect on health to a greater or lesser extent. Nonetheless, the explanatory power of materialist explanations is still compromised because, even when material deprivation is controlled, ethnic differences in health remain (Nazroo 1997; Nazroo and Williams 2006; Taylor and Field 2007).

So what can be concluded from the discussions of these explanations? Most apparent is that no single explanation is adequate in itself and that there are many issues that need to be addressed to ensure the rigour of any theory about ethnic variations in health. The fact that ethnic health inequalities are the outcome of interactions between a range of factors at the macro and micro levels, including other social divisions, needs to be acknowledged. Another issue is that it is necessary to recognize that mediating factors affecting health are at work. An example is the way in which the socially integrating effects of culture within minority groups can counteract some of the adverse effects of other factors – one such factor being material deprivation. Finally, the composition of our minority ethnic groups is not static. A major predicted change is that the number of older people within ethnic minority groups will double between 2004 and 2026 (Parliamentary Office of Science and Technology 2007). Therefore, explanations need to be able to accommodate evolutions in the groups who are the subject of their theorizing.

Activity 4.4

The following three quotes are taken from the work of Sir Liam Donaldson, the UK's chief adviser on health issues (see Department of Health 2008c). In these he echoes some of the main points made in this chapter. To help you clarify your own thinking about the issues raised, see if you can identify the links between the content of the different sections of the chapter and the quotations below. There are some ideas to help you in the 'Activity feedback' chapter on page 228.

(**1**) *Contemporary European and American research on race, ethnicity, and health uses poorly defined labels to describe study populations. The search for accurate terminology remains controversial, for scientific and social reasons.*

(American Journal of Public Health, 1998, 88: 1303)

(**2**) *Although, given the size and young age structure of the Asian population, absolute numbers of cases were small, a significant excess of Asian cases (compared with the expected) occurred for cancer of the tongue, oral cavity, pharynx, and oesophagus. For most sites there were fewer Asian cases than would be expected, particularly so for the stomach, testis, and skin. The results indicate the need for formal epidemiological study to test specific aetiological hypotheses which may account for these apparent differences.*

(Journal of Epidemiology and Community Health, 1984, 84: 203–7)

(**3**) *Those preparing health education materials for ethnic minorities need to have a sound understanding of the history, culture and development of the ethnic minority community they serve.*

(Health Education Journal, 1988, 47: 137–40)

Conclusions

As you will have seen in this chapter, ethnic inequalities in health pose many challenges, not least of which is obtaining accurate and up-to-date data and developing viable explanations so that they can be addressed effectively. Mention has been made of some of the successes of policy initiatives, but there is a need for many more, targeted and creative in their approaches to the health inequalities experienced by the diverse and changing minority ethnic groups in society. In order to implement such initiatives, more extensive and rigorous research into this particular social aspect of health is required.

Key points

■ Those who belong to a minority ethnic group in this country are more vulnerable in general to ill health than the white British population.

■ There are also significant differences in the types of physical and mental illnesses they experience.

■ There are many influences on the complex relationship between ethnicity and health – for example, income and poverty, housing, and healthcare.

■ While there are several explanations of the relationship between ethnicity and health, continuing racism is an underlying cause.

Discussion points

■ In what ways do you think that the concepts of 'race' and 'ethnicity' overlap?

■ To what extent do you agree with the statement, 'the relationship between ethnicity and health is a very complex and changing one' (Taylor and Field 2007: 75)?

■ Which of the explanations of the relationship between ethnicity and health do you find most convincing and why?

Suggestions for further study

■ Up-to-date statistics on ethnic minority groups can be found in the Focus On series produced by the Office for National Statistics (www.statistics.gov.uk/focuson/ethnicity).

■ For a more in-depth discussion of the physical and mental health of those in ethnic minority groups, see Chapters 2 and 3 in Culley and Dyson (2001) and the Department of Health website (www.dh.gov.uk). The latter also provides details of current policies.

■ The Joseph Rowntree Foundation has recently produced several studies about poverty rates among ethnic groups and these can be found on their website (www.jrf.org.uk).

■ Nazroo (2001) provides more details about the range of explanations regarding the relationship between ethnicity and health.

Ageing and health

. . . inequalities over the life course may cast a long shadow and lead to inequalities in health that persist into retirement.

(Higgs and Rees Jones 2009: 8)

Overview

Introduction

The final chapter of this section explores the relationship between age and health. The systematic inequalities in the life chances and material circumstances between people of different ages means that 'age' is now recognized as a distinct social division (Jamieson and Victor 2002; Vincent 2006). The relationship between age and health is very topical, hence it is important that this is addressed in order to complete your understanding of the potential influence of social divisions within the study of the social aspects of health.

Some of the key themes that have emerged about this relationship are presented in this chapter. It begins by exploring the social processes involved in the concept of 'age' *per se*. Data about health across the different phases of the life course are then be examined and the patterns that can be identified are explained. One of the most important issues for our society to emerge from the data is the way that older people have a higher incidence of ill health compared to the rest of the population. Therefore the last part of the chapter focuses on the health and healthcare of older people.

The chapter draws mainly on the life course perspective as this has been applied to a wide range of issues within the literature on age and health. It offers insights into many of the areas addressed in this chapter, such as the construction of age differentiation across the life course and the relationship between ageing and health. The age categories used for official statistical gathering purposes have been adopted throughout the chapter.

The meaning of 'age'

The varying constructions of 'age'

'Age' has different meanings between cultures and across time, and these varying constructions are reflected in the ways age is used to differentiate between people. For instance, studies have shown that in foraging societies (for example the Mbuti people of the Congo) there is minimal social differentiation in terms of age. In contrast, the structure of more traditional societies, such as that of a tribal society and in rural India, tends to be based around rigid age criteria with older people having considerable power over younger people. Although western societies do not tend to have age boundaries fixed by any objective criteria in this way, there are broadly defined social statuses, roles and patterns of appropriate behaviour which are linked to different chronological stages in our life course. Terms which correspond with particular age groups are used to identify these stages, for example, 'childhood', 'adolescence', 'middle age' and 'old age'. There are also rituals to mark the passage from one age to another, such as eighteenth birthday celebrations and retirement parties. Furthermore, age categories are used for statistical purposes (Vincent 2003; Hunt 2005).

However, the literature on age in European societies has highlighted the way that such terms, categories and rituals change over time. For instance, with reference to childhood in medieval Europe, this was not a distinct stage of life in most cultures in that children were not regarded as significantly different from adults. They were integrated into adult working and social life, and were treated and dressed as miniature adults who gradually assumed adult roles and slowly matured into adulthood. Children in the lower classes worked at a very early age and for the same long hours as adults (Ariès 1962). There are those who argue that in many societies the recognized number of life stages has increased and now also include engagement, home-ownership, parenthood and grandparenthood. The ways in which these are ritualized has changed in that the extent to which they are associated with distinctive consumption patterns has increased (Hareven 1995).

The life course perspective and 'age'

Evidence about the variations in life experiences across cultures and time have been used within the life course perspective (see Chapter 3) to argue that life stages are not biologically fixed, standardized, chronological, sequential or gendered. Instead, they are socially constructed through a range of social, cultural, political and economic processes (Hareven 1995; Hunt 2005; Vera-Sanso 2006). Hence, in addition to its biological element, this perspective argues that 'age' is also socially and culturally determined. Indeed, this view has led to the concept of an age-determined life course being challenged.

Explanations of the life stage of 'old age' developed by those who adopt a life course perspective illustrate these social constructionist elements (see Chapter 1) in the arguments put forward. In its account of old age, the life course perspective identifies the sources and nature of the 'socio-economic and cultural changes' (Hareven 1995: 132) that have culminated in the emergence of old age as a life stage. It argues that certain social, demographic, cultural and economic changes which occurred as a result of industrialization were highly influential – old age as a life stage did not exist in pre-industrial society. As communities were self-sufficient and older people were still land and property owners, everyone worked for most of their lifetime and there was far less of a distinction between those in their middle years and those in their later years. Families were also large and individual members were closely engaged with each other. Thus older people were afforded considerable economic, social and familial power. However, during industrialization the move from the land to the cities for work meant that older people lost the status previously derived from their work, land and property. There was also a reduction in family size and these smaller families were likely to live in the cities. Consequently, older people became socially and economically segregated. Life course explanations maintain that it was this constellation of changes that gradually led to their differentiation from other age groups and created a recognized formal phase of life for older people in society that was not soley related to biological ageing (Cohen 1987; Hareven 1995; Hockey and James 2003; Hunt 2005).

As indicated, these changes also impacted negatively on the lives and experiences of older people. According to the life course perspective, other social and cultural changes occurred that had further negative implications for this group in society. These included the proliferation of negative stereotypes about older people, the growth in the literature on gerontology which highlighted the psychological and social problems of old age, and the establishment of mandatory retirement and its concomitant association with dependency on social security (Hareven 1995).

The life course perspective also argues that more recently, further socioeconomic and cultural changes have led to the dissolution of some of the life course patterns associated with old age. For example, the raising of the retirement age, the increase in workforce participation rates of older people, changing patterns of marriage and cohabitation and the increasing choice of lifestyles available to older people (Hunt 2005; Vincent 2006).

Some of those working within the life course perspective place particular emphasis on the role of the individual, and the interplay between private lives and public events. An example of this type of approach is the work by Holstein and Gubrium. Their view is that within the constraints of social, cultural and historical circumstances, individuals continuously construct their own life course; they argue that we are the 'everyday authors of our own lives' within 'circumstantial constraints' (Holstein and Gubrium 2000: 182).

The life course perspective in general has been accused of being 'vague at the theoretical level' (Arber and Ginn 1995: 28) and not contributing to sociological theory. The justifications put forward for these accusations are that while material influences on the transitions in social life are highlighted, their sociological significance (such as their relative power) is not addressed. Nonetheless, despite these criticisms, the life course perspective and the different approaches within it do help to increase our understanding of the social construction of 'age'.

The preceding discussion has shown the socially constructed nature of 'age' means that the life course is not static. Consequently, the relationship between our age and other aspects of our lives can be uncertain. Nonetheless, there is evidence that although it is a complex one, there is a relationship between our health and our age and it is to this that we now turn.

Health across the life course

Activity 5.1

As you read through this section, make a note of any conclusions you feel can be drawn about the relationship between health and the life course. Compare your conclusions with those presented after the discussion of mental illness on page 88.

Differences in health across the life course have been assessed by a using variety of indicators, such as self-reported health, indicators of health service use, **acute** and **chronic** sickness rates and incidence of mental illness. These show that the relationship between our health and our life course is not straightforward (Larkin 2009). Each of the aforementioned indicators is examined below to illustrate the complexities of this relationship.

Self-reported health

Table 5.1 shows that the percentage of both males and females in the population reporting 'good' general health declines across the life course as age increases. In addition, those reporting 'not good' health increases with advancing years, with the most significant increase being for those aged 75 and over. Therefore, Table 5.1 indicates that people *report* their level of health progressively deteriorating as their chronological age increases. However, analysis of the data on the incidence of acute, chronic and mental illness[1] shows different patterns of relationship between our health and our life course.

Acute illness

Table 5.2 indicates that for both males and females, acute illness tends to decrease between the ages of 5 and 15 and then increase from 16 onwards, with the sharpest increases occurring after the age of 45.

Chronic illness

Two categories for chronic illness were used in the sources of data drawn upon for this chapter. One was 'chronic longstanding illness' which refers to longstanding illness or disability. The other was 'chronic limiting longstanding illness' which is used for longstanding illness or disability which

---

[1] Tables 5.2–5.4 have been compiled using data from a number of General Household Surveys with the aim of showing trends over a minimum of five years. The range of calendar years and the age cohorts included within each table depended on the availability of comparable data.

Table 5.1 Self-reported health in Great Britain, by age and sex, 2006 (%)

	Good	*Fairly good*	*Not good*
Males			
0–15	85	12	2
16–24	83	14	3
25–44	74	20	6
45–64	58	28	14
65–74	44	36	19
75 and over	33	43	24
All ages	68	23	9
Females			
0–15	87	11	2
16–24	78	18	3
25–44	70	21	8
45–64	59	26	15
65–74	43	38	19
75 and over	33	39	28
All ages	66	23	11

Source: Office for National Statistics (2008b)

Table 5.2 Acute sickness: average number of restricted activity days per person per year, by sex and age, 2003–7

	2003	*2004*	*2005*	*2006*	*2007*
Males					
0–4	16	12	13	9	10
5–15	11	13	11	10	8
16–44	18	17	16	16	17
45–64	36	36	35	35	29
65–74	47	45	40	41	40
75 and over	56	59	54	56	45
Females					
0–4	14	16	11	10	10
5–15	11	8	8	11	7
16–44	22	22	24	21	21
45–64	42	41	37	40	37
65–74	57	52	57	55	43
75 and over	70	76	70	70	59

Source: adapted from Office for National Statistics (2005, 2006b, 2007b, 2008b, 2009)

limits an individual's activity. Tables 5.3 and 5.4 show that increasing age brings with it a greater incidence of chronic illness for males and females, be it chronic longstanding illness or chronic limiting longstanding illness and disability, particularly among those over 65.

Mental illness

The level of mental health problems within the population is usually measured in terms of life satisfaction. While the incidence of different types of mental illnesses does vary, as Figure 5.1 shows the

Table 5.3 Percentage reporting chronic longstanding illness, 2003–7

	2003	2004	2005	2006	2007
Males					
0–15	17	18	17	16	15
16–44	20	20	22	21	20
45–64	41	43	44	45	43
65+	62	60	61	66	62
Females					
0–15	15	14	14	14	13
16–44	22	32	24	23	22
45–64	41	62	43	44	41
65+	66	50	61	67	60

Source: adapted from Office for National Statistics (2005, 2006b, 2007b, 2008b, 2009)

Table 5.4 Percentage reporting chronic limiting longstanding illness, 2003–7

	2003	2004	2005	2006	2007
Males					
0–15	6	7	7	6	5
16–44	10	10	11	10	11
45–64	24	26	26	23	25
65+	39	37	39	41	41
Females					
0–15	6	6	6	5	5
16–44	11	12	13	12	12
45–64	25	24	26	27	25
65+	41	40	43	45	42

Source: adapted from Office for National Statistics (2005, 2006b, 2007b, 2008c, 2009)

Figure 5.1 Average life satisfaction score by age group

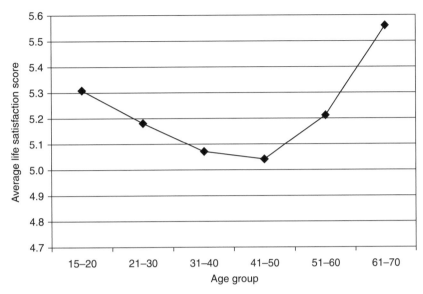

Source: Allen (2008)

relationship between the incidence of mental health problems and age is U-shaped. This is because mental distress is now higher in childhood, young adulthood and very old age than in middle age (Rogers and Pilgrim 2003; Pilgrim 2007; Allen 2008).

Let's look at this U-shape in more detail. With reference specifically to the mental health of the under-16s, 'measures of health seem to indicate that it is a difficult phase' with up to a quarter manifesting 'distress or dysfunction' (Pilgrim 2007: 194). Levels of mental health problems, particularly among boys under 16, have also been rising since the Second World War. This has been attributed to factors such as the increasing exam culture (Bradshaw *et al.* 2006; Pilgrim 2007).

Contrary to cultural assumptions about increased levels of mental distress in middle age because of phenomena such as 'mid-life crises' and the 'empty nest syndrome', this is the life phase where we experience our best mental health (Rogers and Pilgrim 2003; Pilgrim 2007). As Figure 5.1 shows, the prevalence of mental health problems does not start to increase until around 55, but from then on rises sharply. This is supported by other research which has found that the sharpest increases are in older people, especially those over 85. As many mental health problems among older people remain undiagnosed and untreated (more so than for other groups in the population), this side of the U-curve may be even steeper than shown (Davison *et al.* 2007; Age Concern 2008). In addition, there is likely to be a rise in the number of older people who experience mental ill health. For instance, new health problems have emerged with developments in medicine. The earlier diagnosis and more effective therapies that slow the progression of dementia mean that older people will remain in the early stages of dementia for longer. Although independent living is possible, they do experience considerable emotional turmoil and problems with cognitive loss in these early stages (Steeman *et al.* 2007; Wolf *et al.* 2007; Allen 2008; McCrone *et al.* 2008).

The complexities of the relationship between our health and our life course
The different indicators highlight some significant variations and illustrate the complex relationship between our health and our life course. Nonetheless, two main conclusions emerge from the data presented above:

- there is a linear correlation between age and both mental and physical health from around 40, which results in our mental and physical health worsening as we age from then onwards;

- the worst health is experienced by those over 65, but particularly by those over 75.

These trends need to be considered in conjunction with other evidence and arguments to gain a comprehensive appreciation of health across the life course. A development that has been recently identified is the emergence of new health issues among children and young people which means the data presented in this section are subject to change. Examples of these new health issues are the rises in chronic illnesses and obesity rates in those under 16. The greatest relative rise in the prevalence of chronic illnesses, such as Type 1 (or insulin-dependent) diabetes and asthma, has been among those under 16 years. With regard to obesity rates in 1995, fewer than 10 per cent of primary school children were classified as obese. In 2007, obesity rates had jumped to 16.9 per cent of boys and 16.8 per cent of girls aged between 2 and 10, with a third of all children leaving primary school overweight. It is now estimated that 24 per cent of boys and 32 per cent of girls will be overweight by 2025. Both of these changes have implications for future trends in child and adult health. For instance, apart from the fact that obesity is a disease in its own right, as children who are overweight tend to carry obesity into later life, it can also cause many chronic diseases in adulthood. These include heart disease, cancer, diabetes, strokes, high blood pressure, high cholesterol levels and mental illness (Finch and Searle 2005; Foresight 2007).

In addition, although the most striking and consistent trend to emerge from the health indicators discussed in this section is the higher incidence of ill health among the over 65s, and especially the over 75s, this also requires further evaluation. While several studies of older people's health have supported this conclusion, for example, a recent survey of people over 65 funded as part of the ESRC Growing Older Progamme found that 'ageing was most definitely seen in terms of deteriorating health' (Victor *et al.* 2009: 88), there is also evidence that a significant proportion of older people, particularly those under 74, enjoy good health and lead healthy, active lives (Home Office 2003; Allender *et al.* 2006; Sayce 2009). Indeed, as Tables 5.3 and 5.4 show, on average just under 40 per cent of those over 65 do not have a chronic longstanding illness and over 50 per cent do not suffer from a chronic limiting longstanding illness.

Adopting a critical approach to the conclusions drawn about the relationship between age and health is therefore important. Moreover, integral to their critical evaluation is an examination of explanations of this relationship which have been put forward within the study of the social aspects of health. Some of these explanations are discussed in the next section.

Explaining the relationship between age and health

We all know that biological processes contribute to poorer health as we get older but, as already indicated in the discussions in this chapter, there are other influences, both throughout the life course *and* during old age itself which affect our health. This section will explore the above two trends using explanations which are not purely physiological. The first trend about the way our level of health gradually decreases after the age of 40 is addressed under the heading 'Ageing and health' and the second under 'Older people's health'.

Ageing and health

The theoretical perspective that has made one of the most substantial contributions to our understanding of the relationship between ageing and health within the study of the social aspects of health is the life course perspective. As demonstrated in the discussions about approaches to the social class gradient in health in Chapter 3, the emphasis in life course explanations of health is on the way that adverse health effects accumulate across the various stages of the life course. We also saw in Chapter 3 how the interrelated concepts of 'biographical time' (personal events in our lives) and 'historical time' (social and economic events that occur in the course of a person's life) are central to these explanations.

Therefore, in relation to ageing and health, the life course perspective argues that the health of a person involves the interaction between both a biographical element and a historical element. The former accounts for the different ways that people age as individuals and how features of their personal biographies influence their health as they age. Such features include type of employment undertaken and personality. For instance, employment based mainly around manual labour can lead to osteoarthritis from middle age onwards. With reference to personality, studies have shown how specific childhood personality attributes, such as conscientiousness, distress-proneness and behavioural inhibition influence adult physical health (Friedman *et al.* 1993; Sanders *et al.* 2002; Kubzansky *et al.* 2009).

The examples just given relate to how certain aspects of our personal biographies can impact on physical health during the course of our lives. With reference to mental health specifically, psychological theories have long emphasized how experiences in childhood influence the incidence of mental health problems throughout the life course. Family environment has received much attention. Although there is an interaction with social class position, children who are subject to neglect and/or abuse are significantly more likely to be distressed or dysfunctional and experience increased rates of mental health problems as they progress through their adult lives (Pilgrim 2007).

The concept of 'historical time' within this approach provides an understanding of how people's adult health is influenced by the particular generation or age cohort to which they belong. Influential factors include the standards of nutrition associated with particular generations – for example, the possible effects of the current 0–15 cohort's dietary habits on their physical and mental health in later life was discussed in the previous section. Attitudes to health and life have also been found to be shaped by medical, economic, political and social developments when younger. A medical development that is frequently cited to illustrate this point is the realization in the 1960s that cigarette smoking was actually a serious threat to health. Consequently, the lack of knowledge about the dangers of smoking meant that preceding age cohorts had an increased vulnerability to the associated health risks. Studies into the other types of developments have shown how, for instance, those who experienced radical social changes in their youth see life as meaningful and want to stay physically and mentally active for as long as possible as they age. In addition, those who lived through the privations of the Second World War have been found to be more prone to self-denial and able to cope with life's problems in adulthood (Vincent 2006; Gunnarsson 2009).

As explained, the life course perspective argues that the beneficial and damaging effects of 'biographical' and 'historical' time are cumulatively stored within the human body throughout the course of life. This has two key implications for the relationship between ageing and health. The better health of young people can be accounted for by the fact that any damaging factors are stored but do not manifest themselves during youth. The way the damaging effects of 'biographical' and 'historical' time gradually accumulate over the life course means that the longer someone lives the more chance they have of these impacting negatively on their health. Hence, the life course perspective supplements more biologically-based explanations of the linear correlation between age and ill health post-40. It can also be used to explain current and future variations in the adult health of particular age cohorts (Blane *et al.* 2004).

Those working within the life course perspective who use **epidemiological** data adopt a slightly different approach. They focus on what are referred to as 'critical periods' or 'sensitive periods' in our early lives when certain influences can have more permanent and longer-lasting effects than in later periods of our lives. The following quotation illustrates the nature of the arguments within this strand of the life course perspective about the relationship between ageing and health:

> *Fetuses, infants, children and adolescents pass through many critical and sensitive periods as they develop to maturity, particularly between conception and early childhood. This makes not only pregnancy but also childhood and adolescence, particularly in the early years, an unparalleled time during which external influences, both good and bad, can influence an individual's health and well-being across their whole life.*

> (Graham 2009: 26)

Despite the divergence in views with those who use the concepts of 'biographical' and 'historical' time, this approach provides insights into why health can deteriorate after the first decades of life.

Older people's health

Most of the theoretical perspectives on old age itself do not explicitly address the health of older people. For instance, within Marxist theory, the poorer health of older people is seen as part of the more general dependency of older people that is 'constructed' by capitalist society. This approach argues that one of the consequences of the constant search for greater profits and the maximization of profit inherent in capitalism is that the cost and productivity of workers are closely scrutinized. In the early part of the twentieth century, it not only became apparent that older workers were more expensive than younger ones but also that their ability to maintain high levels of productivity was questionable. Thus, fixed age retirement policies (initially at age 60) were introduced to reduce the cost of paying older workers, and optimize productivity. The exclusion of those over 60 from work considerably reduced the income of people in that age group and also institutionalized a generally lower social and economic status for older people. In combination with pensions and social services policies, this exclusion from work also legitimated and enforced the dependency of older people on the state and others for support. This increased economic and social dependence in turn contributed to physical and mental dependence (Walker 1992; Vincent 2006).

The evidence about the experiences of older people in the UK is more useful in showing that their health is not solely associated with the physiology of ageing. Some of the main influences and their varying effects that have been identified are as follows.

Income

Older people's incomes have improved considerably in recent years. Pensioner poverty has also reduced since 1997. However, despite these improvements, 21 per cent of pensioners in the UK currently still live in income poverty. In addition, some groups of pensioners are still much more badly off than others, such as older pensioners and women. Pensioner poverty levels are predicted to remain at their current level until 2018 (Brewer *et al.* 2007; Department for Work and Pensions 2008; Leicester *et al.* 2008).

The persistence of lower incomes for some older people has implications for their health. For example, low income often leads to fuel poverty and older people not keeping warm enough. Consequently, they are vulnerable to cold-related illnesses, and between 2001 and 2006, 31,000 older people died of such illnesses (O'Neill *et al.* 2006; Shelter 2007). Low incomes and benefit dependency among the elderly have also been associated with a greater likelihood of having emotional and mental health problems (Evans *et al.* 2003; Allen 2008).

Living arrangements
Demographic and political changes that have occurred during recent decades have affected older people's living arrangements. With reference to the former, there has been a decline in intergenerational households. One of the main reasons for this is geographical mobility, both in the search for jobs and as a result of social mobility, which increases the chances of children moving away from their parents. Other reasons are the decline in fertility (the average family size is now standardizing at one or two children) and the increase in voluntary childlessness. These two trends mean that the elderly are more likely to have fewer children to call upon for help than in previous generations, and possibly no children at all. The final trend is the higher incidence of marital breakdown; those parents who are not awarded custody may have weaker links with their children and therefore their risk of being isolated in their old age is greater (Phillipson 1998; Vincent 2006; Williams *et al.* 2007). As a result of the decline in intergenerational households, only 5 per cent of the over 65s now live with an adult child (McCarthy and Thomas 2004).

The political swing to community care since the 1980s and the subsequent increase in intensive home care and community-based services (see Chapter 10) has meant that more older people have been able to live in their own homes and there has been a reduction of older people needing to enter residential care (Baggott 2004; Social Exclusion Unit 2005; Patsios 2006).

One of the consequences of these changes is that most older people now live in their own homes and a significant number of 'older' old people live in residential establishments. In 2001, among those aged 90 and over, 34 per cent of women and 20 per cent of men were in residential care. The corresponding figures for those aged 75–84 were only 5.2 and 3.2 per cent respectively (Stewart and Vaitilingham 2004; Department for Work and Pensions 2005; National Statistics 2005a).

Both of these living arrangements can adversely affect the health of older people. For instance, living in your own home in your old age can also mean living alone – 60 per cent of women over 75 and 29 per cent of men of the same age still live alone (Tomassini *et al.* 2004). As mentioned above, older people in general experience reduced social contact and social support. Those living alone spend 70–90 per cent of their time in their home and are at much greater risk of becoming socially isolated, particularly older men and those in rural areas. Indeed, it is estimated that 1 in 10 are currently chronically lonely and by 2021 nearly 2.2 million of the over 65s will be socially isolated (Davidson *et al.* 2003; McCarthy and Thomas 2004; Riddell 2007). Social isolation and lack of social support can increase vulnerability to poorer physical and mental health (Berkman and Syme 1979; Penninx *et al.* 1997; Berkman *et al.* 2000; Department for Work and Pensions 2005; National Statistics 2005b).

Being able to live in his or her own home often depends on an older person having an **unpaid carer**. Those who care for older people are usually spouses or adult children. Spousal carers of older people are likely to be retired, and increases in longevity mean that many of those adult children caring for the over 85s are also 65 and over (Social Exclusion Unit 2005; Pickard *et al.* 2007). Although carers may choose to care, and there has been a considerable increase in the support for such people over the past two decades. As explained in Chapter 2 (see also Chapter 10), caring negatively affects carers' physical and psychological health and such negative affects are compounded for those caring for older people because their own advancing years means they are more likely to have a pre-existing medical condition (Bandeira *et al.* 2007; Chun *et al.* 2007; Hanratty *et al.* 2007). Therefore, the increase in older people who need support living in their own homes can have adverse consequences on the health of those older people in our society caring for them (Allen 2008; McCrone *et al.* 2008).

Moreover, a third of older people live in 'non-decent homes' (as defined by the Decent Homes Standard 2000). This is a much higher proportion than other groups in the population and means that older people's houses are more likely to lack central heating, and have damp and infestation problems. Thus, when older people live in their own homes there is a higher than average possibility of them living in poor quality accommodation which in turn puts their mental and physical health at risk (see Chapter 1, page 27) (Social Exclusion Unit 2005; Shelter 2007).

The second type of living arrangement – residential care – is associated with high levels of depression and those with moderate cognitive impairments are more likely to be depressed than other residents. Furthermore, less than half of those suffering from depression in residential homes receive any form of treatment (Davison *et al.* 2007; Age Concern 2008). Both treated and untreated depression, together with the lack of privacy, loss of independence and exclusion from everyday life that are inevitable consequences of living in such establishments have been cited as contributing to the fact that nearly half of older people admitted to residential or nursing home care die within 18 months of admission (Biggs 2000; Gott 2005; Social Exclusion Unit 2005).

Wherever older people live, there is a further major threat to their health – abuse. Elder abuse can include physical, psychological, financial or sexual abuse, and neglect. Accurate statistics are difficult to obtain because elder abuse is often unreported, but it is estimated that 5 per cent of older people suffer psychological abuse and 2 per cent suffer physical abuse. Perpetrators are commonly partners, family members, neighbours and domiciliary care workers. Those aged 70 and over (particularly women over 70) are most vulnerable to abuse. However, those living in their own homes, particularly those living on their own, are more vulnerable, and a recent analysis of calls made to the Action on Elder Abuse Helpline showed that 64 per cent of cases of abuse had occurred in an individual's own home and 23 per cent had occurred in a residential care home (Action on Elder Abuse 2004, 2007; Department of Health 2004a; Pritchard 2006).

Although these discussions have shown that older people are vulnerable to ill health whether they live on their own or in a residential establishment, when evaluating such findings it is important not to romanticize the living arrangements of the elderly in the past. These evolved as a result of different demographic, historical and cultural factors and there is no 'ideal' system, as every form of living arrangement for older people will have its drawbacks.

Healthcare
The way that mental health problems among older people are often undiagnosed and untreated was mentioned above. Other examples of failings identified in the provision of healthcare for older people which have negative consequences for older people's health are:

- the continuation of age discrimination in healthcare – for instance, there are age restrictions on screening and cardiac care;

- shortfalls in receipt of basic recommended healthcare by adults aged 50 or more with common health conditions, particularly those in residential and nursing homes;

- evidence that many dementia sufferers are not being diagnosed early enough and are often deprived of the specialist care they need;

- the less favourable treatment older people receive from professionals working in health and social care;

- inadequate access to GPs (Roberts 2000; Dixon-Woods 2005; Degnen 2007; National Audit Office 2007; Steel *et al.* 2008; Harrop and Potter 2009).

With reference to community and residential establishments specifically, research has shown that older people experience poorer quality healthcare in both of these settings. Taking the community first, although the move to community care (referred to above) is viewed as a positive development, it does not necessarily have positive outcomes for all those affected by the changes that have occurred. Despite the initiatives to improve the availability and quality of support, many problematic issues can arise for both older people living in their own homes and those who care for them. Failures in the delivery of appropriate care and support and the damaging implications these have are well documented. These failures include the inflexibility and lack of integration of services, poor standards, confusion over the roles of volunteers and professionals, and difficult relationships experienced with some professionals. There have also been concerns about gaps between quality and level of provision and user needs, and the geographical variations in these gaps. These have increased with recent rationing and the changes in eligibility criteria used by local authorities. Further variations in services identified have been linked to an older person's race, class and level of education. Indeed, social care arrangements for older people in their own homes compare unfavourably with several other European countries (Chamberlayne and King 2000; Miller 2003; Evandrou and Falkingham 2005; Social Exclusion Unit 2005; Larsson *et al.* 2006; Leutz and Capitman 2007; Shelter 2007).

Activity 5.2

The vignette about Lily, below, illustrates many of the points made in the previous sections about older people's health and healthcare. Read it through and answer the questions that follow it. Thinking about and answering these will help you to revisit and consolidate your understanding of important issues that have been raised. More help is available in the 'Activity feedback' chapter on page 229.

Lily, an 86-year-old widow whose husband died 10 years ago, lives alone in the downstairs of her run-down nineteenth-century terraced house. Managing on her pension is a struggle and she often economizes on the heating. She suffers from both arthritis and glaucoma and rarely leaves her home. This is partly because of physical difficulties she experiences and partly because she has suffered from depression since the death of her husband. Despite exhortation from her daughter and son, she refuses to talk to her GP about this. Apart from a neighbour who calls in every couple of days, there are very few other visitors to the house. As a result Lily often spends hours on her own.

Although her children do their best to support her, they both live over an hour's drive away and have families of their own. She refused to move from the home which she has lived in since she was married so they contacted social services to see what support was available to her. An assessment was carried out and it was concluded that Lily needed help with preparing her meals and taking her medication. A meeting between Lily, her daughter, the social worker appointed to Lily's case and the homecare organizer followed during which it was agreed that a package which involved a home carer coming in twice a day would be appropriate.

However, there were disputes over who should administer the eye drops Lily has to take for her glaucoma; the home care organizer felt that this was an invasive procedure which an untrained home carer should not undertake. When the district nurse was contacted, she refused to do it as she felt that Lily could do this as long as she was supervised by the home carer. Throughout the heated exchanges that ensued, both the district nurse and the home care organizer supported their stance by referring to the same locally agreed policy document about job demarcations negotiated by the local authority and the local NHS. A solution to the impasse that developed proved impossible. Therefore, Lily's daughter and son made their own private arrangements for an ex-neighbour to come in to administer Lily's eye drops.

(**1**) Lily has arthritis, glaucoma and depression. What type of illnesses are these?

(**2**) What effects do Lily's health problems have on her quality of life?

(**3**) What factors could be influencing her health?

(**4**) What healthcare issues does this vignette highlight?

Older people and the provision of healthcare in an ageing society

Although there are variations in the health of older people and some do remain in relatively good health, it is a fact that older people in our society, particularly those over 85 who experience the highest rates of ill health, 'are significant consumers of healthcare' (Timonen 2008: 47). The cost of providing for the healthcare needs of old people has been a major social and political concern, particularly in the light of the fact that there are more and more older people in our society and their number will increase. This phenomenon is referred to as our 'ageing society', and it has been estimated that there will be a dramatic rise of 87 per cent in the healthcare needs of those aged 65 and over between 2002 and 2051 (Allen 2008).

The concept of our ageing society is explained in more detail at the beginning of this section. It will be followed by a discussion of the steps that are being taken to address the increasing healthcare costs that are predicted in the light of the move to an ageing society in the UK.

Our ageing society

Activity 5.3

Examine Figure 5.2 and answer the following questions.

(**1**) Which age group in the UK is getting smaller?

(**2**) Which age groups in the UK are increasing in size?

> (3) Which age group in the UK is predicted to expand the most?
>
> Now read the text that immediately follows Figure 5.2.

Figure 5.2 Age structure of UK population

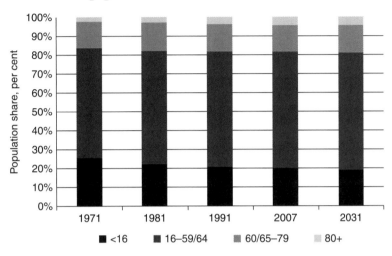

Population: by age, United Kingdom

Source: Office for National Statistics (2008c)

As you can see from Figure 5.2, since 1971 the percentage of the population aged under 16 has been declining while the percentage of those over 65 has increased. These trends are predicted to continue and the fastest growing age group in the UK population will remain the over 65s. Moreover, within this group, the numbers of those aged 85 years and over will increase the most; this age group more than doubled between 1971 and 2007 and, as shown in Figure 5.2, is predicted to rise further.

These trends are mainly due to the decline in fertility referred to in the previous section and the increase in life expectancy. As we saw in both Chapters 2 and 3, while there are variations between socioeconomic groups, life expectancy has increased dramatically over the past 100 years for both males and females. In 1901 it was 45 for males and 49 for females. By 2002 it was 76 and 81 for males and females respectively, and these figures are projected to rise to 79 and 84 respectively by 2020 (Stewart and Vaitilingham 2004; National Statistics 2006a).

A consequence of such changes is that since 2007 there have been less people under 16 in the UK than there are over 65. In addition, far more people in the population are over 65; their numbers have doubled since 1931 with the result that they currently make up around 18 per cent of the population. This figure is predicted to rise to 20 per cent (1 in 5 of the population) in 2020. The decline in the under-16s and increase in those aged 65 and over is likely to continue until 2050. Thus, the UK's population is ageing and the phrase 'ageing society' is now widely used (National Statistics 2006a, 2008; Vincent 2006; Allen 2008).

The UK is not alone in having an ageing society – ageing populations are an international phenomenon for the same reasons as discussed above in relation to this country. For example, some European countries, such as Germany and Italy, also have higher ratios of those over 65 to those under 16 in their populations (Allen 2008).

Addressing healthcare costs in our ageing society

Analyses of the themes in policy responses to concerns about the extent of the cost implications of our ageing society show that they are aligned to some of the issues addressed in this chapter. For instance, a life course approach is evident in the steps that have been taken to prevent higher levels of mental and physical ill health among older people by promoting healthy living at all ages, which should lay the foundations for better health in old age (Department of Health 2004b, 2004c; Department for Work and Pensions 2005). There is also a commitment to reducing some of the negative life experiences of older people in our society, such as improving the delivery of health and social care services. One of the main drivers is the the *National Service Framework* (NSF) *for Older People* (Department of Health 2001). This was published in March 2001 as a 10-year programme and aimed to deliver higher quality services to older people. It set national standards and service models of care across health and social services for all older people, whether they live at home, in residential care or are being looked after in hospital. The progress achieved since the publication of the NSF is being built upon through a programme supporting system redesign for older people. There have been many postive outcomes: with reference to health services specifically, services for old-age conditions are being strengthened by increasing their flexibility, making them more person-centred and ensuring that they provide better management for complex and longstanding condi-tions. For those older people who are living in their own homes with the support of community-based services, there is an ongoing commitment to improving and expanding these services. There is both more choice and opportunities for user involvement, together with increased levels of housing-related services (such as good neighbour and handymen networks). More home adaptations and improvements are also being provided to enable older people to stay in their own homes. Additional support is now available for those who care for older people in their own homes; steps are being taken to further protect carers' income and to encourage wider neighbourhood support for them by promoting more active citizenship within communities (Department of Health 2001, 2008d; Department for Work and Pensions 2005; Social Exclusion Unit 2005).

There is clear evidence that costs are reduced by the types of intervention just described. For instance, the development of health services so that more older people can receive healthcare in their own homes has reduced the length of costly hospital stays and the number of admissions to long-term care (Social Exclusion Unit 2005; Holmes 2007). When the weekly costs of adaptations to older people's houses in order to help them live in their own homes were compared to keeping an older person in residential care, the former worked out at around 1.5 per cent of the average cost of the latter (Heywood 2001).

Conclusions

This chapter has used relevant research and theoretical perspectives as well as statistical evidence to show that the relationship between age and health is not just based on physiology and that many other factors are influential. These include the way age itself is constructed in our society, our life experiences and healthcare. Mention has also been made of the role of other social divisions, such as gender and class. The influence of the social categories of gender, class, race and age on health have been addressed in separate chapters in this first section of the book. However, as shown in these chapters, in order to fully understand the relationship between social categories and health, it is necessary to acknowledge the extent of the interaction between all of them in shaping our health across the life course.

Key points

- There are varying constructions of 'age' and its socially constructed nature means that the life course is not static.

- Although there is a complex relationship between our health and our life course, analyses of health data show that physical and mental health tend to worsen from 40 onwards and older people have a higher incidence of ill health compared to the rest of the population.

- The main influences on older people's health are income poverty, their living arrangements and the healthcare they receive.

- Demographic changes mean that 18 per cent of the population are now over 65 and the increase in the size of this age group is predicted to continue. As a result, we live in what is referred to as an 'ageing society'.

Discussion points

- To what extent is 'age' socially constructed?

- What are the main problems of an ageing society?

- What do you think are the main issues that will impact on health throughout the life course in the future?

- In the light of your reading around this subject and your own experiences, develop your own theory of ageing and health.

Suggestions for further study

- Chapter 1 in Hunt (2005) provides a useful account of the development of the life course perspective and gives details of recent changes within this perspective.

- For a highly readable account of the social construction of old age, read Hareven (1995). Although this is written from an American perspective, it explains the process and factors involved in the creation of this life stage very well.

- An in-depth discussion of life course influences on the health of older people can be found in Part 1 of Graham's *Understanding Health Inequalities* (2009).

- If you want to explore issues around health and social care provision for older people, see Glasby and Littlechild, *The Health and Social Care Divide: The Experiences of Older People* (2004).

The experience of health and illness

Introduction to Section 2

This section will now move on to the second theme identified within the social aspects of health, 'The experience of health and illness'. The topics within this theme are:

- Experiencing illness

- Experiencing mental illness

- Experiencing disability

- Dying, death and grieving

Each of these topics is dealt with in a separate chapter and hence there are four chapters. The emphasis in Chapter 6 is on the experience of illness *in general*. More specific experiences of illness, such as mental illness, disability and terminal illness are now recognized as separate subject areas within the social aspects of health. Hence, these are addressed in Chapters 7, 8 and 9 respectively. Although the chapters can be read independently, you should refer to both the Glossary at the end of the book and to the outlines of the theoretical perspectives that inform the study of the social aspects of health to help you fully understand each topic.

Experiencing illness

Illness, like other forms of misfortune, can arrive in the midst of an orderly life without warning, and this is troublesome not only to the ill person but also to those around him.

(Bradby 2009: 109)

Introduction

Most of us have experienced illness at some point in our lives, but, how many of us appreciate the extent to which our experiences of illness are attributable to the wider social context and not solely to illness *per se*? The increasing focus on the social aspects of health has meant that it is now recognized that illness is not just located within the individual but also that being ill is a *social state*. This is as a result of the acknowledgment that, in addition to biological and physiological changes, our experiences of illness are shaped by a range of social processes, including the definition of social reality, both at a societal and an individual level. Any course of study involving the social aspects of health therefore requires an exploration of these social dimensions of the experiences of illness.

Several key theoretical insights into the experience of illness as a social state have been developed. These have focused on both acute and chronic illness. Although these concepts have been mentioned in earlier chapters, this chapter starts with a detailed distinction between acute and chronic illness and then moves on to explore one main theoretical approach to the experience of each type of illness. These theoretical approaches have been chosen in order to illustrate the variation that exists in explanations of the role and type of social processes in the experience of illness. Functionalism is used as an example of the former and symbolic interactionism for the latter. The last two sections of the chapter address the role of the changing definitions of illness on our experience of it, and consider some of the social processes involved in defining illnesses and diseases as such, together with the experiential impacts of these definitions. A further feature of this chapter that requires clarification is that the exploration of theoretical perspectives is more central to the discussions of the topic than in preceding chapters.

The nature of illness

Illnesses can be either acute or chronic. Acute illnesses are those which are short-term and curable, such as colds and sickness bugs. Recovery occurs within a few days, with or without medical intervention. Chronic illnesses are ongoing, long-term and non-communicable health disorders. They are also emergent in nature, and the stages in their progress can be unpredictable. They usually have an 'insiduous onset' (Bury 1982: 168) and although symptoms may fluctuate and treatments are available, there are no known medical cures or chances of returning to a pre-morbid state. These types of illness require continuous medical intervention and often interfere with social interaction, the ability to carry out everyday roles and the capacity to fulfil social obligations. Examples are cardiovascular diseases, certain types of cancer, asthma, multiple sclerosis, diabetes, Parkinson's, hypertension, rheumatoid arthritis, migraine, epilepsy, psoriasis and senile dementia. Furthermore, people can simultaneously suffer from two or more chronic illnesses. This is referred to as co-morbidity and examples of co-morbid chronic conditions are diabetes, Alzheimer's, asthma and cardiovascular disease. Several 'new' chronic illnesses have also been relatively recently identified. Among these are HIV/AIDS, stress, anorexia nervosa, bulimia, and obesity (Bury 1991; Bradby 2009; Jowsey *et al.* 2009).

According to recent reports, the frequency of illness in the UK in general has fallen. As the then Public Health Minister, Gillian Merron, said in her introduction to the latest profile of the nation's health:

> *The health of the nation is improving, thanks to excellent work by dedicated people throughout the NHS and local authorities, underpinned by Government action and the means to do the job. It is*

good to see that people can expect to live longer, that early deaths from heart disease, cancer and smoking-related diseases are decreasing.

(Department of Health 2009a: 3)

However, such findings do not present a complete picture of the nature of illness in this country. Over the last two centuries, there has been an increasing shift in the burden of disease from acute to chronic illness, with the result that 'the predominant disease pattern in England and in most other developed countries is now one of chronic or long-term illness rather than acute disease' (Department of Health 2007a: 6). Chronic diseases now account for nearly 60 per cent of deaths worldwide. Although these diseases cannot not be cured, medical advances in their treatment mean that more and more people are living for a greater proportion of their lives with a chronic illness and its consequences than ever before. Indeed, many people live with such illnesses from middle through to old age. The concept of 'remission society' has been used to describe this phenomenon and its financial consequences in terms of health and social care have been the subject of considerable political concern (Department of Health 2007a; Taylor and Field 2007).

Much illness, be it acute or chronic, is unreported, as most of us do not visit the doctor when we feel ill. This is referred to as the 'clinical iceberg' or 'symptom iceberg'. A study by Rogers *et al.* (1999) shed further light on this phenomenon. It suggested that while one third of those experiencing symptoms do consult a doctor, one third do nothing and one third self-medicate or seeks alternative therapies. Furthermore, more patients with minor symptoms consult their GPs than patients with significant symptoms, which means that those who do consult their doctors are not those who are necessarily the sickest. These findings show that illness is therefore not a simple matter of biological definition but is the product of actions taken by individuals in relation to it. Such actions are called **illness behaviour**. Many of the complex factors which influence this behaviour have been identified in the literature over the past four decades and include the extent to which the symptoms are visible and familiar, the impact on an individual's life and relationships, an individual's anxiety levels and the extent to which their actions are being sanctioned by others (Zola 1973; Petrie and Weinman 1997).

Acute illness – the 'sick role'

As mentioned in the Introduction to this chapter, functionalism has been chosen as an example of a theoretical perspective which has provided insights into the experience of acute illness as a social state. The most well-known work on acute illness within this perspective is that of Parsons (1964). He developed the concept of the 'sick role' which he used to explain how the experience of having an acute illness is socially, and not primarily biologically or physiologically, defined.

> **Activity 6.1**
>
> As explained, Parsons' 'sick role' is framed within functionalism. This was outlined in Chapter 1. Try to recall the main ideas within functionalism before reading through the rest of this section. A summary of this perspective can be found in the 'Activity feedback' chapter on page 230.

The functionalist emphasis on social order and shared cultural and social expectations about the way social roles should be carried out is strongly reflected in Parsons' model. He argued that sickness is a form of **deviance** because when an individual becomes 'sick' he or she is unable to fulfil his or her normal function and role in society and therefore cannot contribute towards its solidarity and stability. When individuals become 'sick' they are also adopting a socially defined role and, like any other role in society, this is subject to societal expectations. In order that social stability and social order can be maintained, when in the 'sick role', the sick person has certain socially determined rights and obligations. These are set out below. As you can see, they involve the role of medical care. Indeed, Parsons saw the medical profession as 'policing' entry to, and exit from, the 'sick role', because its members decide who is really 'ill' and therefore who can adopt the 'sick role'.

Parsons' rights and obligations of the sick role

The rights of a sick person are:

- legitimate exemption from normal activities and responsibilities, such as those associated with family and work roles;

- not to be held responsible for their sickness;

- the expectation of assistance from others.

The obligations of a sick person are:

- to want to get better and get out of the sick role as soon as possible;

- to get better in an appropriate manner – for example staying in bed;

- to seek appropriate medical care and comply with advice given.

If these social expectations are met, the disruption caused by illness to the normal functioning of society is minimal and equilibrium is maintained but when they are unmet, societal dysfunction occurs. Therefore, the existence of the 'sick role' ensures the smooth functioning of society.

As mentioned in Chapter 1, functionalism has been criticized in general for its assumptions about shared and static meanings and the extent to which individuals passively carry out their roles. Although Parsons' sick role theory has made a significant contribution to the understanding of illness as a social state and has inspired research, it is not without its critics either. For example, it has been criticized for approaching illness solely from a western viewpoint in that it fails to address alternative forms of healthcare and healing. Furthermore, given the findings about illness behaviour (outlined in the previous section) and the fact that only a minority of people seek medical help when ill, it would seem that it is more of an explanation of the 'patient role' than the 'sick role' (Gallagher 1976; Shilling 2002).

It is apparent from the distinction made between acute and chronic illness above that these two types have different temporal structures and hence chronic illness involves far more than entry into, and exit from, the 'sick role'. As we shall see in the next section, one of the consequences is that explanations of the experience of a chronic illness as a social state are more complex.

Chronic illness – disruption and coping

Many of those contributing to the literature that now exists about experiencing chronic illness have adopted a symbolic interactionist perspective. As you will recall from Chapter 1, symbolic interactionism focuses on how individuals, as social actors, make and define their own reality through their perceptions and interpretations of the social world that arise from their interactions with each other. Hence, the literature on the experience of chronic illness emphasizes how individuals' experiences of chronic illnesses are not only defined by the physiological consequences of their illness but are also the product of the way that individuals themselves create their own reality in the face of their chronic illness. One of the outcomes of this approach is that it has helped to direct attention away from the medical focus on the difficulties associated with chronic illnesses and towards the positive actions people take when faced with these illnesses. The themes in this literature are the disruption chronic illnesses cause to people's lives and the ways in which individuals cope with this disruption. These are both discussed below.

Chronic illness and disruption
Two types of disruption have been identified. One is called 'biographical disruption' and the other is that caused by the impact of treatments for chronic illnesses.

Biographical disruption
Bury (1982, 1991, 1997) argued that life can be seen as a narrative about which we construct our own personal biography in terms of what has happened in our lives and what we hope will happen. He developed the concept of biographical disruption to describe how chronic illness radically disrupts this biography: 'illness, and especially chronic illness, is precisely that kind of experience where the structure of everyday life and the forms of knowledge which underpin them are disrupted . . . the development of a chronic illness is most usefully regarded as . . . a form of biographical disruption' (Bury 1982: 169).

The disruption occurs at several different levels of an individual's taken-for-granted world: it disrupts their sense of identity, their everyday life and their hopes for the future. During the experience of the first of these, there is a 'loss of self' as the body fails and the individual experiences a disjuncture between the healthy self and the ill self. This demands a fundamental rethinking of a person's relationship with their body – their self-concept – and a search for explanations.

Everyday life has to be reorganized because of the effects of chronic illness on the type of activities a person can undertake, such as employment and leisure pursuits. The growing physical and emotional dependence caused by chronic illness means that existing relationships also have to be renegotiated and new relationships associated with the care now required have to be forged. With reference to existing relationships, research has shown that long-term illness invariably adds strain to relations between family members; marriages are at greater risk following the onset of chronic illness and, while families can be a source of support, they can also be a source of strain as different family members have different ways of coming to terms with the illness (Bury 1997; Williams 2000; Thorpe 2009).

Chronic illness also raises questions about quality of life during the rest of an individual's life course. This, in combination with the aforementioned re-evaluation of employment prospects and relationships, means that any continuity between past and future biographies constructed within individuals' **narratives** can no longer be assured. Consequently, future hopes and plans require re-examination and often cannot be reformulated because of the increased unpredictability of life that chronic illness brings.

Hence, biographical disruption brings change and uncertainty. The extent of the disruption caused by a chronic illness is also influenced by the **stigma** associated with certain diseases which leads to them being less than fully accepted by others. One of the most well-known sociologists who studied stigma was Goffman (1968a). He maintained that the negative reactions of others to us can affect our identity because they can cause us to doubt ourselves. These reactions can ultimately 'spoil' our identity in that we lose all confidence in ourselves, our self-image crumbles, and we feel depressed. Goffman argued that the degree to which certain chronic diseases are more stigmatizing than others and hence 'spoil' our identity depends on several factors. These are as follows.

- The *visibility* of the symptoms of the disease. For instance, psoriasis is a continually evident condition and would therefore be more visible than, say, hypertension.

- The extent to which others are *aware* of the illness. Using diabetes as an example, it is possible when this is well managed for those who work with a diabetic to be unaware that they have the condition.

- The degree to which the illness affects the *interaction* between the person who has the illness and others. For example, senile dementia impedes normal communication and interaction with other people.

Therefore, the nature of some chronic illnesses makes them more stigmatizing than others because they produce different reactions in other people around us. It is these reactions that spoil identity to a greater or lesser extent and lead to stigma. Experiencing stigma can potentially be the cause of withdrawal from social participation, especially in public places (Goffman 1968a).

Despite the persuasiveness of Goffman's work, it has been criticized for ignoring the social and cultural contexts of stigma which are important in understanding the symbolic meanings attached to it in different situations. Other dimensions to the concept of stigma have also been identified. These were not acknowledged by Goffman and are 'enacted stigma' and 'felt stigma'. The former is used to denote actual stigmatizing reactions from others, while the latter refers to the personal shame individuals feel about their condition and can result in their concealment of it from those close to them. Interestingly, 'felt stigma' was found to be more disruptive to the lives of those with a chronic illness than 'enacted stigma' (Taylor and Field 2007).

Moreover, the argument that the onset of a chronic illness always brings biographical disruption has been challenged. Age has been found to influence the disruptive impact of chronic illness; those who are affected by it when young are more likely to be depressed, whereas older people tend to expect and accept such illnesses as part of ageing. The context of someone's life also has a bearing on how disruptive a chronic illness is for them. Research has shown that those who already have several health problems see yet another illness as part of their 'biographical flow' (Williams 2000). On a more philosophical level, in view of the fact that change and uncertainty are the norm in contemporary western societies, there are those who have questioned the extent to which the change and uncertainty that accompanies chronic illness is truly disruptive. According to this view, chronic illness is just another source of uncertainty to cope with in an uncertain world (Thorpe 2009).

Impact of treatment
Clinical treatment and chronic illness are inextricably linked. Treatments vary widely in form – for example, some people may have to face thrice-weekly dialysis sessions while others may only have to take daily medication. While acknowledging the therapeutic impact of treatments, the literature about experiencing chronic illness has highlighted the variation in the extent to which treatments disrupt the lives of those affected. In addition, although there is some overlap between them, the literature has identified two main disruptive impacts. One set are 'affective'. This refers to the way

treatment alters the way people see themselves in relation to their past biographies and in relation to others, particularly if the treatment is stigmatizing. Affective impacts include the 'medical merry-go round' involved, and the way that this causes 'expectations of what can be offered to alleviate symptoms to rise and fall' and 'hope and frustration [to] alternate' (Bury 1991: 457). The other set of impacts are more instrumental in nature. Examples are the reorganization of time that attending clinical appointments necessitates, and learning to manage any technology and medication within treatment regimens.

Chronic illness and coping

As mentioned above, the second theme in the work in this area is that individuals develop ways of coping with the disruptive effects of chronic illness. Studies have shown that when people face a chronic illness they make positive attempts to 'manage, mitigate, or adapt to it' (Bury 1991: 452) and maintain some sense of their self and identity.

Let's first look at coping with biographical disruption. Bury (1997) argues that individuals overcome biographical disruption in two ways and thereby deal with the consequences and significance of their illness. One is by constructing their own explanations of their condition and the other is through the achievement of legitimacy by acknowledging that their chronic illness has changed their lifestyle, and absorbing those changes into their daily lives and interactions with others. These twin processes enable individuals to create a meaningful story about their condition and minimize the biographical disruption that has occurred. Similarly, people incorporate the instrumental impacts of treatments for chronic illnesses into their restructured everyday lives. This may involve negotiation between medical staff where patients have a particular perception of how they see their treatment working in the overall context of their life and chosen lifestyle. For instance, a diabetic who has a very active social life may decide to ignore dietary advice about controlling blood sugar levels on more occasions than other less sociable diabetics. The ways in which people cope with the affective impacts include searching for information themselves, making use of self-help groups and using complementary medicine (Bury 1991; Bennett *et al.* 2008; Thorpe 2009).

More generally, other positive action individuals can take when they experience a chronic illness involves adopting what have been referred to as 'coping strategies'. While they are contiguous to some extent, three have been used to distinguish between their different dimensions. These are as follows.

- **Coping:** refers to the 'cognitive' processes which individuals work through in order to tolerate or put up with the effects of the illness and to maintain their sense of worth in the face of an altered situation and altered body. For instance, they may try to come to terms with the illness by focusing on what they can *still* do – such as work, albeit for a reduced number of hours – as opposed to what they *cannot* do. There are strong emotional dimensions to this strategy and its outcomes in terms of success vary considerably according to individual values and social circumstances.

- **Strategy:** the term used to describe the sort of actions that people take or resources they use to manage the disruptive effects of their illness on their personal and social lives and 'maximise favourable outcomes' (Bury 1991: 462). There are a broad range of such actions. Some people decide to do as much as they can before their condition worsens and, say, travel to countries they have never visited. Others adopt very different approaches. These include trying to avoid the general public to minimize the risk of stigma, living as 'normally' as possible, hiding their symptoms or breaking the day down into 'manageable chunks'. Strategies may also be altered during the course of the illness, depending on changes in an individual's condition and social situation.

- **Style:** this is how the person with chronic illness chooses to socially present themselves in order to maintain their self-identity. For example, cancer patients who have chemotherapy may have their hair cut short so they look 'normal' and thereby integrate their disorder into an altered public identity. 'Styles' adopted can also be influenced by social class and culture (Bury 1991, 1997).

Although this work on chronic illness and coping has been commended for promoting the idea of 'positive action' in the face of chronic illness, questions have been raised about the extent of the choices available to people when coping with life as a chronically ill individual. They can be restricted by a variety of factors including the physical effects of their illness, 'financial resources, time, energy level and other roles such as employment, study and parenting' (Thorpe 2009: 385). Co-morbidity can cause additional problems which also reduce people's ability to manage their everyday lives (Jowsey *et al.* 2009). However, one of the most significant outcomes of the recognition of the agency of people with chronic illnesses is the acknowledgement that they themselves develop expertise in their condition and treatment. This has been publicly acknowledged through the development of initiatives such as the Expert Patients Programme (see Chapter 10). Such initiatives are aimed specifically at people living with long-term conditions and encouraging them to use their own skills and the information they have gathered to help them in the self-management of their diseases (Department of Health 2007a).

Activity 6.2

Ruth Picardie, a journalist, was only 32 when she was diagnosed as having breast cancer in 1996. She described the progress of her illness in a series of articles written for a Sunday newspaper (*The Observer*) before she died in 1997 at 33. Her articles were put together in a book, posthumously. Set out below is an extract from one of them which illustrates the themes about experiencing a chronic illness discussed in this section. Once you have read through the extract, think about the questions that follow it. Some ideas to help you can be found in the 'Activity feedback' chapter on page 230.

"You're 32, a stone-and-a-half overweight, depressed by the stains on the sofa and have never come to terms with having piggy eyes but, still, life is pretty great: you've got a husband who can make squid ink pasta and has all his own hair, your one-year-old twins are sleeping through the night and, as for your career - well, you might be interviewing George Clooney next week.

And that lump in your left breast, the one you noticed after you stopped breastfeeding last summer? In the squid-ink/Clooney-filled scheme of things, the hospital would smile and tell you not to worry, it was the harmless fibroadenoma they'd found in 1994. But this is the fat, stained, piggy-eyed parallel world of illness, and your lump, I'm sorry to say, is actually cancer. Or should we say lumps, because, oops, it's spread to the lymph nodes under your arm and in your neck, which means it's stage three cancer and you've a 50:50 chance of living five years. As you'd expect, the diagnosis turns you into a grumpy, bitter, envious old cow. After a fourth acquaintance tells you their aunt has breast cancer, you realise you don't feel sorry for any post-menopausal woman who has the disease because fiftysomething isn't a bad crack at life, especially if your kids have grown up. You start feeling resentful about the amount of money that goes into HIV research and complaining about having a non-glamorous illness. (AIDS = pretty men who die young. Breast cancer = old ladies in wigs.) You ram a non-organic carrot up the arse of the next person who advises you to start drinking homeopathic frogs' urine. Appeals for the seahorse conservation project go straight in the bin. The strange thing is that, alongside all this anger, the

Clooney-luvin' Pollyanna inside you just won't give in. OK, so the cancer has spread to the lymph system but, because surgery is now futile, at least you don't have to have a mastectomy and then die anyway, breastless, five years down the line. All right, the chemotherapy means you have to hoover your hair off the pillow every morning, but it's finally forced you to have your bush cropped, which would look fabulously Jean Seberg if you weighed less than 10 stone. And, hey, it's not food combining, but perhaps chemotherapy will help you lose weight.

Then, in February, when the disease spreads to your bones, your oncologist tells you that this is the 'best' secondary breast cancer to have, because the skeleton isn't a vital organ and you can live with it for years. Also, there's nothing like terminal illness for not getting divorced. As for not seeing your babies grow up, better to have had half a life with your beautiful children than a whole life without. Finally, in May, seven months after the original diagnosis and five days after your 33rd birthday, you learn the disease has spread to your liver and lungs. Abruptly, you enter the bleakly euphemistic world of palliative care. Pollyanna commits suicide. Your chic crop turns into a toilet brush. You're so grumpy and depressed you start believing your children would be better off without you, sooner rather than later."

(Picardie, 1998:38)

(1) What evidence of 'biographical disruption' can you find?

(2) This extract does not really address the instrumental impact of the treatment that Ruth had to endure but there are some examples of the affective impacts of her illness. Try to identify them.

(3) What examples of 'coping strategies' does Ruth seem to adopt?

You can find suggested responses in the 'Activity feedback' chapter on page 230.

The 'medicalization thesis'

The discussions in the last two sections about acute and chronic illness show the limitations of the extent to which biological and physiological processes shape our experiences. They also assume a consensus about what 'illness' is. However, our conceptions of illness and disease change over time. Another set of arguments about illness being a social state focus on the role of social processes in these changing conceptions. Central to these arguments are the 'medicalization thesis' and a phenomenon that has occurred as a result of medicalization: health surveillance. This section explores the medicalization thesis and the next section examines how the rise of health surveillance has led to an ever-increasing focus on 'illness'. Both sections highlight the unique insights these changing constructions provide into the construction of illness and the implications they have for our experiences of health and illness.

Medicalization

The concept of medicalization was originally developed in the 1970s, mainly through the work of Zola (1973) and Illich (1976). It is used to refer to the way that medicine gradually defines human conditions and behaviours as medical issues or problems requiring medical explanation and medical intervention. Examples of medicalized human conditions are menstruation, pregnancy, menopause, infertility, baldness, jet lag and insomnia. Behaviours that have been medicalized include shyness, hyperactivity, over-indulgence in food and/or alcohol, spending habits, smoking and nail-biting. In other words, during medicalization 'if anything can be shown in some way to affect the workings of the body and to a lesser extent the mind, then it can be labelled a "medical problem"' (Zola 1973: 261).

There is a lack of agreement over the exact nature of the aforementioned role of medicine within medicalization. Some argue that the expansion of medical jurisdiction over an increasing range of human processes and behaviours is indicative of the medical profession exerting its power in order to extend its professional dominance. Others see medicalization as being one of the consequences of the medical profession responding to broader social processes, such as industrialization, the development of complex bureaucratic systems and an increasing reliance on 'the expert' (Zola 1972; Illich 1976).

Although both Zola and Illich were critical of medicalization, it was Illich who was its most vociferous opponent. He put forward the theory of iatrogenesis to refer to the harmful and detrimental effects that medical interventions can have on us. This theory was integral to his critique of medicalization as he maintained that it was inherently iatrogenic. He identified three different types of iatrogenesis that human beings experience as result of medicalization. These are as follows.

- **Clinical iatrogenesis:** this is the direct harm caused by medicine through medical treatment, adverse reactions to treatment and drug therapy, medical accidents and negligence, hospital-induced infections and injuries, and complications following surgery. It is estimated that some 10 per cent of all people admitted to hospital suffer some form of clinical iatrogenic complication.

- **Social iatrogenesis:** the expansion of medicalization into social life means there is a blind belief in medical progress and expertise, and an institutionalization of medicine as an industry that commodifies and sells health. Those working in the medical establishment and the medical industry promote the consumption of medical products as the only means of realizing people's health expectations. Hence, 'medical practice sponsors sickness . . . reinforcing a morbid society that encourages people to become consumers of curative, preventative, industrial and environ-mental medicine' (Illich 1976: 42). Consequently, through social iatrogenesis, 'the responsibility for health has been appropriated from individuals by medicine and the medical industry' (Illich 1976: 49), and people no longer take responsibility for their health problems.

- **Cultural iatrogenesis:** this last form refers to the fact that medicialization robs people of the ability to cope with any 'normal' conditions they or others experience that cause pain and suffering. As this renders them unable to care for themselves and others, they are dependent on medical attention and treatments whenever they are ill. In Illich's words, they are 'unable to suffer their own reality', they 'unlearn the acceptance of suffering' and 'learn to interpret every ache as an indicator of their need for padding and pampering' (Illich 1976: 133).

The 'medicalization of life'

The above outline of medicalization shows how this development has redefined numerous natural life processes as deviant and now pervades our everyday lives. Indeed, Illich (1976) went on to develop the concept of 'medicalization of life'. His rationale for putting forward this concept was that 'experiences once seen as a normal part of the human condition, such as childbirth, pregnancy, unhappiness, loss of sexual function in later life, ageing and dying, have now been brought under medical scrutiny and control' (Illich 1976: 56).

Hence, ordinary life experiences are now deemed to be 'medical problems' and to require the use of medical knowledge and/or medical technology in a hospital environment. As so much of our human existence is now viewed as medically problematic, medicalization has made us all 'patients', irrespective of whether we actually have an illness or not. Criticisms of the 'medicalization of life' centre around the extent to which it is a form of social control and its negative impact on women's lives. These are both explained further below.

The 'medicalization of life' as a form of social control
Zola and Illich, as well as subsequent writers on medicalization, have been critical of the way that the medicalization of life increases the potential for the exertion of social control. Zola (1973) felt that ultimately it would result in *all* human habits becoming the concern of the medical profession, both physically and psychologically. The plethora of medical advice that currently exists about our everyday habits and lifestyles, such as how much we drink, our diet, sexual activity, levels of exercise and cleanliness, provides evidence to support his argument. To illustrate this point, some of the latest advice is set out in the panel below.

An A–Z medicalization of our everyday lives

Alcohol consumption
> *A man should not regularly drink more than 3–4 units a day and a woman should not regularly exceed 2–3 units a day . . . One unit is 10ml or 8g of pure alcohol. This equals one 25ml single measure of whisky (ABV 40%), or a third of a pint of beer (ABV 5–6%) or half a standard (175ml) glass of red wine (ABV 12%).*
>
> (www.drinkaware.co.uk/tips-and-tools/drink-diary/)

Diet
> *A healthy balanced diet contains a variety of foods including plenty of fruit and vegetables, plenty of starchy foods such as wholegrain bread, pasta and rice, some protein-rich foods such as meat, fish, eggs and lentils and some dairy foods. It should also be low in fat (especially saturated fat), salt and sugar.*
>
> (Food Standards Agency 2009, www.food.gov.uk)

Dish-washing
> *Dish cloths and tea towels should be frequently washed (and preferably boiled). If the water is hot enough and the crockery/cutlery rinsed in clean water, the tea towel can be dispensed with to a large extent, dishes etc. being dried in the plate rack.*
>
> (www.babyclothingcentral.co.uk)

Exercise
> *Half an hour of moderate activity every day, such as brisk walking, can be enough to improve health and fitness.*
>
> (www.nhs.uk/conditions/exercise/Pages/Introduction.aspx)

Household hygiene
> *Disinfect the lavatory pan, the seat and the handle of the flush mechanism – dangerous germs are so easily passed round.*
>
> (www.babyclothingcentral.co.uk)

Fluid intake

In climates such as the UK, we should drink approximately 1.2 litres (six to eight glasses) of fluid every day to stop us getting dehydrated.

(Food Standards Agency 2009, www.food.gov.uk)

Personal hygiene

The use of an anti-perspirant deodorant is very useful for keeping excessive sweating of the underarms at bay. There are many varieties to choose from, some un-perfumed, others for sensitive skin; try a variety until you find a brand that is suitable for you. The removal of excess hair helps to reduce the areas on which bacteria can breed; shaving during the summer months can help with feeling refreshed and clean and reduces the event of odours developing.

(www.hygieneexpert.co.uk)

Salt consumption

Adults should eat no more than 6gm per day.

(Food Standards Agency 2009, www.food.gov.uk)

Sleep

Sleep is essential to maintaining normal levels of cognitive skills such as speech, memory, innovative and flexible thinking. In other words, sleep plays a significant role in brain development. There is no set amount of time that everyone needs to sleep, since it varies from person to person. Research indicates that people like to sleep anywhere between 5 and 11 hours, with the average being 7.75 hours. Jim Horne from Loughborough University's Sleep Research Centre has a simple answer though: 'The amount of sleep we require is what we need not to be sleepy in the daytime.'

(www.bbc.co.uk/science/humanbody/sleep/articles/whatissleep.shtml)

Sex

Safer sex involves using condoms correctly every time you have sex. If you don't use a condom you are more at risk of getting a sexually transmitted infection.

(www.fpa.org.uk/Information)

Smoking

Cigarette smoking is the greatest single cause of illness and premature death in the UK. About 106,000 people in the UK die each year due to smoking. Smoking-related deaths are mainly due to cancers, COPD (chronic obstructive pulmonary disease) and heart disease.

(www.patient.co.uk/health/Smoking-The-Facts.htm)

Sunshine exposure

Spend time in the shade between 11am and 3pm. Make sure you never burn. Aim to cover up with a T-shirt, hat and sunglasses. Remember to take extra care with children. Then use factor 15+ sunscreen.

(www.nhs.uk/Livewell/Summerhealth)

In contrast to Zola, Illich (1976) focused on the 'coping' mechanisms and support systems communities developed which empowered them and enabled them to be independent of medicine or medical practice. For Illich, the 'medicalization of life' led to these being stripped away and replaced by sanitized, technological medical interventions. Using childbirth as an example, Illich argues that throughout history medical intervention was unnecessary because local women would help with any birth that took place, using their own expertise. Medicalization meant that the medical profession took control of childbirth and in most cases it became a matter for hospitalization. Individuals and societies were unable to fight back against such processes and were consequently rendered defenceless and under medical control. Illich therefore concluded that the medicalization of our lives is a form of social control.

Other arguments are based on the tangential relationship with biological functioning in many medicalized phenomena. There is a distinctive rationale in these accusations. It is argued that this relationship is characteristic of medicalization because the defining and labelling of diseases and illnesses it involves is often not the outcome of biological malfunctioning. Rather, it is the product of social expectations about appropriate behaviour. The recent changes in the definition of public drunkenness illustrate this point. Until recently such behaviour was dealt with as a criminal offence but, increasingly, it is being seen as a matter for referral to psychiatric services for treatment. Within this critique, the change in definition from criminal to medical is seen as an indication of medicalization and the outcome of a change in the societal response to this type of 'deviant' behaviour, rather than a biological imperative. Hence, because of medicalization, failure to conform to social expectations about behaviour in public by, for example, being drunk outside of the private domain, may now result in being labelled as being ill. This in itself is seen as a form of social control, as is the use of legally sanctioned chemical, surgical or electrical treatments following diagnosis to control behaviour in public and ensure conformity to societal expectations (Szasz 1961; Zola 1972; Conrad 1992).

The medicalization of women's lives
Reference has already been made to some of the effects of medicalization on the experience of childbirth. Since the 1980s feminist writers have claimed that the medicalization of life has had a greater impact on women's lives than men's. This is mainly because of women's biological role in terms of reproduction. The widespread dominance of biomedicine and the increased use of medical technology meant that the 'natural' processes of pregnancy, childbirth and the menopause were subject to medical control and seen as requiring 'expert' medical attention and intervention. As it was mainly male, white and middle-class health professionals who had such expertise, these feminists argued that women were subjected to patriarchal and social domination in their reproductive healthcare. Such domination in this area of their lives was seen as symbolic of their wider oppression in society (Oakley 1980, 1984; Miles 1991; Conrad 1992).

More recently, debates about the medicalization of women's lives have focused on the huge increase in the amount of advice given to women with regard to their reproductive health. In the next panel there is an extract from a Department of Health book about pregnancy (Department of Health 2007b). As you can see, it illustrates the depth and complexity of the dietary advice currently provided. Such examples have been used to show that medicalization evolves and can take different forms, all of which are equally intrusive into women's lives. Alongside these developments in the medicalization thesis there has been an acknowledgement that the medicalization of women's lives does have some benefits. For instance, many women welcome technological interventions in childbirth and both maternal and infant deaths as a result of childbirth have significantly decreased. Moreover, as the body of literature on the medicalization of men's bodies has grown and highlighted the political emphasis on governing men's health, there has been a recognition that it is not only women's lives that are medicialized (Cahill 2001; Crawshaw 2007; Gatrell 2008; Halpin *et al.* 2009).

The dangers of eating when pregnant

Besides eating a wide variety of foods, there are certain precautions you should take in order to safeguard your baby's well-being as well as your own.

- *Cook all meat and poultry thoroughly so that there is no trace of pink or blood and wash all surfaces and utensils after preparing raw meat. This will help to avoid infection with Toxoplasma, which may cause toxoplasmosis and can harm your baby.*

- *Wash fruit, vegetables and salads to remove all traces of soil which may contain Toxoplasma.*

- *Make sure eggs are thoroughly cooked until the whites and yolks are solid, to prevent the risk of Salmonella food poisoning. Avoid foods containing raw and undercooked eggs like homemade mayonnaise, ice-cream, cheesecake or mousse.*

- *Avoid eating all types of paté, including vegetable patés, and mould-ripened soft cheese, like Brie and Camembert, and similar blue-veined varieties, like Stilton or Danish blue, because of the risk of Listeria infection. You can eat hard cheeses such as cheddar and parmesan, and other cheeses made from pasteurised milk such as cottage cheese, mozzarella cheese and cheese spreads. Although Listeria is a very rare disease, it is important to take special precautions during pregnancy because even the mild form of the illness can lead to miscarriage, stillbirth or severe illness in the newborn.*

- *Drink only pasteurised or UHT milk which has had the harmful germs destroyed. If only raw or green-top milk is available, boil it first. Don't drink unpasteurised goats' or sheep's milk or eat their milk products.*

- *Don't eat liver or liver products, like liver paté or liver sausage, as they may contain a lot of vitamin A. Too much vitamin A could harm your baby. You should also avoid high-dose multivitamin supplements, fish liver oil supplements or any supplements containing vitamin A.*

- *Avoid eating peanuts and foods containing peanut products (e.g. peanut butter, peanut oil, some snacks, etc.) if you or your baby's father or any previous children have a history of hayfever, asthma, eczema or other allergies. Read food labels carefully and, if you are still in doubt about the contents, avoid these foods.*

- *Avoid eating shark, marlin and swordfish and limit the amount of tuna you eat, as these types of fish contain high levels of mercury which can damage your baby's developing nervous system. Limit tuna to two steaks or four cans (each of 140g drained weight) per week. This also applies if you are breastfeeding.*

(Department of Health 2007b)

Activity 6.3

① How would you feel if you were one of the recipients of the advice from the Department of Health?

② To what extent do you think this advice is intrusive into women's lives?

Is medicalization all bad?

Illich (1976) concludes his critique of medicalisation by calling for the abolition of our dependence on medicine and medical practice and its monopolistic control over our everyday lives. However, the negative picture of medicalization that he paints has been challenged. There are those who argue that he overemphasizes human compliance in the face of medicalization and ignores the role of human agency. An example of this view is that 'in this world of uncertain times, one thing remains clear: namely people are not simply passive or active, dependent or independent, believers or sceptics, rather they are a complex mixture of all these things (and much more besides)' (Williams and Calnan 1996: 1619).

Furthermore, as indicated in the discussion of the medicalization of women's lives above, there are positive aspects to medicalization. In addition to those briefly mentioned, clinically it has lead to spectacular improvements in both the treatment of diseases such as cancer and heart disease and the quality of people's lives. The emphasis on advice about disease prevention in our everyday lives has led to people being better informed about health risks and empowered in situations where they discuss health issues with professionals. Medicalization is also a two-way process in that just as some healthy processes become medicialized, others become demedicalized. Such demedicalization has had positive effects – for example, the demedicalization of homosexuality in 1973, and the gradual demedicalization of disability with the introduction of the social model (see Chapter 8) (Conrad 1992; Earle 2005).

Health surveillance

What is health surveillance?

The concept of health surveillance has also been used within the study of the social aspects of health to show how conceptions of illness can vary. This is seen as an extension of medicalization and is most often referred to in the context of the swing from curative to preventative medicine that is central to the contemporary public health movement (see Chapter 1). Health surveillance is used to describe activities devised following direct and indirect scrutiny and observation of health behaviour at both the individual and societal level. These activities aim to prevent illness and improve the health of the population. They include providing health professionals and the public with information about risks to their health and achieving good health, collecting information about assessing health risks and health needs, identifying 'at risk' groups, screening, and developing and evaluating interventions to improve the health status of the population. Such activities started to emerge from the middle of the twentieth century, and subsequent use of technological advances has increased their sophistication and contributed to their recognition. They now dominate health and medical care and are called 'surveillance medicine' (Armstrong 1995).

The rise of health surveillance means that illness has been constructed as being highly preventable as well as treatable. One of the consequences of this is that everyone is targeted, irrespective of whether they are ill – for example, as in mass screening programmes for breast and cervical cancer and mass public health campaigns. In addition, there is an increased focus on 'illness' as opposed to 'health' which can lead to life itself becoming an illness. Indeed it has been argued that health surveillance means that 'your body becomes an enemy of your health' (Reinharz 2001: 438). The identification of more and more threats to our health in our everyday lives also causes anxiety and what can prove to be unfounded 'health panics' (Armstrong 1995; Link and Phelan 1995).

Explaining the rise of health surveillance

Explanations of the rise of 'surveillance medicine' have been informed by the social constructionist perspective adopted by the French sociologist Foucault, and more specifically, have made use of his concept of the 'clinical gaze'. You will recall from Chapter 1 that social constructionism is a strand of postmodernism.

Activity 6.4

List the main points about social constructionism. Check your ideas against the outline of this perspective on page 24 of Chapter 1 and the brief summary below.

As we have seen, social constructionist perspectives emphasize the subjectivity and contestable nature of social reality. This is because they argue that our social world is not 'natural' or biological, but actively constructed by individuals and groups. Foucault (1973, 1979) applied these arguments to the human body and showed how conceptualizations of our own and others' bodies have emerged and changed over time. In his earlier work, he focused on how the rise of biomedicine, with its assumptions about the importance of anatomy and physiology and the need for a scientific understanding of the biological causes of disease, led to the 'clinical gaze'. Foucault used this term to refer to how the processes of observation and interpretation that characterized biomedicine resulted in particular ways of 'seeing and knowing' the body in terms of an 'anatomical atlas' which showed 'the distribution of disease'. He maintained that this view of the human body was not 'natural' and provided an example of yet another 'fabrication' which replaced previous fabrications and would be superseded in time by others.

According to Foucault, the construction of the human body within the 'clinical gaze' also represented power and control; the 'mutation in medical knowledge' that occurred meant that health professionals now required extensive training and knowledge in order to use the 'anatomical atlas'. This gave them considerable power over patients and led to the development of treatment regimes which enabled them to monitor and control patients and their bodies.

Those who have applied Foucauldian ideas to 'surveillance medicine' see the expansion of health surveillance as an evolution of the 'clinical gaze' to the 'community gaze'. By this they mean that the former now not only involves the surveillance of sick people in hospitals but also encompasses healthy people who may be 'at risk' in the community (Conrad 1992; Armstrong 1993, 1995). As such, this move to social surveillance has been seen to be beneficial by some. For instance, it means a reduction in medical control, in that individuals, families and communities are more actively involved in their health. However, others argue that it simply represents more subtle forms of power, control and regulation. Among these are the Foucauldian feminists in their work on public health programmes (such as the mass screening for cervical and breast cancer already mentioned) which are integral to 'surveillance medicine'. This group of feminists view these programmes negatively as they see them as being linked to both patriarchy and the medicalization of women's bodies. To support their case, Foucauldian feminists point to the fact that such programmes do not exist to such an extent for male diseases.

Despite their extensive use in the study of the construction of illness, Foucauldian analyses of health surveillance have not escaped criticism. They have been accused of neither acknowledging the fact that individuals can resist and challenge dominant ideas, or the frequency of non-compliance with medical advice (Diamond and Quinby 1988; Macleod and Durrheim 2002; Marshall 2006).

Conclusions

The discussions in this chapter have shown that the experience of illness is subject to a host of social processes, including continually changing definitions of what it is to be ill. Indeed 'illness' is not an objective phenomenon.

Both the experience of illness and illness itself have been analysed using several explanations that are well established within the study of the social aspects of health. As demonstrated, all of the explanations explored have weaknesses. Indeed, it is questionable as to whether the experience of illness can ever be captured effectively because its very nature means that so many of its dimensions are not articulated (Frank 2001). However, this chapter has shown that that being ill is as much a 'social experience' as it is a 'biological experience'. We shall see how similar arguments apply the same to the experience of disability, the topic of the next chapter.

Key points

- Illnesses can be either acute or chronic. Acute illnesses are those which are short-term and curable. Chronic illnesses are ongoing, long-term and non-communicable.

- Over the last two centuries, there has been an increasing shift in the burden of disease from acute to chronic illness.

- Both types of illness are shaped not only by biological and physiological processeses but also by a range of social processes.

- Functionalism has informed the study of acute illness and symbolic interactionism the work on chronic illness. We now have a much better understanding of the experience of both types of illness, particularly chronic illness.

- Conceptions of illness and disease change over time. The social processes central to these changing conceptions are medicalization and health surveillance.

Discussion points

■ Why do you think a 'clinical iceberg' exists?

■ Is the concept of the 'sick role' still relevant today?

■ What can be done to help people minimize the effects of the 'biographical disruption' that occurs at the onset of a chronic illness?

■ Identify and list some examples of clinical, social and cultural iatrogenesis. You may like to draw on your own experiences as well as relevant literature.

■ Next time you go to your GP surgery pick up some of the leaflets offering health advice. Assess these in the light of the concept of 'health surveillance'.

Suggestions for further study

■ For further information about specific chronic illnesses, it is worth visiting the websites of the different organizations and charities set up to support people with specific conditions such as Asthma UK, the Multiple Sclerosis Society, Diabetes.co.uk and Arthritis Care.

■ If you want to read Parsons' original work on the sick role, see Parsons (1964).

■ For an in-depth exploration of biographical disruption see Bury's work (1982, 1991, 1997).

■ Various aspects of medicalizataion are explored in the following articles by Conrad and Schneider: Conrad (1992, 2005) and Conrad and Schneider (1980, 1992).

■ Armstrong's work (1993, 1995) provides some very interesting ideas about the expansion of health surveillance.

Experiencing mental illness

7

Psychiatrists 'can no longer claim any privileged understanding of madness, alienation or distress'.

(Bracken and Thomas 1998: 17)

Introduction

The profile of mental health has increased significantly in recent years. This can be attributed to a variety of factors. One has been the growing recognition of the importance of mental health to physical health and that there is 'no health without mental health'. The way that well-known figures such as Stephen Fry, Alistair Campbell and Patsy Palmer have publically acknowledged their mental health problems has also helped to promote more positive social attitudes towards mental illness and a greater openness about mental health issues in general.

A consequence of these developments is that there is now a better and more holistic understanding of the experience of mental illness and extent to which it can severely blight the lives of both those who suffer from it and those around them. The study of the social aspects of health has contributed to this understanding by extending the search for explanations of mental illness and its effects on sufferers' quality of life (Rogers and Pilgrim 2005; Ahlström *et al.* 2009). These two areas are therefore the main focus of this chapter and their exploration will help to increase the reader's understanding of the social dimensions of the experiences of illness that was started in Chapter 6.

In order to provide a comprehensive account of the experience of mental illness, the chapter begins with a discussion of the extent of mental illness in the UK. It then moves on to the two main types of explanations of mental illness found within the study of the social aspects of health. The second half of the chapter explores the many and varying effects of mental illness on many people's lives. While several theoretical approaches are drawn upon, the main one is social constructionism and, as in Chapter 6, any theoretical discussions are integrated into the issues addressed within the chapter.

Mental illness and its incidence

There are many different types of mental illnesses and disorders which range considerably in their degree of seriousness. Examples include anxiety disorders, depression, bipolar disorder, schizophrenia, dementia, personality disorders, anorexia nervosa and bulimia. A brief description of these examples is set out below.

Examples of mental illnesses and disorders

- *Anxiety disorders:* people with these disorders experience constant worry and fear that interferes with their normal functioning. There are many different types of anxiety disorder and they include panic disorder, obsessive-compulsive disorder, post-traumatic stress disorder, social anxiety disorder, specific phobias and generalized anxiety disorder.

- *Depression:* this is when feelings of sadness, worthlessness and loneliness are very intense and last for long periods of time. This illness is also referred to as unipolar depression.

- *Bipolar disorder:* this involves elevated mood states (known as 'hypomania') alternating with depression. Nearly 60 per cent of people with bipolar disorder also misuse drugs or alcohol which makes accurate diagnosis difficult.

- *Schizophrenia:* this has been linked to unusual activity of chemicals (neurotransmitters) in the brain which leads to those parts of the brain responsible for emotion and sensation not working properly. Thought processes become distorted and, when severe, sufferers experience intense panic, anger, over-activity, hallucinations and delusions. As a result, schizophrenia may prevent a person from living a normal life and lead to their withdrawal from those around them.

■ *Dementia:* this is a syndrome that is associated with ongoing damage to the structure of the brain. Hence an individual's ability to understand, speak, remember, control their emotions and behave appropriately in social situations declines. Aspects of personality may also change.

■ *Personality disorders:* these result in recurrent and enduring disturbances in conduct (such as being abnormally rigid and maladaptive) and are associated with dysfunctional interpersonal relationships. There are many different types of personality disorder, for example, paranoid, schizoid, obsessive-compulsive and histrionic.

■ *Anorexia nervosa:* this is a condition whereby people develop an obsession about food and their weight. This causes people to think they are fat when they are actually very underweight. Anorexia seriously damages health and can be fatal.

■ *Bulimia:* another eating disorder in which people go on eating binges and then force themselves to vomit the food they have eaten or use diet pills, laxatives or diuretics to prevent themselves from gaining weight. These binge-and-purge episodes typically occur at least twice a week.

Sources: American Psychiatric Association (2004);
Pilgrim (2007); Conrad and White (2010)

The *Diagnostic and Statistical Manual of Mental Disorders* (DSM) is widely used by mental health professionals as a diagnosis guide and an evidence-based reference point to classify mental disorders. Classification is carried out on the basis of manifest symptoms, which are organized into subtypes of psychiatric disorders. The original version, DSM-I, was produced in 1952 and has been revised subsequently many times; DSM-II was produced in 1968, DSM-III in 1980, DSM-IV in 1994 and it is anticipated that the next version, DSM-V, will be published in 2011. In order to reflect research and changes in knowledge, it is not uncommon for interim revised versions to be produced, for instance there was a DSM-III-R, and DSM-IV-TR was published in May 2000.

Statistics show that the incidence of mental ill health is high. For instance, it has been estimated that around 1 in 4 adults experience at least one diagnosable mental health problem in any one year, and as many as 1 in 6 experiences a diagnosable mental health problem at any given time. Furthermore, 1 in 7 have considered suicide at some point in their lives and 1 in 200 have a psychotic disorder such as psychosis and schizophrenia (Office for National Statistics 2001; Allen 2008).

Several indicators also show that the number of those suffering from mental ill health has risen. One set of indicators are those measuring psychological distress. Figure 7.1 shows how levels of psychological distress have risen since 1991. Other indicators include the number of people claiming incapacity benefit and severe disablement allowance on the grounds of mental illness and behavioural disorders. This increased from 31 per cent in 2001 to 41 per cent in 2007 (Dunnell 2008). There is also evidence that these numbers will continue to rise.

One of the most common forms of mental illness is depression. As Figure 7.2 shows, although there are variations between groups, the overall trend is that those experiencing depression will increase between 2007 and 2026. In addition, there is evidence that there is a global growth in the number of people suffering from a mental illness (Allen 2008; McCrone *et al.* 2008).

Figure 7.1 Average levels of psychological distress

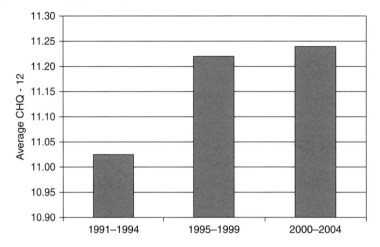

Source: Allen (2008)

Figure 7.2 Projected change in number of people with depression, 2007–26

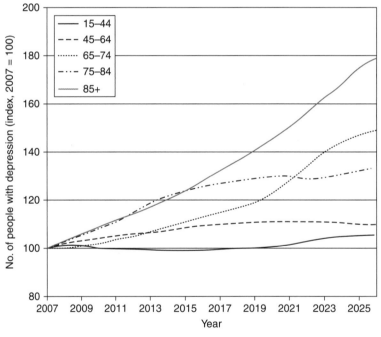

Source: McCrone *et al.* (2008)

When discussing the incidence of mental illness, it is important to consider the way that it persists across generations. The children of those with a mental illness may also experience mental ill health because untreated mental illness in a parent can affect their children's social and mental development. This in turn leads to emotional problems and educational failure, both of which can adversely affect future employment. These factors increase their own risk of mental illness in their later lives (Social Exclusion Unit 2004b; Payne 2006).

In addition, mental illness has negative economic consequences through lost employment, and it is now the most expensive health problem of all. Furthermore, the predicted rise in the numbers of those suffering from mental ill health means that mental health service costs are projected to increase by 45 per cent by 2026 (McCrone *et al.* 2008; World Health Organization 2008; Molarius *et al.* 2009).

However, the accuracy of the figures about mental illness rates has been challenged. This is mainly because of the definitional problems associated with mental illness – the nature of mental illness itself is contested and its meaning, classification and measurement change over time, across cultures and between disciplines. Another reason why the accuracy of mental illness figures has been questioned is that there are often no clear-cut objective signs that someone is suffering from a mental illness and diagnostic tools vary in terms of their effectiveness. Indeed, many people have real psychiatric problems but remain undiagnosed and untreated (Shulman and Hammer 1988; Floyd 1997; McCrone *et al.* 2008). Nonetheless, despite controversies over mental health statistics, the study of the social aspects of health has played an important role in furthering the under-standing of the intricacies of the social processes behind mental illness. One of the areas on which it has had a significant contribution is in explaining what causes mental illness. This is addressed in the next section.

Explanations of mental illness

It is widely acknowledged that 'explanations for mental health problems remain varied' (Pilgrim 2007: 193). Mental health professionals tend to opt for biological or medical explanations which argue that mental illness is a physical disease like polio or cancer. The emphasis in such explanations is on the recurring behaviour, or 'pathological symptoms', of a disease as well as 'diagnosis' and 'treatment with drugs' as in physical medicine. For example, low serotonin levels are associated with depression and hence this has been treated with pharmaceutical interventions such as SSRIs (selective serotonin reuptake inhibitors).

Psychological explanations are also used. These attribute mental distress and disorder to patients' experiences – usually childhood experiences. One of the most well-known theories about the childhood origins of mental ill health is psychoanalytical theory. This is based on the work of Freud and argues that mental illness occurs when children have failed to pass through the various stages of psychosexual development that are identified within this theory (Davar 2001; Rogers and Pilgrim 2005).

The role of social processes and the social and cultural environment have been explored as well. Such factors started to be related to explanations of mental health problems at the beginning of the twentieth century. This initially occurred in the USA where leading psychiatrists linked the alarming increases in mental illness to the American preoccupation with social mobility. Following this, concerns were voiced in the UK about the way that the increasing complexity of life was causing more chronic and less curable mental illnesses. As a result, explanations of mental illness which include social factors and processes have been developed (Rogers and Pilgrim 2005; Ahlström *et al.* 2009).

Although biological and psychological arguments are recognized in explanations of mental illness within the study of the social aspects of health, the role of social influences and processes are the main focus. These explanations fall into two broad camps – those that look at the way society 'constructs' mental illness and those that look at the range of 'causes' of mental illness. While it is acknowledged that 'there has been no official adjudication that one position is more compelling than the other' (Rogers and Pilgrim 2003: 23) they both offer significant insight into mental illness. Hence, they are both addressed in this section.

The 'construction' of mental illness

The view that mental illness is socially constructed has been influenced by the work of Foucault (1973). As we saw in Chapter 6, Foucault argues that there is no single incontestable truth as both individuals and powerful groups construct society through their ideas and conceptualizations. Central to his argument about mental illness is the notion of discourse which he uses to describe the accepted conceptualizations about mental illnesses that are constructed by powerful groups, such as psychiatrists. Like other discourses, these can remain dominant in society over a period of time.

More generally, those who adopt a social constructionist approach to mental illness point to the historical and cultural variations in the way mental disorder is defined. With reference to historical variations, in the Middle Ages mental illness was constructed as being caused by demonic forces at work in the brain. Mentally ill people were often killed or tortured. During the eighteenth century, people thought to be mad were regarded as deviant and incarcerated with other 'deviants' such as criminals and paupers. Treatment was punitive. Even now, when we have a more humanitarian social construction of mental illness, the assessment of it lacks objectivity and still varies over time – changing classification systems, inadequate diagnostic concepts, and the role of values in the diagnosis of mental illness have been found to lead to disagreement among psychiatrists in around 54 per cent of cases (Pilgrim and Bentall 1999; Rogers and Pilgrim 2005).

Furthermore, the anti-psychiatry movement in the 1960s and 1970s accused psychiatry of being a fraudulent medical speciality as it only uses symptoms (i.e. what people say and do) and not clinical evidence, as in other areas of medicine (Rogers and Pilgrim 2005). Szasz (1974) went as far as accusing psychiatry of manufacturing the criteria on which behaviour is evaluated and used the term 'the myth of mental illness'. He and others within the anti-psychiatry movement also argued that mental disorder involves **labelling**. Central to their argument is the view that there are no brain changes in madness. Instead, mental illness is the result of socially powerless individuals committing deviant acts similar to those committed by everyone at one time or another during a lifetime (e.g. losing their temper really badly or getting very drunk) and being caught by socially powerful others. Once caught, they are then given the label of 'mentally ill' because the type of behaviour they have displayed is *viewed* as mental illness. In other words, the fact of the illness is inferred from the behaviour so that the behaviour itself is the illness. Thus, although individuals may only have failed to manage their lives within the demands of the social environment, they are labelled as mentally ill because their behaviour violates prescribed norms.

In relation to changes in the numbers of those diagnosed with a mental illness, this approach would argue that these are due to changes in the way that mental illness is constructed, as opposed to actual decreases or increases in the incidence of mental ill health. Hence the rises in the incidence of mental illness as reported in the first section in this chapter would be attributed to factors such as differences in discourses over time and between cultures, which in turn led to amendments being made to classification systems and the criteria used to diagnose mental illnesses.

Activity 7.1

The following is an extract from a journal article about depression, one of the most common forms of mental illness. The extract illustrates the arguments presented by those who believe that mental illness is socially constructed. As you read it, try to identify which points relate to a social constructionist approach to mental illness. There are some suggestions for you to consider in the 'Activity feedback' chapter on page 231.

> *Within the psychiatric and clinical psychology literature, there are a variety of positions taken about what constitutes depression. In some texts, no working definition is offered at all, although a range of symptoms are explored. This approach is evident in the writings of some biological theorists . . . as well as some who are more psychologically oriented . . . this failure to provide a clear definition implies that the concept of depression has a self-evident validity. However, closer inspection reveals that different authors assign primacy to different psychological phenomena when writing about depression. For example, some texts insist that it is primarily a disturbance of mood and that all associated phenomena are secondary to this affective state . . . others focus primarily on cognitive features. Perhaps most influential in this latter respect has been Beck and his colleagues, who have argued that the depressive experience is character- ised by a negative view of the self, the world and the future . . . in an attempt to avoid assigning primacy to one particular feature of depression some writers have argued that depression is a 'Syndrome not a symptom and this syndrome requires the presence of several symptoms' (Montgomery, 1990: 31). In accord with this assumption, DSM-IV . . . requires the presence of depressed mood and four other symptoms before 'major depression' can be diagnosed. Other psychiatric definitions include looser or more arbitrary inclusion criteria.*
>
> (Pilgrim and Bentall 1999: 262)

The 'causes' of mental illness

There are two different types of explanation of the 'causes' of mental illness: one group of explana- tions puts forward models of the causes and the other group uses the concepts of social integration and social support. These explanations are outlined below.

Models of the 'causes' of mental illness

As discussed in Chapters 2, 3 and 4, gender, class and ethnicity all influence mental illness rates. Models have been developed to explain how such social factors play a causal role in mental ill health, and the nature of the processes involved in the relationship between them and mental health. This is illustrated in the examples of two such models set out in Figures 7.3 and 7.4.

Melzer *et al.* (2004) developed the model in Figure 7.3 from the results of a re-examination of recent large studies from developed countries to clarify the nature of the relationship between common mental disorders and social position. As shown, social position is seen as encompassing the overlapping dimensions of occupational status, education and income/wealth. There is a causal relationship between most of the other factors identified. For instance, social position was found to be associated with childhood and early influences, which in turn affect 'biological and other uniden- tified factors'. The latter are linked to known risk factors for common mental disorders, such as physical illness and stressful life events. These known risk factors also impact on social position. As you can see, these causal relationships are not simple and their complexity is further compounded by the fact that most of the linking arrows point in both directions.

Another model is presented in Figure 7.4. This was produced by Brown and Harris (1978) following their studies about the relationship between social class, gender and depression. When they compared working-class and middle-class women with children living in London, about a quarter of the working-class women suffered from depression whereas the middle-class women suffered depression at only a quarter of the working-class rate. Their model is therefore based on the factors they identified as being involved in bringing about depression.

Figure 7.3 The potential influences on prevalence rates of the common mental disorders

Source: Melzer *et al.* (2004)

Figure 7.4 Brown and Harris's model (adapted)

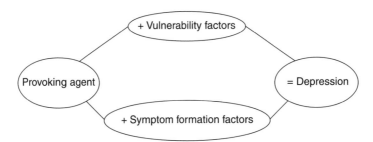

Brown and Harris used the term *provoking agents* to denote those life events such as severe diffi-culties or life-threatening events (e.g. the threat of eviction or being the victim of physical violence) which provoke depression. However, these provoking agents do not necessarily cause depression unless two other sets of factors are present. These are *vulnerability factors* and *symptom formation factors*. The former include the absence of an intimate relationship with a husband or boyfriend, having three or more children under the age of 15 years at home, unemployment and loss of mother before the age of 11 years. Their presence greatly increases the chances of breakdown in the face of provoking agents. Symptom formation factors include other past losses of close rela-tives in childhood and adolescence and they influence the type and severity of depression. For example, loss by death is strongly associated with psychotic-like depressive symptoms, whereas loss by other means (such as parents separating) leads to neurotic-like symptoms. Brown and Harris claimed that because of their social class, working-class women experience more untoward life events and difficulties (provoking agents) and have an excess of vulnerability factors which explains why they have higher rates of depression.

Both models have their flaws. The model in Figure 7.3 can be criticized for the amorphous nature of its categories; many factors can be subsumed by these categories, for instance, 'stressful life events' could include discrimination, domestic violence, political conflict and war. All of these vary considerably in terms of their effects on individuals. Similarly, other known factors, such as being unemployed or economically inactive can be subsumed under 'work circumstances' but again can have significantly different impacts from, say, being self-employed (Davar 2001; Melzer *et al.* 2004; Pilgrim 2007; Merritt 2008). Different studies have identified different interactions between the varying factors from those identified in this model. For instance, Taylor and Gunn (1999) found that people who have a physical illness *and* two or more recent adverse life events are six times more likely to have a mental illness than people without physical illness, and three times more in the case of adverse life events.

Brown and Harris's model in Figure 7.4 has been criticized for omitting men, but also for not including a broader analysis of society. Indeed, as we saw in Chapter 2, feminists have argued that the higher rates of mental illness among women are attributable to the operation of patriarchal power in contemporary society (Showalter 1987; Ussher 1991).

The discussions of these two models show that no single causation model of mental illness can accurately represent the full range of influences, their impacts and the complexities of the relationships between them that shape the connection between social factors and mental health. In addition, it is also clear that in causation models of mental illness the emphasis is on a *range* of causal factors. Decreases and increases in the incidence of mental illness are accounted for in terms of changes in the number and intensity of their identified causes and their impact on individuals, groups and societies.

Activity 7.2	
Compare the two models in Figures 7.3 and 7.4 and complete the table below.	
Similarities	
Differences	
The 'Activity feedback' chapter has some suggested responses, on page 231.	

Social integration, social support and mental illness
There are also explanations of the causes of mental illness that do not involve models as such. The concepts of social integration and social support have already been briefly mentioned in connection with their influence on the mental health of older people and minority ethnic groups. Given the insights both provide about the causes of mental illness, it is appropriate to explore them further in this chapter.

The concept of social integration was originally developed by Durkheim (1968) and is about the relationships between individuals and institutions in society. It focuses on societal relationships, which are those between individuals and societal institutions in society, such as the family, employment and religious, political, community and voluntary groups. Durkheim argued that integration into these societal institutions helps people to cope when facing stressful life events: 'There is a constant inter-change of ideas and feelings from all to each and each to all, something like a mutual moral support, which instead of throwing the individual on his own resources, leads him to share in the collective energy and supports his own when exhausted' (Durkheim 1968: 210).

Thus when individuals are socially integrated in this way they do not have to depend solely on themselves. Durkheim hypothesized that the more people were socially integrated, the more they were able to cope with stress and were 'protected' during life's crises and ultimately from mental ill health (Durkheim 1968; Freund and McGuire 1995). However, criticisms of Durkheim's work include the way that he does not acknowledge the physical and mental states of individual actors and their influence on the degree to which social integration is efficacious (Gerhardt 1989).

Although the concept of social support is similar, there are important differences. Berkman *et al.* (2000) locate the concept of social support in Bowlby's work on attachment theory (developed in the 1960s and 1970s) because it articulates individuals' 'needs for secure attachment for its own sake' (Berkman *et al.* 2000: 845). Many studies carried out in the past four decades on social networks, kinship and community have also used the concept of social support. In contrast to the concept of social integration, it focuses on the interpersonal relationships individuals have in particular contexts at the micro level, such as in relationships between friends, as opposed to relationships at a societal level. However, its effects are similar to those of social integration in that social support can also act as a mediator for stress, as well as offer resources in tackling life's troubles and maintaining good mental health. There are different explanations of the effects of social support. These include the way these interrelationships enhance our 'sense of security and self esteem' (Berkman *et al.* 2000: 845), 'empower individuals' and are 'a source of self-validation' (Freund and McGuire 1995: 114) (see also Whelan 1993; Berkman 1995; Penninx *et al.* 1997; Gabe *et al.* 2004).

Living with a mental illness

Understanding the social dimensions of the experiences of mental illness also involves an appreciation of what it is to live with a mental illness. The examples presented below have been selected to give as realistic a picture as possible and to demonstrate the complicated and often interlocking relationships between the various factors.

Quality of care

Two developments within service delivery have been highly significant in the care of people with a mental illness. The first was the introduction of community care in the 1980s. This signalled a move away from institutional care to community-based care for people with mental illnesses. Various theoretical perspectives have proffered critiques of institutional care. An example of a social constructionist approach is Foucault's critique of institutions. He argues that the development of asylums for the mentally ill that began in the eighteenth century was portrayed as being a move to more humanitarian treatment. Prior to this, treatment was punitive and physical with the emphasis on controlling what was regarded as a problematic group in society. However, for Foucault, asylum or institutional care meant that the mentally ill were still subject to constant control and regulation. Therefore, such institutions merely represented a move from one form of control to another – from physical control to moral control (Rogers and Pilgrim 2005).

Those writing from a Marxist perspective have argued that asylums and institutions were useful 'dumping grounds' for those who could not cope with the demands of capitalism and/or were not required within the capitalist system. The legitimate removal of these people from society contributed to the smooth operation of capitalism and the maximization of profits (Scull 1979).

The shift to community-based care (see Chapter 10) has meant that most people with a mental illness, including those with serious illnesses, are now cared for in the community. The major concerns about institutional care mean that this change has been welcomed and, indeed, there were and are many positive aspects to these developments (Means *et al.* 2008). Attempts have also been made to improve service delivery by ensuring there are national standards in mental health services, and the rights of those with mental illness have been strengthened through, for example, the growth of user involvement and engagement. Despite these moves, criticisms of the quality, comprehensiveness and continuity of care provided for people with mental illnesses continue to be made. For instance, according to a recent report, many people with mental disorders are either not in contact with services or are in contact but are not receiving treatment. It is estimated, for example, that 35 per cent of those with depression and 51 per cent of those with anxiety disorders are not in contact with services, and many conduct disorders and eating disorders among children and adolescents are undiagnosed and untreated (McCrone *et al.* 2008).

These criticisms have been directed at both hospital and community-based care. Reports focus on overflowing hospital wards which are dangerous environments, how the staff working in them are exhausted and overworked, and the ways that the pressures of inadequate resources mean that many patients do not receive the appropriate levels of care. In the community, piecemeal development, lack of funds and failures of partnership working have contributed to individual neglect, oversights and allegations that patients 'fall through the net'. Early intervention work, such as helping people to stay in work and maintain their social contacts, often does not always take place, leading to an escalation of less serious mental health problems (Rogers and Pilgrim 2003; Lester and Glasby 2006; McCrone *et al.* 2008).

Discrimination

There have been many initiatives designed to tackle stigma and discrimination connected with mental health issues. Although attitudes to mental illness have become more positive in the past couple of decades and there is a greater openness about mental health issues in general, the stigma attached to mental illness remains (Corrigan 2007; Department of Health 2009b). As discussed in Chapter 6, Goffman (1968a) produced seminal work about stigma; he maintained that stigmatization involves the association of socially constructed negative characteristics with members of a particular social group. This stereotyping produces negative emotional reactions in others which include contempt, disgust and fear. Such reactions make those who are stigmatized feel disempowered, rejected and depersonalized. This leads to self-doubt and a crumbling of self-image, which can ultimately 'spoil' the self-identity of those experiencing the stigma.

Those that argue that the media is culpable for the aforementioned ongoing stigmatization point to discriminatory reporting that reinforces and maintains public hostility towards people with mental health problems. For instance, despite recent efforts to adopt a more considered approach to mental health matters, two-thirds of all British press coverage of mental health has been found to include a link with violence. In addition, 40 per cent of daily tabloids and nearly half of the Sunday tabloids were found to contain derogatory headlines such as 'schizophrenic kills' and references to 'nutters' and 'loonies'. Media stereotypes have been further fuelled by several high profile and brutal murders. Nonetheless, there is much evidence that these negative stereotypes are unfounded; although the rates of violence and arrest among the mentally ill may be higher when compared to the general population, since 1957 statistics show very few people with mental illnesses commit homicides and there is little fluctuation in the numbers. The discharge from long-stay institutions means that this also represents a fall of 3 per cent in the overall homicide rate for people with mental illnesses. Indeed, people with mental illnesses are more likely to be the *victims* of crime (Social Exclusion Unit 2004b; Lester and Glasby 2006; Markowitz 2006; Pilgrim 2007).

Whatever the cause(s) of this stigma, it manifests itself in the continued discrimination against those who have a mental illness; people with mental health problems are attributed with qualities such as violence and unintelligibility, and fewer than 4 in 10 employers say they would consider someone with mental health problems. Indeed, it is estimated that as many as 9 out of 10 mentally ill people experience discrimination (Rogers and Pilgrim 2003; Social Exclusion Unit 2004b; Kelly 2006).

The ongoing stigma associated with mental illness can also result in a reluctance to seek help, which in turn contributes to the lack of diagnosis and treatment of many mental health problems (Rogers and Pilgrim 2005; Barney *et al.* 2009). This has been shown to be a particular problem among older people (see Chapter 5), who seem to be more sensitive to discriminatory attitudes to mental ill health than other groups in society.

Poverty and employment

Mental illness is also associated with living in poverty. This has mainly been attributed to the fact that many of those with mental health problems do not undertake paid employment. While there is evidence that 90 per cent of users of mental health services want to work, those with a mental illness have the lowest employment rate of any of the main groups of disabled people. The employment rates are worse for those who have been out of work for the longest periods of time. Even when they have a job, their chance of losing it is twice that of others and on average and they only earn two-thirds of the national hourly rate. Benefit dependency is also high; recent statistics show that 34 per cent of Incapacity Benefit claimants have a mental health problem (Meltzer *et al.* 2002; Kelly 2006; Payne 2006; Schneider *et al.* 2009).

Initiatives have been introduced to support people with mental health problems to find and retain work. These include specialist agency support, re-vocational training that helps prepare individuals for paid work, and supported employment (i.e. on-the-job support). More individualized approaches have been found to be the most successful. Moreover, there is evidence that paid work for people with mental health problems brings 'greater financial satisfaction' and higher 'levels of well-being (self-esteem and hope) . . . with the greatest increases shown by those moving into work' (Schneider *et al.* 2009: 157) (see also Department for Work and Pensions 2007; National Social Inclusion Programme 2007).

However, at a more general level, the value of employment for those with a mental illness has been questioned. There are several reasons why it may not be a simple protection against poor mental health and social exclusion. One reason is that it has variable effects on mental health – for example, mental health is affected by the level and status of the paid employment. Another reason is that if it involves antisocial hours, it restricts social activities outside of work and consequently increases, as opposed to reduces, social isolation. The negative effects of social isolation on mental health are well established (Marmot *et al.* 2001; Goodwin and Kennedy 2005). Therefore, for employment to be effective in improving mental health, it needs to meet certain criteria such as improving status and reducing isolation.

Housing

One of the consequences of living in poverty is that those with poor mental health, particularly those with more severe mental illnesses, are less likely to have a stable home than other groups in society. They also tend live in poor-quality accommodation that is inadequate, noisy and crowded, and located in undesirable neighbourhoods characterized by high deprivation and unemployment rates (Payne 2006; Kyle and Dunn 2008).

Social isolation

People with mental illnesses have fewer social and family networks than average; many of their contacts are related to health services rather than to employment (as discussed above), family, friends, leisure, social and community activities. In addition, they experience considerable difficulties in establishing and maintaining long-term intimate partner relationships. The relationships of those with serious mental illnesses in particular tend to be characterized by a lack of intimacy and commitment. One of the consequences is that those with a mental illness are three times as likely to be divorced (Perry and Wright 2006; Wright *et al.* 2007). As mentioned above, the social isolation that results from this lack of social networks and personal relationships can also contribute to a further deterioration in mental health (Meltzer *et al.* 2002; Huxley and Thornicroft 2003).

Increased morbidity

Mental ill health often goes hand-in-hand with poorer physical health. There are several reasons for this. First of all, links have been established between the chronic stress experienced as a result of some mental illnesses and cardiovascular disease, as well as between serious mental illness and an increased risk of cancer (Pandiani *et al.* 2006). Another reason is that the clinical treatments for some mental illnesses can have adverse physical effects. An example is the use of antipsychotics for treating schizophrenia. Some antipsychotic drugs are known to increase the risk of hyperpro-lactinaemia (the excessive production of prolactin which can suppress ovulation and the produc-tion of the thyroid hormone) in women, and the risk of diabetes in both men and women (Briggs *et al.* 2008). Mental illness is also associated with more risky health-related behaviour, such as smoking, which increases the chances of physical health problems (Lawrence *et al.* 2009).

The relationship between social isolation and relative lack of personal and social support to poorer physical and mental health has been addressed in other chapters in this book. Given the findings reported above, it is therefore unsurprising that another reason put forward for the decrease in the physical health of those with a mental illness is the concomitant isolation that mental ill health often entails (Pilgrim 2007; Allen 2008).

The research discussed so far about the reasons for the coexistence of poor mental and physical health has focused on how mental illness can lead to poorer physical health. There is also evidence of this relationship in reverse. Some physical illnesses or acquired disabilities, such as a cancer diagnosis or amputation, can lead to severe emotional distress and personality changes. Drugs used to treat a physical illness can also cause temporary psychological disturbances (National Statistics 2004b; Pilgrim 2007).

Increased mortality

Those with a mental illness have higher rates of mortality than those who do not. Mortality rates do vary with the nature of the illness – for example, people suffering from schizophrenia or an eating disorder are more at risk than those with depression. However, much of this mortality profile can be attributed to the generally raised suicide rates among the mentally ill (McCusker *et al.* 2006).

Social exclusion

The discussions in this section of the experiences of those living with a mental illness show that multiple interlocking and reinforcing processes can contribute to exclusion from many aspects of life, such as employment, social activities and community involvement, that others take for granted. The loss of confidence, impaired social relations and well-being that this engenders can lead to the development of what Goffman terms a 'spoiled identity'. Furthermore, research has shown that many people with a mental illness now living in our communities experience social exclusion in that their participation in society is considerably constrained by discrimination, lack of material resources, geographical location and – last but not least – their ill health. Those with more serious mental illnesses are more likely to be socially excluded than those with less serious problems. Indeed, these people have been found to be among the most excluded in British society (Social Exclusion Unit 2004b; Lester and Glasby 2006; Merritt 2008).

Case example: Ben's story

The following case study illustrates many of the points made above about what life can be like for those with a mental illness.

Ben had always been a very sensitive person; right from when he was young his parents were amazed at how he reacted so emotionally to events and to people. He was extremely bright and was often teased at school for being a 'swot' and a 'geek'. He had never had any friends but during adolescence he became increasingly reclusive, often spending the whole day in his room and only coming downstairs for meals. He got into a local university and although he initially coped he found the social side of university life very stressful. Although other students tried to include him, as he consistently declined their offers, they eventually gave up. He withdrew into himself even more and started missing teaching sessions and assignment deadlines. Things came to a head when he did not turn up for an essential field trip that was part of his assessment for one module. After having to remove the door of his room because he had barricaded himself in, university staff found him weeping in his bed. He was subsequently diagnosed as having a breakdown. He returned home, and despite support from his GP and parents decided to leave university.

Following this point in Ben's life, he often became aggressive and acted violently for no apparent reason, and his parents found it impossible to have him live with them. He managed to get a part-time bar job and found a bedsit in a run-down part of his home town. Without parental support, he frequently missed his medication and medical appointments made to monitor his illness. He also started to drink heavily and this problem was exacerbated by the fact that he worked in a bar. After an incident where he was drunk and abusive at work, he was sacked from his job. His parents tried to keep up contact with him but he rarely wanted to see them. He then had a series of low paid part-time jobs with none of them lasting more than a few months because of his 'odd' and often drink-fuelled behaviour. Meanwhile, his physical health also deteriorated as a result of the excessive drinking and the fact that he did not bother to eat properly. A row with another tenant led to his eviction from his bedsit. Upon finding that he was no longer in his bedsit, his parents finally managed to find him in a caravan park just outside town. He would not allow them into the caravan and refused all offers of professional help. Two months later he was found dead in the caravan, having committed suicide.

Activity 7.3

What approach do you think symbolic interactionism would take to explaining the experiences of those who live with a mental illness? The sections on symbolic interactionsim in Chapter 1 and in Chapter 6 will help you with this activity. Compare your thoughts with the account provided in the 'Activity feedback' chapter on page 231.

Conclusions

This chapter has shown that while there are definitional and measurement issues around mental illness, it is clear that there is a high incidence of mental ill health in our society, and that it is increasing and likely to continue to do so. Many explanations of mental illness have been developed. While all of these make a contribution to the understanding of this complex health problem, they need to be critically considered in combination to be of real benefit. The exploration of the experience of living with a mental illness showed that mental ill health has many negative effects on sufferers' lives and they are at an increased risk of social exclusion.

Addressing social exclusion in the context of mental illness is highly problematic. One of the main issues of concern within policies has been the persistence of mental ill health across generations. As a result, many mental health initiatives not only promote the social inclusion of those with a mental illness but also aim to reduce social exclusion across the life course. The emphasis in these is on integration of policy areas, such as housing and employment, and close collaboration across government departments and with the private and voluntary sectors (Kelly 2006; Payne 2006). The increase in the numbers of those experiencing mental ill health and both the quantifiable and unquantifiable costs to society identified mean that this social problem will retain political prominence. More importantly, unless solutions are found, the mentally ill will continue to be denied their right to full participation in society.

Key points

■ The incidence of mental ill health is high and increasing.

■ The explanations of mental illness within the study of the social aspects of health fall into two broad camps – those that look at the way society 'constructs' mental illness and those that look at the way society 'causes' mental illness.

■ Explanations which focus on the way society 'constructs' mental illness argue that definitions of mental illness vary historically and culturally.

■ Those explanations which argue society 'causes' mental illness focus on a range of factors which are known to cause poorer mental health. Examples are social class, gender, education, income, early life influences, stressful life events, physical illnesses and lack of social support and integration.

■ Living with a mental illness involves many negative experiences which include discrimination, poverty, unemployment, poor-quality housing, social isolation, increased morbidity and mortality and ultimately social exclusion.

Discussion points

- Why do you think some groups in society are more likely to suffer from mental ill health than others?

- To what extent do you think that 'social processes are crucial to the understanding of mental health and disorder' (Busfield 2000b: 544).

- Discuss the main similarities and differences between the two explanations of mental illness presented in this chapter.

Suggestions for further study

- Any of the mental health charity websites will provide you with further and more detailed data on the incidence of mental health. Publications by Pilgrim and Rogers are excellent for an in-depth understanding of mental illness, its causes and the experiences of those who live with it.

- Highly recommended are *Key Concepts in Mental Health* (Pilgrim 2007), *Mental Health and Inequality* and *A Sociology of Mental Health and Illness* (Rogers and Pilgrim 2003, 2010).

- For a further exploration of the anti-psychiatry movement, see work by Schell, Szasz and Laing.

- Lester and Glasby (2006) provides a readable and useful overview of mental health services and both past and current policy developments.

Experiencing disability

Disability is something imposed on top of our impairments by the way we are unnecessarily isolated and excluded from full participation in society.

(Oliver 1996: 22)

Overview

Introduction

Although around 21 per cent of the adult population in the UK is disabled, interest in disability waxes and wanes (Disability Rights Commission 2006). For instance, disability issues were frequently in the headlines in the late 1990s when changes to benefits were being proposed. During one incident, disabled activists besieged Downing Street, paint was thrown, wheelchairs were padlocked to the railings, and some of the activists lay down in the road to protest (Hughes 1998). More recently there has been a surge of interest in the experiences of people with disabilities because of the increase in the number of hate crimes reported in the media. Within the study of the social aspects of health, the commitment to extending knowledge about disability and the experiences of the significant numbers of people in our society who are disabled is ongoing. An overview of the insights that have been produced will therefore add to the understandings gleaned from other chapters in this section of the book about the social dimensions of the experience of illness.

One of the consequences of the interest in disability is that there has been a longstanding recognition of the fact that people with disabilities face more negative life experiences and inequalities, such as poverty and welfare dependency, and exclusion from employment, than many other groups (Humphrey 2000; Gardiner and Millar 2006; Gannon and Nolan 2007). An understanding of the relative disadvantages experienced by those who live with a disability requires the exploration of the concept of disability, the changes in the way that disability has been constructed in our society and the lived experiences of people with disabilities. These issues are therefore addressed in this chapter. The term 'disability' is used in its broadest sense and refers to disabilities caused by both physical and mental impairments, or diseases which result in functional and activity limitations, as well as conditions which cause learning disabilities, such as Down's syndrome. The main theoretical approach adopted in the analyses is social constructionism.

The concept of disability

> **Activity 8.1**
>
> Write down all the terms that you can think of that have been and/or are used when referring to disability or people with a disability. Once you have done this, divide them into those that would be unacceptable and acceptable today. Now read the rest of this section.

Many different terms have been used in the past to define disability. Most of these were either offensive or depersonalizing. Examples of the former are 'imbecile', 'cripple', 'spastic', 'feeble-minded', 'retarded', 'mentally deficient' and 'mongol' (Hughes 1998; Beckett 2009). The latter include 'physically handicapped', 'mentally handicapped', 'blind' and 'deaf'. Moreover, not only do these terms have negative connotations but they also infer that those to whom they are applied are innately inferior. Since the 1970s there has been a move away from such 'disablist' terminology, as more recent definitions, such as those set out below below, demonstrate.

> **Definitions of disability**
>
> [disability is] *the disadvantage or restriction of activity caused by a contemporary social organisation which takes no or little account of people who have physical impairments and thus excludes them from the mainstream of social activities.*
>
> (Union of the Physically Impaired Against Segregation 1976: 14)

[disability is] *the functional limitation within the individual caused by physical, mental or sensory impairment.*

(Disabled People's International 1982: 105)

a person has a disability for the purposes of this Act if he has a physical or mental impairment which has a substantial and long-term adverse effect on his ability to carry out normal day-to-day activities.

(HM Government 1995)

The ICF [International Classification of Functioning, Disability and Health] *puts the notions of 'health' and 'disability' in a new light. It acknowledges that every human being can experience a decrement in health and thereby experience some degree of disability. Disability is not something that only happens to a minority of humanity. The ICF thus 'mainstreams' the experience of disability and recognises it as a universal human experience. By shifting the focus from cause to impact it places all health conditions on an equal footing allowing them to be compared using a common metric – the ruler of health and disability. Furthermore ICF takes into account the social aspects of disability and does not see disability only as a 'medical' or 'biological' dysfunction. By including contextual factors, in which environmental factors are listed, ICF* [allows the recording of] *the impact of the environment on the person's functioning.*

(World Health Organization 2009)

Although the previous negativity is absent from the above definitions of disability they are problematic in that they are inherently contradictory. For instance, disability is defined as an impairment which imposes functional limitations on individuals and results in them being unable to perform 'normal' activities. This type of definition portrays disability as being ultimately reducible to the individual and physiological pathology, and hence medicalizes and individualizes the problems of disability. In contrast, other definitions acknowledge that there are social dimensions to disability, and locate the causes within society and social organization.

These different approaches to defining disability indicate that the concept is more of a question of social definition than objective truth. Indeed, there are those who argue that the concept of 'disability' is socially constructed. As we have seen in other chapters, this refers to the way that aspects of society or behaviour are actively 'constructed' as a result of social relations and human agency at particular points in time, in particular cultures, rather than being 'natural' or biological in origin.

Oliver (1990, 1996, 1998) has written extensively on the social construction of disability. He maintains that disability has been socially constructed through the activities of powerful groups, vested interests, historical and cultural developments and language which is heavily influenced by ideology. Consequently, the way disability is constructed has changed over time. The argument that disability is socially constructed is supported by evidence of historical changes in the way people with disabilities have been viewed and treated. It is to this evidence that we now turn.

The social construction of disability

In order to provide the reader with a comprehensive understanding of the social construction of disability, four models of disability will be discussed in this section: evolutionary, medical, social and cultural.

The evolution of disability
Finkelstein, a wheelchair user himself, was responsible for some of the original work on the social construction of disability. Writing in the late 1970s and early 1980s, he developed an evolutionary model of disability which linked changing social constructions of those with disabilities with three different phases in history (Finkelstein 1981). These are as follows.

Phase 1
In pre-industrial Britain, the economy was based on feudalism which meant work was rurally based, cooperative and small scale. Disabled people were able to participate and therefore had a role, albeit limited in some cases, in the production process. The small and isolated communities that existed at that time also meant that people with disabilities could more easily be absorbed into the life of communities without special provision. Furthermore, the uncongested rural surroundings posed less problems for disabled people compared to the towns and cities that developed during industrialization. Although the disabled were often regarded as being one of the groups at the lower end of the social hierarchy, for the reasons just outlined, Finkelstein argues that disabled people were not segregated or excluded from the rest of society.

Phase 2
Changes that occurred during industrialization and the period after it led to a change in the way that disabled people were socially constructed. During industrialization there was a move to large-scale industrial production which was 'geared to able bodied norms' (Finklestein 1981: 7). The implications for disabled people were significant because, as capitalism developed, they increasingly found it harder to meet the demands of industrial production processes. They were seen as slower and less productive and the result was that 'the operation of the labour market in the 19th century effectively depressed handicapped people of all kinds to the bottom of the market' (Morris 1969: 9).

Disabled people were gradually excluded from paid labour and became 'unemployable'. This exclusion from the workforce also contributed to their ultimate segregation from their communities. In the eighteenth and nineteenth centuries, unemployed people in the cities came to be regarded as a 'social problem' for civil authorities. Unemployable disabled people were treated in the same way as those who were unemployed – that is, they were put into large-scale institutions and workhouses, and therefore segregated from mainstream social life.

However, the segregation of disabled people was not just limited to those who were unemployable – it gradually became universal throughout industrialization. Finkelstein attributes this to the rise of biomedicine. As we have seen, biomedicine rests on an assumption that all causes of disease – mental disorders as well as physical disease – are understood in biological terms and it views disease and sickness as deviations from normal functioning which medicine has the power to put right with its scientific knowledge and understanding of the human body. Finkelstein's argument is that the rise of biomedicine meant that from the nineteenth century disability became medicalized; disabled people were viewed as medical problems who needed to be 'helped' by the medical profession. According to Finkelstein, a further consequence of the rise of biomedicine that played an important role in the segregation of disabled people was the growth of hospital-based medicine. Synthesizing these points, he developed his argument that from the early 1800s onwards, both the medicalization of disability and the growth of hospital-based medicine meant disabled people were treated in secure long-stay institutions, such as special schools, colonies and asylums. Not only did these sorts of institutions segregate disabled people from the rest of society, they also frequently subjected them to regimes of moral management and custodial forms of discipline.

Finkelstein concludes that it was the institutionalization to which disabled people were subjected during and following industrialization that caused their subsequent reconstruction as dependent, needy and passive.

Phase 3

Finkelstein saw this phase as beginning in the last quarter of the twentieth century and was hopeful that it would bring an end to the social oppression of disabled people. For him, this was the era of the introduction of new technologies and collaboration between professional and disabled people in working towards common goals. Developments in both these areas would enable disabled people to lead independent lives in the community and segregative practices would eventually cease. Hence, this phase would mark the beginning of the liberation of disabled people and their inclusion in society once more. Moreover, disability would no longer be constructed as a social restriction.

Beyond the evolutionary model of disability

Finkelstein's work has been criticized for being over-simplistic and over-optimistic in that it ideal- izes the 'community' in Phase 1 and implies that attitudes towards, and treatment of, disabled people were somehow positive. The extent of the social inclusion of disabled people Finkelstein predicted in Phase 3 has also been questioned (Oliver 1990). Nonetheless, his ideas did stimulate further theorizing on the social processes behind the oppression of disabled people. For instance, Oliver developed the themes in Finkelstein's model into an account of how disability was 'produced' by the economic, political and social changes that occurred during the transition from feudalism to capitalism in western societies. His analysis is essentially Marxist, with the emphasis on the role of changes in the mode of production in creating disability. Oliver links such changes to shifts in the 'modes of thought' about disability. These involved the move to the individualization and patholo- gization of any form of impairment by medicine, and the acceptance of the view that impairment is a question of 'personal tragedy' rather than the result of social and structural relations. As such, 'disability' and the social oppression of disabled people is fundamentally bound up with the ideology and relations of production in capitalist society.

Activity 8.2

The following is taken from Chapter 6 in Michael Oliver's influential mongraph *The Politics of Disablement* in which he develops Finkelstein's model, as mentioned above. Read it through and then think about the questions at the end. A discussion of can be found in the 'Activity feedback' chapter on page 232.

Work is central to industrial societies not simply because it produces the goods to sustain life but also because it creates particular forms of social relations. Thus anyone unable to work, for whatever reason, is likely to experience difficulties both in acquiring the necessities to sustain life physically, and in establishing a set of satisfactory social relationships. Disabled people have not always been excluded from working but the arrival of industrial society has created partic- ular problems . . . disabled people often being excluded from the work process, because of the changes in the methods of working and the new industrial discipline continuing to make meaningful participation in work difficult, if not impossible.

The onset of industrial society did not simply change ways of working, but also had a profound effect on social relations with the creation of the industrial proletariat and the gradual erosion of

existing communities, as labour moved to the new towns. Industrialisation had profound conse-
quences for disabled people therefore, both in the ways that they were less able to participate in
the work process and also because many previously acceptable social roles, such as begging or
village idiot, were disappearing.

The new mechanism for controlling economically unproductive people was the workhouse
or the asylum, and over the years a whole range of specialised institutions grew up to contain
these groups. These establishments were undoubtedly successful in controlling individuals who
would not or could not work. These also performed a particular ideological function, standing
as visible monuments to the fate of others who might no longer choose to subjugate themselves
to the disciplinary requirements of the new work system. There were problems too in that it was
soon recognised that these institutions not only created dependency in individuals but also
created dependent groups.

(Oliver 1990: 85–6)

(1)   Can you see any parallels with Finkelstein's model ?

(2)   What evidence is there of a Marxist perspective in this extract?

In addition to being the impetus for theoretical developments, this evolutionary approach has led to other interpretations of the construction of disability. The most significant is that the increased integration of disabled people into society is a sign of the underlying change from a medical model of disability to the adoption of a social model.

The medical model of disability

As mentioned above, the rise of biomedicine meant that from the nineteenth century disability was medicalized and disabled people were constructed as being medical problems who, if not curable, needed to be 'helped' and were dependent on medical care and the medical profession. This approach to disability is called the 'medical' model of disability and is illustrated in Figure 8.1.

This individualistic model has dominated disability during the last two centuries. It involves medicine colonizing disability and the individualization of disability in terms of individual pathology; impairments are classified and those with disabilities treated as patients. Thus, the emphasis is on the impairment rather than the person. In addition, the impairment is regarded as being their individual problem and requiring rehabilitative medical intervention. The role of the environment in which disabled people live is ignored in this model because of the exclusive focus on the association between impairment and disability. Disabled people are also labelled as abnormal.

As disablement can only be treated by medical intervention, the power to decide how the person with the disability is treated resides with the medical profession (see Chapter 12) and other allied professions. This means that disabled people are treated as passive objects of 'intervention, treatment and rehabilitation' (Oliver 1990: 50). Furthermore, they are not involved in decisions that have major implications for their quality of life in that they cannot, for example, determine the extent and quality of their education and whether they can work or not.

The medical model has been adopted in legislation about the disabled and disability. Policy interventions based on medicalized and individualized views of disability have focused on individuals' impairments and vulnerabilities rather than the social constraints to social participation for people

Figure 8.1 The medical model of disability

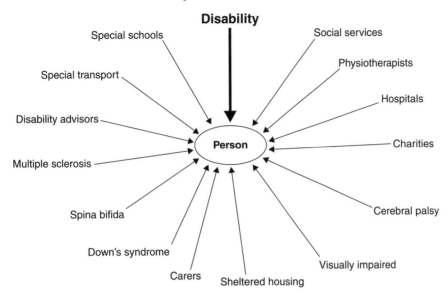

with disabilities. Many different services have been developed by able-bodied people to address disabled people's needs and functional rehabilitation.

Therefore, not only does this model ignore the experiential, social and situational components of disability, but it also has lifelong and oppressive consequences for disabled people (Oliver 1990, 1996; Hughes 1998; Hyde 2006a). Unsurprisingly, the hegemony of the medical model has been challenged. Since the 1990s, disability has gradually been demedicalized and a new conceptual framework for understanding disability has emerged – the social model.

The social model of disability

The origins of the social model can be traced back to a meeting of the Union of the Physically Impaired Against Segregation (UPIAS) in 1976. It was at this meeting that the following definition of disability was put forward, part of which was cited earlier in the chapter:

> it is society which disables physically impaired people. Disability is something imposed on top of our impairment by the way we are necessarily isolated and excluded from full participation in society. Disabled people are therefore an oppressed group in society. Thus we define impairment as lacking part or all of a limb, organs or mechanism of the body and disability as the disadvantage or restriction of activity caused by a contemporary social organisation which takes no or little account of people who have physical impairments and thus excludes them from the mainstream of social activities.

(Union of the Physically Impaired Against Segregation 1976: 14)

This definition has now been broadened to include the full range of impairments – that is, physical, sensory and intellectual. It has also been officially adopted. The recognition of the 'centrality of institutional, ideological, structural and material disabling barriers within society' (Barton 2004: 287) was the main stimulus for the development of the social model of disability or, as it is sometimes called, the social barriers model of disability (see Figure 8.2). This constructs disability in a

Figure 8.2 The social model of disability

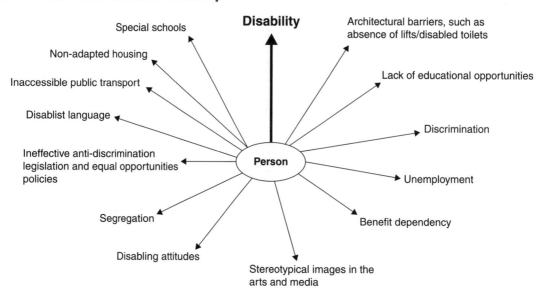

radically different way from the medical model. It argues that disability is not the problem of an individual's impairment but it is the attitudinal, cultural, social and environmental constraints imposed by a society geared towards a norm of able-bodiedness that oppresses disabled people and curtails their opportunities and capabilities.

The social model concentrates on what society does to construct disability. Integral to this focus is an examination of how society needs to change in order to emancipate disabled people so that they can participate in society and are empowered as citizens with rights. Adoption of the social model has resulted in a distinct set of policies which have aimed to abolish the fixed notion of 'normality' that disabled people have to aspire to and to make the physical, cultural and economic environment accessible and less discriminatory for people with disabilities. Consequently, there have been changes such as ramps and chairlifts, and equal opportunities policies. There have also been policies to alleviate the oppression of disabled people. Examples are the legislation in the 1970s and 1980s to reclassify people once regarded as idiots, mongols, retarded, mentally deficient, mentally handicapped and so forth. In addition, there have been policies to involve them in decision-making about their own lives, integrate them into ordinary life, make them more independent and equip them with social and practical skills (Oliver 1990, 2004; Fawcett 2000; Hyde 2006b).

Although this change in approach to disability, heralded by the emergence of the social model, has been popular with many, it has also been subject to criticism. Those working within the sociology of the body have argued that the social model focuses solely on disability in terms of social discrimination and social oppression. Therefore, it does not acknowledge the role of physical impairment in disability, and the way that the implications of bodily impairment can impact on disabled people's ability to engage in everyday life as much as, say, discrimination. This point has been developed further by those who argue that the social model overlooks the fact that whatever modifications are made to the environment, the nature of some disabilities severely limits the performance of any activities. Recent criticisms have also focused on the way that the social model does not engage with the breadth of experience that 'disability' encompasses (Oliver 2004; Hyde 2006a;

Matthewman *et al.* 2007). These criticisms are illustrated further in the discussion of the 'deaf culture' model of disability that follows and the exploration of the experiential dimensions of disability in our society today in the third section of the chapter.

The 'deaf culture' model of 'disability'

The term 'deaf culture' was first put forward in the 1970s to reflect the fact that deaf communities have 'their own ways of life mediated through their sign languages' (Ladd 2003: xvii) which are distinct from the hearing world. The idea has been developed and applied to a range of issues about disability that have subsequently emerged. Those active within the 'deaf culture' have been among the most vociferous critics of the social model of disability and have rejected it, arguing that it is not applicable to deafness. This is because they maintain that deaf people are not disabled but are a 'linguistic minority' (Corker 2000: 452) who use other forms of communication, such as sign language and internet-based communication. These forms of communication delineate their identity and enable them to participate fully within the deaf community, in which there is a strong sense of kinship and shared culture. Indeed, deaf activists assert the validity of 'deaf culture' and emphasize the fact that, in terms of cultural comparison, mainstream hearing culture is neither 'normative', nor does it have a privileged status. One of the consequences of these beliefs is that they oppose attempts to help deaf people integrate into the mainstream world (such as medical cures and oralist education) because the latter is not superior or preferable to belonging to the deaf world.

Some of the critics of this model have focused on the impossibility of proving that 'deaf culture' actually exists. Others have highlighted the fact that the model may not be applicable to all deaf people because some forms of deafness cannot be overcome by alternative forms of communication, resulting in some being unable to be part of 'deaf culture' (Corker 2000; Ladd 2003).

Activity 8.3

The following quote comes from Baroness Jane Campbell, co-chair of the All Party Parliamentary Disability Group:

> *Most reports on our experiences as disabled people focus on the barriers and problems we face. But if we focus first on problems, we often forget what is possible – we become pessimists. For me as a disabled member of the House of Lords I know it was my dreams that took me there, and the inspiration of others who had gone before me. That hope and optimism gave me the motivation to overcome the barriers in my path. If I had thought mainly about the barriers (and heaven knows there were many of them) I would have given up long ago.*
>
> (Sayce 2009: 2)

Which of the theoretical perspectives in Chapter 1 can explain this approach to disability? For a discussion of this question see the 'Activity feedback' chapter, page 232.

Experiencing life as a disabled person

Although the adoption of the social model over the past two decades has had many positive outcomes for disabled people, it has not addressed the full range of experiences of those who are disabled (Tregakis 2002). As mentioned at the beginning of the chapter, those who are disabled still experience many inequalities in their lives. An understanding of these inequalities is essential to the understanding of the experience of disability in contemporary society. Some are illustrated in the case study below and the in-depth exploration of specific inequalities that follows illustrates the way they overlap and interact with each other as well as with other social divisions.

Case example: Simon's story

Simon was aged 55 and lived for most of his life in an ex-mining community in the North East of England. Childhood poliomyelitis (polio) had left him with a partially paralysed left leg which meant that he walked with a pronounced limp. He had often been teased about the way he walked as a child and he had endured some of the local children imitating his gait. Although he was academically able and had passed his 11-plus examination to go to the grammar school in the next town, his parents could not afford to send him there. When he left school, he got a clerical job with the then National Coal Board. Simon enjoyed his job and managed his finances carefully so that he could buy himself a terraced house near to his parents. He lived alone and never married or had a long-term relationship.

Simon had progressed to the position of team leader when the decline of the mining industry started and sadly he was made redundant at the age of 40. Age started to worsen his disability and although he could still walk unaided, his mobility was much reduced. He found that he was repeatedly unsuccessful with job applications and unemployment led to him having to default on his mortgage repayments. His house was repossessed and he was offered social housing in a run-down part of another town, several miles away from his home. Simon did not visit his parents on a regular basis because his dependency on benefits meant that he could not afford the bus fares. As his parents were now elderly, he saw less and less of them. Lack of money meant that he could not socialize and he gradually became more and more socially isolated. Whereas he had been known to the local services in his home town, this was not the case in the town in which he had been housed. Consequently, he did not receive any support until he was picked up by paramedics after he tripped and fell in the local shopping centre.

Prejudice and discrimination

The fact that there has been a reduction in the more blatant forms of prejudice and discrimination towards disabled people is mainly due to successful campaigning by the disability movement throughout the 1980s. The growth in the size and power of this movement started in the 1960s. In addition to a high-profile political agenda, it now has a well-developed group consciousness and identity. It has challenged the dominant definitions of disability and the use of negative language in relation to disability. It has mobilized mass support and taken action that has been of a direct, collective and political nature. This movement has also played a major role in shaping initiatives and legislation at both national and European level which have promoted the equalization of opportunities for, and the elimination of discrimination against, disabled people. Furthermore, the shift from a medical model of disability to a social model has been attributed to the disability movement.

Another influence on levels of prejudice and discrimination is the growth of an increasingly respected body of literature written by activists in the disability movement since the early 1990s, such as the work of Michael Oliver. There have also been many attempts to counter the dominant discourse of dependence in the arts and media, and challenges to the use of disablist language (Hughes 1998; Corker 2002).

However, although these developments are to be welcomed, prejudice and discrimination against disabled people is still common and negatively affects many areas of their lives. It has been argued that among the most notable causes are professionals' 'disabling attitudes' (Foster *et al.* 2006). There is also evidence that more subtle forms of prejudice exist in the mass media. For instance, publicity campaigns by disability charities have presented images of disabled people as helpless and pitiable in order to attract public donations. The absence of images of disabled people taking part in everyday life, such as working and taking an active role in their families, has led to negative views of the extent of their capabilities (Wates 2004; Deal 2007). The inevitable internalization of such stereotyping can cause much distress for disabled people. For example, Grue and Laerum's (2002) study of physically disabled mothers found that they felt constant pressure to show that they were managing 'normally' and feared that their children would be taken from them if they did not appear to live up to societal expectations of being an 'ordinary' mother.

Moreover, the disability movement itself has been accused of not being truly representative of all disabled people and 'running out of steam' (Hyde 2006a). The former accusation is compounded by the fact that many people do not see themselves as disabled or identify themselves as a disabled person. Consequently, they do not take part in the movement (Watson 2002). These criticisms naturally raise questions about the movement's ability to effectively campaign to reduce the discrimination experienced by disabled people.

Employment

Many disabled people want to work and in the UK New Labour (1997–2010) introduced a plethora of initiatives to increase their workforce participation. Nonetheless, disabled people still experience high rates of unemployment. Figures show that they are about twice as likely to be unemployed as non-disabled people. When they are in paid employment they are more likely to do part-time work which generally has lower status and pay, less job security and fewer employment rights. Furthermore, although career aspirations have been found to be equal between disabled and non-disabled people, the former face many disadvantages in terms of career progression. For example, a recent study found that disabled people are 'a third as likely as nondisabled people to earn £80,000 or above; and less than half as likely to be a board level Director' (Sayce 2009: 6).

Studies have shown that age, gender and ethnicity interact with disability in this aspect of disabled people's lives; levels of their labour market disadvantage increase from middle age onwards and are greater for disabled women and disabled people from ethnic minority groups. These findings have been partly explained by the fact that many disabled people face a number of potential barriers to employment such as concerns about benefit entitlements, lack of relevant experience or skills and discrimination from employers. With reference to the latter, research has shown that employers often misunderstand disability and associate it with 'risk and uncertainty' (Heenan 2002: 387). Despite legislation to counteract this (e.g. the Disability Discrimination Act 2005), there is evidence that such discrimination is still widespread. For instance, disabled people are six times more likely to be refused an interview than a non-disabled person with similar skills and qualifications (Heenan 2002; Bailey 2004; Sapey 2004; Bambra 2005).

Health and healthcare

People with a disability often suffer from multiple conditions. In addition, disability increases the probability of experiencing further health problems (Hyde 2006a; Beckett 2009). Therefore, disabled people inevitably experience significant health inequalities compared to non-disabled people. They also experience barriers when accessing healthcare, for example, health professionals' discriminatory attitudes, lack of knowledge and understanding of their health issues, delays in receiving services and inconsistencies in service delivery (Gulliford 2003; Melville 2005; Slade *et al.* 2009).

Education

Those who are disabled are far more likely to have lower or no academic qualifications than non-disabled people (Smith and Twomey 2002; Disability Rights Commission 2006). This is because of the way they are disadvantaged throughout the education system. Attendance at a special school at primary and secondary levels leads to the segregation of disabled children and possible discrimination. Such schools also deliver a narrower curriculum and the educational attainment of the children who attend them has been shown to be lower than those who are integrated into mainstream schools. In college education, disabled young people are not provided with the opportunities they need to compensate for their lower levels of educational achievement while at school. As a result, their chances of entering university education are much reduced compared to the non-disabled. Indeed, disabled people are still only half as likely as non-disabled people to be qualified to degree level. In addition, despite the significant progress that has been made in the development of provision for disabled students in universities, this pattern of inequality has not changed since 1998 – those who do enter higher education can still face disadvantage and further improvements are required to ensure equalization of opportunities (Tinklin *et al.* 2004; Disability Rights Commission 2006; Hyde 2006b).

Income

Their high unemployment rates, health problems and lack of educational qualifications result in disabled people being the largest group in receipt of benefits – they account for about 25 per cent of benefit expenditure in the UK. Benefit dependency invariably means living on a low income and being at greater risk of poverty; it is estimated that 45 per cent of disabled adults live in poverty. Low income and poverty inevitably impact negatively on many disabled people's socioeconomic position (Bambra *et al.* 2005; Hyde 2006b).

Housing

Despite the introduction of community care, many disabled people are still segregated in residential homes and those who are not face considerable disadvantages in relation to housing. Their choice is limited when it comes to meeting their housing needs and they are also more likely to live in public housing and less likely to rent privately or have a mortgage than non-disabled people (Stevens 2007). A recent study showed how disabled people with mobility problems are often excluded from the owner-occupation market because the design of houses for owner-occupation automatically renders them unsuitable for their needs (Thomas 2004).

Social and personal life

Several factors have negative impacts on the social and personal lives of disabled people: limited disposable income, lack of their own means of transport, inability to use public transport, inaccessibility of buildings and tourist attractions and inadequate provision of suitable leisure activities can all restrict social activities. Consequently the number of their interpersonal relationships is lower than for non-disabled people and this is reflected in the fact that, overall, disabled people are less likely to have the opportunity to have sexual relationships and to have children (O'Grady *et al.* 2004).

There is also much evidence that those who live in the community do not receive adequate support to enable them to participate in mainstream society. This has been attributed to the failure of community services to respond to disabled people's needs because of their inadequate funding, fragmentation, inflexibility and inequitable distribution (Kemp 2002; Gardiner and Millar 2006).

Social exclusion

The combination and continuation of these sorts of experiences and the powerful way in which they interact constitute barriers to the social inclusion of disabled people and have led to inequalities between disabled and non-disabled people in our society. There are those who point to the emergence of new types of inequalities for disabled people created by globalization and the move towards a consumer culture. It is argued that globalization increases the isolation and segregation of disabled people because the global information network does not address their concerns. The emphasis in consumer culture on aesthetics such as choice, beauty and youthfulness conflict with disability and represent yet another form of exclusion for disabled young people in particular (Barton 2004; Hughes *et al.* 2005).

Conclusions

This chapter has shown that approaches to disability have changed considerably over time as well as the extent to which such changes determine the experience of disability. These experiences have varied dramatically, for instance, in relation to whether disabled people are institutionalized or live in the community. Although the experience of disability has improved in recent years, it is clear from the discussions in the chapter that disabled people still have to endure inequalities and exclusion from mainstream society in many areas of their lives.

There are many suggestions in the literature about ways of improving the lives and experiences of those who are disabled in our society. Some propose increasing resources to improve their incomes (regardless of employment status) and service provision. Others propose enhancing the role of disabled people in our society (Van Hoten and Bellemakers 2002; Rummery 2006). Another set of arguments focus on the ways in which the social model should be developed. For example, Tregakis (2002) argues that there is a need to concentrate more on non-disabled people in order to address the persistence of disabling attitudes and encourage them to adopt more inclusive practice. Whereas these sorts of suggestions place the responsibility for change on society, there are also arguments that both individuals with a disability *and* society have a mutual responsibility to work towards greater inclusion (van de Ven *et al.* 2005). Whatever view you empathize with most, the evidence presented in this chapter shows that everyone in society has a responsibility to work towards the goal of improving the experience of disability.

Key points

■ The concept of disability is more a question of social definition than a statement of fact or objective truth.

■ The social construction of disability can be demonstrated by examining models of disability. Those addressed in this chapter were the evolutionary, medical, social and cultural models.

■ Although the adoption of the social model over the past two decades has had many positive outcomes for disabled people, they still have many negative life experiences. These include prejudice and discrimination, health inequalities, low employment rates, lower rates of academic achievement compared to non-disabled people, high benefit dependency, low income, restricted personal and social life and social exclusion.

Discussion points

■ How realistic is Finkelstein's evolutionary model of disability?

■ To what extent has the social model led to the social inclusion of disabled people in mainstream society?

■ To what extent do you think the type of society one lives in structures the experience of disability?

Suggestions for further study

■ The emergence of the social model of disability is well documented in Oliver's work (1990, 1996).

■ Different perspectives on the social model can be found in Chapter 4 in Twigg (2006) and the chapters in Parts 1, 2 and 5 of Swain *et al.* (2004).

■ For recent research on the experiences of those who are disabled, it is worth doing an electronic database search and selecting articles that have appeared during the past five years.

■ Articles in the *Journal of Disability and Society* are particularly useful and informative.

Dying, death and grieving

Mortality may be a universal feature of human societies, but the form it takes and the ways in which we deal with it is complex and reflects the social and cultural diversity amongst and within every human society.

(Howarth 2007: 2)

Introduction

Many people have little exposure to death during their lives. This is because death is no longer part of daily existence. Infant mortality rates are now low and increasing longevity in the western world means that most people live well into old age. Most deaths also take place in relatively segregated environments, such as residential homes, hospitals and hospices, rather than at home. As a result, our understanding of death is often limited (Seale 1998, 2000).

As a result of the development of the sociology of death and dying since the 1970s, the literature on dying and death within the study of the social aspects of health has increased considerably. This body of literature has challenged the common assumption that death occurs when the body ceases to function biologically and one of its key themes is that death and the process of dying cannot be detached from the personal and social contexts in which they take place. While this literature has provided invaluable insights into the personal context of these experiences, the focus has been more on the social context of dying and death. Hence, exploration of the topic within the study of the social aspects of health will complete the reader's understanding of the social dimensions of the experiences of illness.

In order to demonstrate the ways that the study of the social aspects of health has added to knowledge about dying and death, this chapter begins by considering the personal context of dying and death before moving on to the evidence and arguments that our end of life experiences and our departure from this world are very much determined by the social context in which they take place. When discussing both the personal and social contexts of dying and death, grief and grieving are also addressed. This is because very few people's deaths are unmourned by others and therefore grief and grieving are integral to explorations of dying and death.

Seminal texts are drawn upon fairly extensively because they have been so influential on subsequent work and still have contemporary relevance. Several theoretical perspectives are discussed in the course of the chapter and in the final section postmodernism is used to provide additional insights into the issues addressed.

Activity 9.1

As you read through the first two sections of this chapter, make a note of the possible influences on the experiences of a dying person and one of their loved ones. Some of the key factors are discussed in the 'Activity feedback' chapter on page 232.

The personal context of dying, death and grieving

Case example: A personal journey

John was a successful journalist. He often worked long hours, but enjoyed life to the full. He had been married to Sue for 10 years and they had two boys, aged 4 and 6. When he had just turned 38, John started to suffer a persistent nagging pain in his back. These pains increased in intensity and, on his wife's insistence, he went to his GP. A series of tests revealed an inoperable malignant tumour. The prognosis was very bleak and at best John had two years left to live.

Both he and Sue found the news impossible to absorb – this was something that happened to other people, not a fit, relatively young man, with everything to live for. John tried to find an explanation. Was it hereditary? Was it stress-induced? Was it some sort of punishment for his wrongdoings?

Although he was not a particularly religious person, John spent a day at a monastery where he talked to the abbot at length in order to develop a different perspective on his fate. John could not accept the arguments put forward about life after death that were put to him and became very angry.

The endless soul-searching resulted in John becoming very depressed and he retreated into himself, not wishing to work or socialize. His GP prescribed him some antidepressants and once the edge of the depression had started to numb, John was able to make some plans for his future. Together with Sue and their boys, he took a trip to Disneyland Paris. Following a consultation with a financial adviser, he started to work for just two days a week and enjoyed his new work–life balance that enabled him to spend more time with his wife and family. He reluctantly and sadly adapted to the prospect of his considerably shortened lifespan and tried to remind himself that each day was special.

Although the way individuals deal with their own death varies with their personality and culture, there are certain circumstances which are known to affect all personal experiences of dying and death. The main examples include the extent to which death is predictable, the age at which death occurs and personal beliefs. These are addressed under the first three headings below. There are also patterns of grieving that are universally recognized and these are explained under the fourth heading.

Predicted death

While there are many unexpected deaths – for instance, from fatal accidents, suicides and sudden heart attacks – some deaths can be predicted in advance. Examples include cases of extreme old age or when there has been a diagnosis of a terminal illness. Various psychological and emotional processes have been associated with coping with expected death. For instance, the concept of *anticipatory grieving* has been used to capture the nature of these processes (Seale 1998). Kübler-Ross (1973), a psychiatrist who worked extensively with terminally ill patients, identified five progressive stages in individual reactions to the news of predicted death. These are set out below.

The 'five-stage theory of dying' by Kübler-Ross

- *Denial:* this is the first reaction to a terminal diagnosis and involves feelings of denial. Some individuals refuse to accept the news.

- *Anger:* once there is no doubt that the diagnosis is correct, anger then sets in. Death is viewed as an undeserved punishment and the dying person attempts to find someone or something to blame. The sense of anger can be all-consuming.

- *Bargaining:* in this stage, the dying person tries to make some kind of deal with fate or God. For example 'If you let me live, then I will . . .'

- *Depression:* this is the time when patients lose all hope and face the full impact of their impending death. They frequently become very fearful of dying and a preoccupation with a sense of loss is common in this stage.

■ *Acceptance:* in this final stage individuals are able to prepare to let go of life. They often experience a sense of relief, rather than happiness. Depending on the nature of their terminal illness, it can prompt the individual to examine their current way of life and decide what is truly important to them. Consequently, they may decide to take a trip that they have always wanted to take, change careers or stop working altogether.

Source: adapted from Kübler-Ross (1973)

Kübler-Ross's work has been helpful in increasing professional understanding of the anguish suffered by people who are dying, and has also been adapted to create stages of grief (as discussed below). However, this work has also been criticized because it is said to implicitly encourage the labelling of any deviations from these five stages as abnormal and does not acknowledge cultural differences in coping with dying (Littlewood 1993).

Age of death
In general, the experience of dying seems to differ between younger and older people. Studies have shown that younger people who are told they are dying tend to feel cheated of life and fight as hard as they can to stay alive, often displaying impressive determination to live despite the limitations imposed upon them by their illness. There is also evidence that they spend longer in the first four of Kübler-Ross's stages. In contrast, older people are more likely to be resigned to death, accepting it rather than struggling against it (Judd 2000; Howarth 2007).

Personal beliefs
Our reactions to dying and death also depend on our personal beliefs. Those who believe that death is an inevitable consequence of life, such as Jewish people, are likely to be more accepting of their fate than others. Beliefs about the afterlife are also important. Although Freud argued that belief in an afterlife was a sign of unhealthy denial, people with religious convictions about the existence of an afterlife tend to display the least anxiety about death. Interestingly, those with confused religious beliefs show more anxiety than atheists. There have been debates about the extent to which the decline in adherence to established religion and the move to secularization in western societies have impacted on personal levels of anxiety about death. Such debates have evolved to embrace arguments about the simultaneous introduction of eastern religions, such as Hinduism, Sikhism and Buddhism in western secular society. Thus, it has been concluded that it is more accurate to say that there has been a rejection of the established Christian Church rather than a rejection of spiritual concerns as such. By extension of logic, it is therefore the impact of this change that needs to be considered when discussing personal anxiety levels about death as opposed to increased secularization (Katz 2000; Howarth 2008).

Grieving and grief work
The death of a loved one always involves a broad range of feelings, actions and physical and psychological reactions. It can also cause major disruption in our lives and demand significant psychological adjustment, for example where there is a change of role, such as when a parent becomes childless or a wife becomes a widow (Seale 1998; Field and Payne 2004; Hunt 2005). Both the inevitability and the universality of these experiences have been widely acknowledged and

several models developed to capture the phases of mourning that individuals experience. Whichever model is adopted, it is clear that there are stages in the grieving process and that these shape everyone's personal experience of grieving to a greater or lesser extent. One of the best known models is Kübler-Ross's 'grief cycle' model (1973). As mentioned above, this is an adaptation of her five-stage theory of dying and is shown in the panel below.

The 'grief cycle' model by Kübler-Ross

■ *Denial:* this involves a conscious or unconscious refusal to accept the situation concerned, ignoring all evidence to the contrary and continuing on as if the loved one will be coming home. It is a defence mechanism and although this stage usually ends when people are presented with the body or attend the burial or cremation, some become locked within it.

■ *Anger:* people who are grieving experience anger with themselves, and/or with others, such as the medical profession, relatives or friends, the deceased themselves or with their religious deity for allowing the death to occur. This anger can be overwhelming at times.

■ *Bargaining:* as in Kübler-Ross's theory of dying, this stage involves attempting to bargain. The bargaining is usually irrational and can involve, for example, an individual begging for their loved one to be returned to life in exchange for whatever the price of such a bargain. Depression, the next stage of grief, is often the outcome of unsuccessful bargaining.

■ *Depression:* emotions characteristic of this stage are sadness, anxiety, fear, regret and guilt as people start to realize that their situation is irrevocable and they really must continue to live without the presence of the deceased in their lives.

■ *Acceptance:* individuals are most likely to enter the acceptance stage after they have resigned themselves to the fact that the deceased will not be returning to them. Reaching this stage is also broadly an indication that they are able to view the death of their loved one with some degree of emotional detachment and objectivity.

Source: adapted from Kübler-Ross (1973)

Kübler-Ross did not intend her model to present grief as a rigid series of sequential or uniformly timed steps. Indeed she emphasized that people's grief is a very individual journey and its nature and extent can depend on a whole range of factors, such as whether the death was predicted, the personal history of the grieving person and their relationship with the deceased. Her model is intended to be more of a guide to the types of phases people go through when grieving. To illustrate these points, she argued that the experience of the five stages is neither linear nor equal. Furthermore, some stages may be revisited, some may not be experienced at all and transition between them can be more of ebb and flow, rather than a progression. Upon completion of their individual journey through their grief, a person will generally accept their new reality and this enables them to cope.

While Kübler-Ross's grief cycle model has achieved acclaim in both academic and professional circles, critics have highlighted the fact that it views the mourner as passive and ignores the way that mourners often undertake 'grief work' to help themselves. Worden (1983) in particular took up these criticisms in his work on grief counselling. He maintained that mourning involves active participation by the mourners and that there are four 'tasks of mourning' which need to be worked through by the mourners themselves in order to re-establish equilibrium in their lives and for mourning to be completed. Instrumental in helping those who are bereaved to work through these tasks are extended families, cohesive communities and effective counselling. Worden's four tasks are:

- to accept the reality of the loss;

- to experience the pain of grief;

- to adjust to an environment in which the deceased is missing;

- to withdraw emotional energy and reinvest in another relationship.

More recently, 'grief work' has been shown to involve the construction of narratives by bereaved individuals. Such narratives are individuals' own explanations to themselves of what has occurred and how it makes sense in the scheme of things. Such narratives essentially help individuals to deal with their own feelings in the face of their bereavement and are part of the 'work' that is required in order to move on and create a meaningful life in which the deceased no longer features (Seale 1998).

Dying, death and grieving as social experiences

In the explanations of the personal dimensions of dying, death and grieving in the last section, there were unavoidable references to the social context. An example was the inclusion of religious beliefs in the discussion about the influence of personal beliefs in the experience of dying. This highlights the way that dying, death and grieving are simultaneously personal and social events. As mentioned in the introduction to this chapter, within the study of the social aspects of health there is much evidence of the influence of the social context on these experiences. This has led to statements such as 'our experiences of dying, death and bereavement are embedded within our social and cultural worlds' (Howarth 2008: 2).

Since the late 1960s, there has been a considerable amount of work on dying and death as social processes and the social organization involved in these processes. Among the most influential studies are those by Sudnow (1967) and Glaser and Strauss (1965, 1968, 1971). Five topics have been selected for this section to illustrate the ways in which dying, death and grieving are social experiences. The first four include discussions of dying, death and grieving, and outstanding points about grieving specifically are dealt with in the last topic.

The denial of death in contemporary western society

Changes in demographics and the care of the dying in our society mean that far less of us experience much exposure to death during our lifetimes (see also the discussion of the medicalization of death, below). There are those who maintain that we now live in a society that denies death, and claims such as 'ours is a death denying society' (Rayner 1997: 262) frequently appear in the literature. However, this has not always been the case. One of the most well-known writers about the denial of death is Ariès (1981). He argues that before the First World War, death was 'a social and public fact' (Ariès 1981: 559); as illness was not so controlled and dying took place within the home, death was much more visible to everyone. There were many customs associated with a death. Whole communities shared in the care of those who were dying, were involved in the public acknowledgement of a death and participated in the collective ceremonies. It was also the norm for close relatives to wear mourning clothes for decades, Queen Victoria being a notable example. While such traditional attitudes to death still exist in some societies, Ariès maintains that in contemporary western society the generality of death is not so absolute. Death is often solitary and hidden from view in hospitals and other institutions, we no longer openly talk about death or mourn the dead so publically and observe long periods of mourning. Indeed there are arguments that death has become such a taboo subject that it has now replaced sex as unmentionable. Hence Ariès concludes that 'society has banished death' (1981: 559).

In addition to the reasons put forward by Ariès above, the denial of death in contemporary society has been attributed to a variety of other factors. Some argue that advances in epidemiology and medical science mean that death is no longer seen as having random causes, being a matter of fate or under the auspices of God's will. With reference to epidemiology, early death is now largely seen as preventable and within the control of the individual (see Chapter 6). For instance, public health discourses claim that if individuals take appropriate preventative measures in relation to their lifestyles (such as not smoking, eating a healthy diet, drinking in moderation only and exercising regularly) they are ensured of a prolonged lifespan. When we are unable to control personal health risks, medical intervention can now be relied upon to save us. These developments have created what has been referred to as a 'mirage of immortality' which in turns vanquishes death (Howarth 2008: 257; Lupton 2008).

Another factor that has been identified is the decline in the role of religion in western society. However, this has been contested by those who point to the growing tolerance and adoption of non-western religions and the resurgence of alternative forms of spirituality in the West, as discussed in the first section. Evidence about the role of the media has also been used to counter arguments about the denial of death in our society. While direct contact with death has decreased for most people in western society, research has shown that there has actually been an increase in images of death in the media. For example, there has been a proliferation of horrific deaths and fictional violence in films. Death is also a central theme in many TV soaps, especially medical soaps, and documentaries. Moreover, loss and bereavement have re-emerged as matters for public consumption as a result of American-style talk shows. While some contend that the media shapes our attitudes, others argue that it is merely reflecting the values in society at particular times. This debate has been developed further by those who use the **structuration thesis** developed by Giddens to support the view that there is a symbiotic relationship between society and the media in relation to mores surrounding dying, death and bereavement. This thesis is part of the structure versus agency debate (see Chapter 1). It sees structure and agency as being inextricably linked and both having the potential to shape each other. More specifically, structure provides the resources people need to frame their action and is also formed by the consequences of social action taken by individuals collectively. Hence, structure is continuously reproduced by social action as well as simultaneously setting the conditions for social action (Giddens 1984). Therefore, when the structuration thesis is applied to the relationship between the media and dying, death and bereavement, the media is viewed as a resource for these issues which people can selectively adopt and adapt to the context of their everyday lives and social worlds. Changes that occur as a consequence of these actions in turn shape media interpretations and images of dying, death and bereavement (Walter 1999; Howarth, 2008).

Consequently the claim that death has been banished from public discourse has been challenged. Indeed Walter (2006) argues that the media has to some extent replaced religion in helping people to deal with death. This is because it often reaffirms social ties and the strength of our social fabric when reporting disasters by highlighting the extraordinary efforts people make to help and support those affected. An example he gives is the media coverage of the attack on the World Trade Center in 2001.

Activity 9.2

Over the next week, as you read the newspapers, watch television and/or films, think about the images of death that are presented and ask yourself the following questions:

■ How is death portrayed?

■ Does the portrayal vary according to the type of article, television programme or film?

■ What reactions do you have to the different portrayals?

Make brief notes of your answers. At the end of the week, see if your answers accord with the findings about death and the media above.

'Good death' and 'bad death'

Any discussion of death as a social experience is incomplete without reference to the concepts of a 'good death' and a 'bad death'. These concepts are used by people in many different countries to describe a death. Sociologists working within the sociology of death and dying have discovered that although these concepts are culturally and historically specific, there are certain characteristics that are associated with both types of death. In general, a 'good death' is one where people can exert control over events. This sense of control finds expression through mortuary rituals and a denial of the finality of death because it is seen in terms of a rebirth. In contrast, 'bad deaths' are uncontrolled, happen at the wrong place at the wrong time and preclude any chance of rebirth. These characteristics are not unambiguous and there can be overlap between them.

As mentioned, there are variations in the concepts of a 'good death' and 'bad death'. With reference to variations across time, in pre-modern times, most of the population had to endure extreme hardships, such as poverty, injustice and misery. According to Ariès (1981) people made sense of their lives in the context of death because they would be rewarded in heaven where they would experience eternal joy. Therefore, a 'good death' was one where they were aware they were dying and could make spiritual and practical preparations for their departure from this world. Spiritual preparations included visits from a priest who could hear last confessions and administer extreme unction (Ariès 1981; Walter 2003).

Differences between cultures that have been identified include the way that the requirements for a 'good death' in Ugandan tribal society are awareness, preparation, peace, dignity and the segregation of the sexes. Such a death is described thus: 'A man should die in his hut, lying on his bed, with his brothers and sons around him to hear his last words; he should die with his mind still alert and should be able to speak clearly even if only softly; he should die peacefully and with dignity, without bodily discomfort or disturbance' (Middleton, cited in Bradbury 2000: 68).

Evidence that there are also variations in these concepts *within* a culture has been found in western societies. Indeed, studies have shown that multiple 'cultural scripts' of the 'good death' can exist at any one time (Young and Cullen 1996; Long 2004). Those who have traditional Christian views see a 'good death' as one which signals an entry into heaven, with the result that sorrow at the loss of the deceased is tempered with a sense of joy that they are in a better place than they were on Earth. However, as already established, western societies are now typically multicultural and highly secular. Multiculturalism and secularization mean that many do not accept this construction of a 'good death'. For instance, the secular view of a 'good death' is one which is usually expected because of old age and is without fear or pain. Moreover, there are those who argue that 'good deaths' are those which, apart from effective pain relief, take place without medical intervention. Medical intervention in dying and death is our next topic (Walter 2003; Howarth 2008).

The medicalization of death

The way that death for most of us is now removed from everyday life and takes place in some sort of medical setting was explained earlier in this chapter. The increasing medicalization of society (see Chapter 6) has been blamed for this change whereby dying and death, like living, have come under medical jurisdiction and control. The key tenets of arguments put forward by those who have been the main critics of the medicalization of death are set out below. These are followed by an outline of some of the changes that have occurred as a result of these criticisms.

Criticisms of the medicalization of death

The attack on the medicalization of dying was launched in the 1970s by Illich. He argued that 'the medicalisation of society has brought the epoch of natural death to an end . . . technical death has won its victory over dying' (Illich 1976: 207). His critique of the medicalization of dying is summarized below.

Critique of the medicalization of dying by Illich

■ The loss of the capacity to accept death and suffering as meaningful aspects of life.

■ The existence of a state of 'total war' against death at all stages of the life course.

■ The devaluation of personal, family and community care, as well as the traditional rituals surrounding dying and death.

■ A form of social control in which a rejection of 'patienthood' by dying or bereaved people is labelled as a form of deviance.

Source: adapted from Clark (2002)

As you can see, Illich identified many consequences of this extension of medicalization in terms of the experience of dying, death and grieving in his critique. Other implications for the social organization of death in our society have emerged. One is that it is a legal requirement that a member of the medical profession certificates every death and designates whether a death has a legitimate or illegitimate cause. A death from natural causes, such as old age, disease or a random accident is deemed to be legitimate. Deaths that have occurred in unusual or suspicious circumstances are illegitimate. Furthermore, whether we are certified as dead or not is subject to changing medical definitions of death. For instance, prior to the 1950s, someone was defined as dead if their heart had stopped beating. Since then the concept of 'brain death' has been developed because medical research has proved that a person can be dead even though their heart is still beating. Therefore we can now be certified as dead even if our heartbeat can be detected. These examples also illustrate the social nature of defining death (Lupton 2008; Bradby 2009).

More importantly, the ways in which medicalization impacts on the care and management of the dying have been the subject of much research. Up until the middle of the twentieth century, the dying were cared for at home and hence died there too. As a result of medicalization, since that time it has become the norm to be cared for and to die in specialized institutions. This removal of the dying from their homes, families and communities has been much criticized. It means that dying can be a very lonely and disempowering experience during which patients may be cared for inappropriately (Elias 1985). With reference to hospital care of the dying specifically, work carried out by Glaser and Strauss (1965, 1968) and Sudnow (1967) showed that hospitals structure medical professionals' discourses in certain ways which marginalize dying people, socially isolate them and conflict with their needs. One example is the way that the emphasis on care and treatment in hospitals leads to death being perceived as a failure. Dying people are consigned to the dying rooms on wards where, with the exception of staff, they often pass away alone. Glaser and Strauss (1968) argued that medical staff construct a 'dying trajectory' for each patient. Predictions are made about the probable length and nature of the dying process, and when 'there is nothing more that can be done'. Inaccurate predictions and alterations in this trajectory result in a mismatch between the patient's needs and the treatment they receive.

This sequestration of the dying has also been described as **social death** (Sudnow 1967; Seale 1998). This is a term which is used to refer to the process whereby people who are dying are separated and marginalized from the rest of society. It has also been established that the longer the time that they are dying for, the less people see of family and friends. In addition, social death has been applied to the later stages of terminal diseases of the mind, such as dementia and Alzheimer's disease, to reflect how a person can lose their social significance but still exist physically (Sweeting and Gilhooly 1997). Hence social death always precedes **biological death**. Furthermore, the distinction between 'social death' and 'biological death' has been made to reinforce the point that 'the material end of the body is only roughly congruent with the death of the social self' (Seale 1998: 34).

Outcomes of the criticisms of the medicalization of death
Criticisms of the medicalization of death have led to the recognition that hospitals do not provide the most humane environment for people who are dying. Although there has been a general move away from institutionalization in many areas of health and social care (see Chapter 10), this has not been so pronounced in the care of the dying. Alternative forms of care have been developed, the main one being that provided by hospices. The hospice movement was at the forefront of the resistance to medicalization and, since the 1960s, hospice care services have expanded dramatically. Hospices are now integral to the delivery of palliative care in this country and adopt a multidisciplinary and demedicalized approach to dying with an emphasis on 'total care' and death without pain. More recent innovations include homecare programmes. These have a philosophy of holistic and demedicalized care similar to hospices and offer patients a wide range of services, such as counselling, domestic and spiritual services, to enable them to die in their own homes. The emphasis on a non-medical death without fear or pain is congruent with the secular view of the concept of a 'good death'. However, around 66 per cent of terminally ill people still die in a hospital and concerns have been expressed that the increasing institutionalization of hospice care may constitute 'creeping medicalization' (Conway 2007: 200) and compromise the movement's founding ideals. Moreover, the continuing emphasis within medical services on resisting, postponing and avoiding death is

seen as evidence of failure of the challenge to the medicalized approach to death to 'balance technical intervention with a humanistic approach' (Clark 2002: 905) (see also McNamara 1994; Seale 2000; Hunt 2005; Conway 2007).

Nonetheless, the earlier research described above about the medicalization of death has also stimulated changes in medical practice in relation to care of the dying. One of the most influential of these studies was about the experience of dying in hospitals in the USA during which a typology of four states of patient awareness about their death was identified (Glaser and Strauss 1965). These are set out in Table 9.1.

Staff were found to prefer 'closed awareness' contexts. This was because, as mentioned above, death is seen as a failure in medical terms, and medical professionals wanted to hide the terminal nature of the illness from dying patients. They also wanted to protect patients from adverse reactions to disclosure, such as depression and anxiety. Glaser and Strauss's study showed that 'closed awareness' contexts had negative consequences for patients as they led to them feeling betrayed, isolated and actually increased, as opposed to decreased, their anxiety levels. In contrast, 'open awareness' contexts were found to resolve these negative consequences and facilitated patient acceptance of, and psychological preparation for, their death. They also enabled patient and family involvement with the practical management of the death, such as decisions about pain relief. As a result of this study, in western societies there has been a move from closed to open awareness in the care of the dying since the 1970s (MacLeod 2001). However, disclosure of terminal illness diagnoses is not appropriate for all cultures. Studies have shown that in Japan, Italy and Ireland 'closed awareness' is seen as protecting the dying person from distress. Furthermore, increasing cultural diversity in western society means that a blanket approach should not be adopted and there should be sensitivity to cultural preferences about disclosure (Seale 1998).

Although there has been a commitment to open awareness in the UK, the reality is that it does not always occur. Open awareness is more likely to occur with some types of patients than others. Examples of such patients are those who have cancer, are not mentally confused, are of a higher social class or have a respondent who has known for some time that the person is dying (Seale *et al.*

Table 9.1 Awareness contexts by Glaser and Strauss

Closed awareness	This occurs when staff and relatives are aware that the patient is dying but agree that the patient should not be made aware of this. This state of unawareness usually only lasts as long as the signs of impending death remain unrecognized by the patient.
Suspicion awareness	Patients become suspicious when they experience inexplicable bodily changes and continued deterioration in their health. Their suspicions may also be aroused by the way that staff and relatives now behave towards them. At this point, they try to get those around them to confirm their suspicions. This can be destructive for relationships.
Mutual pretence	In this awareness state, although the patient, staff, family and friends know the prognosis, they all refrain from discussing it. This may save each party from confronting the truth but simultaneously prevents the patient from exploring their dying with those close to them.
Open awareness	This fourth state occurs when all the parties concerned acknowledge their awareness of the terminal diagnosis.

1997). Other studies have found that health professionals caring for the dying employ 'conditional' rather than 'full open disclosure'. This is referred to as 'conditional awareness' and involves recognition that patients have the right to open awareness but simultaneously acknowledges that not all patients want, or can cope with, full disclosure (Timmermans 1994; Field and Copp 1999).

Treatment of dead bodies

As explained in Chapter 1, the focus on the body as both a natural phenomenon and a product of social, cultural and environmental factors within sociology led to the development of the sociology of the body. One of the consequences of this sociological interest in the body is that there have been analyses of the cultural variations in how bodies are treated after death and they way these change over time. Hence the reason for using the topic of the treatment of dead bodies as another illustration of the role of social processes in death.

Certain cultural traditions are observed in eastern societies. For example, Muslims prepare the body in the local mosque immediately after death, according to tightly prescribed conventions. The body is washed three times, twice with soap and water and then with camphor or other essences. It is then placed in a shroud and following this the family are invited for their last viewing. The rules about the sexes not mingling are observed with regard to males and females viewing the body (Firth 2000).

In western societies, since the development of pathology in the nineteenth century, dead bodies are considered to be a source of infection and disease. There has been a separation between the living and the dead, with corpses being taken to a mortuary and becoming within the domain of experts. Such experts include morticians and embalmers and they are responsible for rendering the body hygienic. For example, they drain bodily fluids from the cadaver to prevent leakage, replace them with formalin to ensure temporary preservation, close wounds and plug orifices. These processes simultaneously humanize the corpse as they restore colour to the skin and make it appear more lifelike. Other techniques that contribute to this reconstruction of the former self of the deceased are the brushing of hair, application of make-up and shaving. Once these procedures have been completed, relatives are then invited to view the body, which appears to be sleeping peacefully in the coffin. This is usually at the funeral parlour, although this practice does vary between societies in the West. For instance, in Ireland, the standard practice is for the open coffin to be taken to the deceased's home and left there for a few days so that people can come to pay their last respects (Power 2000).

In medieval Europe, decaying corpses were treated very differently. They were not hidden away and reconstructed but foregrounded in funeral practices and used as reminders of mortality, with lifelike effigies of them frequently being used on tomb architecture. Similarly, although the dead body has long been used as a teaching tool in medical training, dissection of corpses was prohibited on moral and religious grounds until the middle of the nineteenth century. Further evidence of the absence of such taboos in contemporary western society is the wide acceptance and perceived altruism of organ donation for transplantation purposes after death (Howarth 2007; Lupton 2008).

Grief and grieving

In the first section we saw how, on one level, grief may appear an intensely private matter. However, analysis of the evidence that exists shows that it is shaped by the social context and social relationships of the bereaved person. Moreover, these social dimensions are central to understanding grief and grieving and are nowhere more obvious than in the considerable variation in cultural beliefs about the appropriate expression of grief and funeral rituals.

In secular western societies, although funerals are now more individualized, they are normally brief and there is limited public manifestation of grief. Again, the exception is Ireland where what are called 'wakes' are held after a death. These include reception of the body into the church the night before the funeral, a full funeral service, and another religious ritual as the coffin is lowered into the grave. This is all followed by a religious service a month to the day after the funeral and each year on the anniversary of the death, when an anniversary notice, accompanied by a personal message written by the mourners, may also be placed in a local newspaper (Power 2000; Hunt 2005; Walter 2005).

Small-scale pre-industrial societies frequently place considerable importance on funeral ceremonies and an accompanying period of mourning. Both often involve many members of the deceased's family and the local community, the observation of elaborate rituals before and after the funeral and more open expression of emotions. Mourning can extend over a long period of time, up to six months in some cases, and can include abstaining from certain foods, readings from sacred books and the giving of gifts to a priest or a charity (Langani 1997; Rosenblatt 1997; Firth 2000).

Various explanations of such differences have been put forward. Hunt (2005) has linked them to religious beliefs and argues that the funeral rituals in pre-industrial societies indicate the religious significance attached to the transition from this world to the next. Others see culture itself as being highly influential. Returning to the example of the Irish wakes, these have been linked to Ireland's history of emigration. These rituals are said to provide 'a degree of comfort, both for a person planning their funeral and for their family' (Power 2000: 25). There are also those that point to the role of medicalization; Elias (1985) asserts that not only has this led to death becoming a private event, it has also resulted in the pain of grief being dealt with away from the public domain through medical or counselling therapy.

Whether ceremonies are short, long, secular or religious, they perfom both the psychological and social function of confirming and reinforcing the fact of death. They also validate the social worth of the deceased and potentially mobilize social support for those who are bereaved (Field and Payne 2004; Hunt 2005).

Social context shapes our personal experiences of dying, death and grieving. We have seen the influence of the denial of death in our society, the social and cultural variations in the concepts of good and bad death, medicalization and changes in medical practice. There are also social and cultural influences on the ways our bodies are dealt with following death and how we grieve for those we have lost. Such evidence can only lead us to concur with Howarth's statement above that 'our experiences of dying, death and bereavement are embedded within our social and cultural worlds' (Howarth 2008: 2).

Theoretical interpretations

Activity 9.3

Think back to the main theoretical approaches that were introduced in Chapter 1. Which ones do you think could be used to explain the evidence and arguments about dying, death and grieving presented in this chapter? Compare your thoughts with the points made in this section.

Given the evidence presented so far, the logical conclusion would be to argue that dying and death are socially constructed because of the role of factors such as social organization, social and cultural processes, religion, secularization, and scientific and medical developments in constructing these life events. Indeed, social constructionist explanations have been applied to this area of study. However, more recently, another perspective has started to be applied to various aspects of the changes in approaches to dying, death and bereavement in contemporary society.

You will remember from Chapter 1 that postmodernism argues that our knowledge about the social world is constantly changing. This is because of the way that human beings as 'agents' construct social life through their everyday interpretations of the world around them rather than having their lives and behaviour prescribed by the society in which they live. Since the 1990s theoretical explanations of dying, death and grieving have used postmodernism to highlight some of the ways that people construct the world around them when coping with dying and death.

In the course of this chapter examples of postmodernist interpretations of death in contemporary society have already been discussed. One of these was with reference to 'grief work' at the end of the first section. This has been shown to involve the construction of narratives by bereaved individuals which help them to make sense of, and come to terms with, their loss. Another was the reference to the media as a potential resource about dying, death and bereavement for people to selectively adopt and adapt to the context of their own everyday lives and experiences.

Within the literature on dying and death, those who have adopted postmodernism as a theoretical perspective have focused on how people now have to search for their own meanings in relation to mortality. Three issues in particular have been addressed. One is the loss of traditions in secular societies. The second is the way that the sequestration of death in our society means that individuals no longer experience the presence of death. The third is the coexistence of multiple 'cultural scripts' of the 'good death'. The following excerpt from Walter (1994: 2) captures this well.

> The medieval ars moriendi *applied to all, king and slave alike . . . in seventeenth-century England, published deathbed accounts told puritans the proper way to die; in the nineteenth century, magazines instructed the various social classes in the appropriate length of mourning for particular categories of loss. What we find today is . . . a babble of voices proclaiming various good deaths.*

It has therefore been argued that the consequent absence of death in our lives and the presence of varying interpretive frameworks about dying and death results in people having to create their own meanings (Walter 1994; Seale 1998; Long 2004).

Postmodernism has also been applied to personal grieving and bereavement. As discussed, grieving is less structured by ceremonies and customs than in the past. Psychological research has also led to the acknowledgement that people should grieve in the way they find suits them. Hence, those using this approach maintain that in our postmodern world there is a culture of grief which accepts that controlling their emotion works for some people whereas expressing their grief is more appropriate for others. Moreover, people have the freedom to choose their preferred style of grieving and this has been referred to as 'postmodern grief' (Walter 2007). However, Walter suggests that this new-found freedom poses another set of problems. For instance, someone may have chosen to grieve in private, which can mean those close to them may be unaware of their need for help and support.

The final issues that have been subject to postmodernist analysis are funeral ceremonies and the public expression of grief. The increased personalization of funeral services was referred to above. This includes 'alternative funerals', where disposal of the body may be away from conventional sites, such as in 'woodland burials'. These developments are seen as allowing people greater flexibility in how they honour their dead. In addition, greater variation in the places where people congregate for public mourning has also been identified. People are just as likely to gather at a church for public mourning as they are in shops and public buildings or at war memorials. The postmodernist interpretation of these changes is that people are exercising their right to greater choice in a postmodern world (Walter 1999, 2001, 2005; Conway 2007).

Despite the fact that these are useful insights on specific aspects of dying, death and grieving, there is clearly a need for a more comprehensive theoretical framework in order to deepen our understanding of this subject area within the study of the social aspects of health. It is of considerable interest to academics and professionals and much relevant research is still generated from year to year. Following the developments that take place will therefore prove fruitful for those who wish to extend their knowledge of this area.

Conclusions

In this chapter we have seen the ways in which the study of the social aspects of health provides insights into both the personal and social context of dying, death and grieving. As well as establishing that these life experiences are personal and social, the extent to which they are *social* experiences has been clearly demonstrated using evidence and arguments from the relevant literature. Topics covered have ranged from societal and cultural attitudes to death, to care of the dying, rituals observed with regard to dead bodies, funeral customs and the expression of grief. The current absence of a coherent theoretical approach was also discussed.

The important role of healthcare and medical practice in shaping dying and death was highlighted in the discussions in the second section of the chapter. It is now a well-established fact that the nature of the healthcare we receive throughout our lives is a major determinant of our quality of life and age of death (Baggott 2004; Graham 2009). This has already been addressed in passing in Chapters 2, 3 and 5 when discussing gender, social class and ageing respectively. It is therefore an appropriate point at which to move on to explore the different ways in which healthcare is delivered in our society and the implications this has for us and our health. The delivery of healthcare is the next and final section of this book.

Key points

- Death and the process of dying cannot be detached from the personal and social contexts in which they take place.

- All personal experiences of dying and death are affected by the extent to which death is predictable, the age at which death occurs, and personal belief and universal patterns of grieving.

- One of the best-known theorists on the personal context of dying and death is Kubler-Ross.

- Five topics were discussed to illustrate the ways in which dying and death are social experiences. These were the way that death is now denied in contemporary western society, the concepsts of 'good death' and 'bad death', the medicalization of death, cultural variations in the treatment of dead bodies and the ways in which grief and grieving are shaped by social processes.

- While social constructionism has been applied to the topic of dying and death, postmodernist explanations have more recently been drawn upon.

Discussion points

■ Compare Kubler-Ross's stage theories of dying and grieving to other non-stage theories about dying and grieving that you have read about.

■ To what extent do you think the media shapes our attitudes to dying, death and bereavement?

■ What are the advantages and disadvantages of the medicalization of death?

Suggestions for further study

■ As mentioned in the Introduction to this chapter, much of the seminal work still has contemporary relevance. It is therefore worth having a look at some of this in order to increase your understanding of particular issues. Some suggestions are as follows: Murray-Parkes *et al.* (1997) for an overview of cultural differences; Elias (1985) on the move to institutional caring for the dying; Sudnow (1967) for the social organization of dying and how it is routinized and moulded to fit into the day-to-day functioning of a hospital; Glaser and Strauss (1965, 1968, 1971) on dying and death as a social process.

■ More recent work includes that by both Seale and Walter.

■ The journals *Death Studies* and *Mortality* are also good sources of current research.

■ For up-to-date information about the hospice movement and developments within it, visit the 'Help the Hospices' website (www.helpthehospices.org.uk). This also has a range of useful publications in its 'publications catalogue'.

Section 3
The delivery of healthcare

Introduction to Section 3

This section will explore the third main theme identified within the social aspects of health, 'The delivery of healthcare'. The three topics within this theme to be addressed are:

- Families, communities and healthcare

- Healthcare organizations

- Health professions

As in the other sections of this book, each of these topics is dealt with in a separate chapter. The first chapter, Chapter 10, starts the exploration of this theme by looking at the roles of families and communities in the delivery of informal healthcare. Chapter 11 addresses the organization and delivery of formal healthcare and Chapter 12 focuses on professional power in healthcare. As explained in the introductions to the other sections of this book, these chapters can be read independently but you should refer to both the Glossary at the end of the book and to the outlines of the theoretical perspectives in Chapter 1 as necessary. The book ends with an 'Afterword' in which the author reflects on the growing significance of global influences on our health and the implications for the future study of the social aspects of health.

10

Families, communities and healthcare

*In recent times . . . there has been a conscious move away from all-encompassing,
state-provided healthcare, to an emphasis on self care and care by the families.*
(Brown and Wilson 2005: 181)

Introduction

Although the treatment of complex acute and chronic health conditions still takes place within hospital settings, over the past three decades there has been a progressive shift to both acutely and chronically ill people being cared for in their communities. While formal services have evolved, there has been an increase in demand for healthcare that is carried out on an unpaid and informal basis, particularly for those with long-term conditions. Therefore, this chapter focuses on this highly significant change in the way contemporary healthcare is delivered and organized and considers the implications in relation to the provision of unpaid and informal care in the community. The chapter begins by looking at the concept of the family and the important role it plays in both maintaining the health of its members and their healthcare. The changes in this role are explained with particular reference to the moves to delivering more of our healthcare outside the formal health sector. In addressing these issues, the concept of 'community' is discussed along with the wider implications of increasing our reliance on unpaid informal care within the community. The theoretical perspectives included in these discussions are functionalism, feminism and postmodernism.

'The family'

In order to provide you with a comprehensive understanding of the concept of the family, this section includes discussions of the different types of family, examples of theoretical approaches to the family and the range of functions carried out by families.

Types of family

A family can be loosely defined as a group of people who are directly linked by kinship ties because they are related by blood or through marriage. As you will be well aware, several different types of families exist.

- **The nuclear family:** two adults and their own or adopted children, living together in a household and connected by mutual affection and support.

- **The extended family:** when the nuclear family is part of a larger kinship network of grandparents, brothers, sisters, aunts, uncles, nieces, nephews and so forth. The nuclear family either lives with or very near these close relatives and has a close and continuous relationship with them.

- **The lone/one-parent family:** a divorced, separated, single or widowed mother or a father living without a spouse (and not cohabiting) but with his or her never-married dependent child or children.

- **The reconstituted family:** a household unit including a step-parent as a consequence of divorce, separation and remarriage. This type of family is created when a new partnership is formed by a mother and/or father who already have dependent children. Since most children remain with their mother following divorce or separation, most stepfamilies have a stepfather rather than a stepmother.

In recent decades, there have been several changes in the numbers of each type of family. One such change is that there has been a move away from traditional nuclear and extended families.

The reasons for this that have been identified include increased geographical mobility, voluntary childlessness, divorce rates and unmarried cohabiting parenthood. Indeed, the latter is now more common with an average of 31 per cent of all parents cohabiting. The second change is the increase in lone parents and reconstituted families. The boundary between these two types of family is fluid; Ermisch and Francesconi (2000) found that although about 40 per cent of mothers will spend some time as a lone parent, the duration of lone parenthood is often short, with one-half remaining lone parents for 4.6 years or less. A reason for this is that about three-quarters of these lone parents will form a stepfamily. However, over one-quarter of stepfamilies dissolve within a year, leading to lone parenthood once more (Stewart and Vaitilingham 2004).

Apart from the changes in the types of family that exist described above, new family forms are emerging. One of these is the increasing number of same-sex partners who now form household units in which they bring up children together. There are also groups who choose to call themselves a 'family' even if their relationships do not accord with conventional understandings of relationships within this concept. Groups such as these that pretend to be kin have been called 'elective families' or 'families of choice'. Their emergence is said to represent the replacement of normative expectations about familial intimacy and obligation with highly individualistic forms of relationships that are much more open and diffuse (Weeks 2002).

In addition to evolving over time, family structures also vary throughout the world. In most western societies, the accepted pattern of marriage is **monogamy** whereby it is illegal for a man or woman to be married to more than one individual at a time. Different forms of monogamy have been identified; the changes described above have led to what has come to be known as **serial monogamy** to signify how it is now common for people to have a number of successive partners during their lifetime, but only one partner at a time. Another pattern of marriage called **polygamy** has been found to exist in some non-western societies. This means that a husband or wife is legally allowed to have more than one spouse and because it can apply to both husbands and wives there are two types; one is **polygyny** in which a man is married to more than one woman and is often found in tribal societies. The other is **polyandry** and refers to a woman being married to more than one husband at any one time. The latter is far less common than the former and is usually found in impoverished societies, such as Nepal and Tibet (Steel and Kidd 2001).

The culturally diverse character of our contemporary society means that there are considerable variations in family and marriage arrangements too. For example, families of West Indian origin living in Britain are more likely than other groups to be headed by a married woman without her husband present. They are also more likely to have extended kinship networks than families headed by white females. South Asian families have very strong familial bonds between extended family members and often live together in the same household (Chamberlain 1999; Giddens 2009).

In the light of the above evidence, it has been argued that families are not objective entities but, on the contrary, are 'dynamic, fluid and open ended groupings and relationships' (Shaw 2007: 389) that are subject to social and cultural practices and changes both in our society and globally. The family has also been subject to a variety of theoretical interpretations.

Activity 10.1

List 10 families that you know. Now try to classify them using the list of family types above. What problems did you encounter when trying to do this? Some examples of such problems and their implications can be found in the 'Activity feedback' chapter on page 233.

Theoretical perspectives and the family

Some of the perspectives discussed in Chapter 1 have produced theories about the family. Functionalism and feminism have been chosen in order to illustrate the differences in theoretical interpretations that exist.

Functionalism

As you will recall from other chapters in this book that have included analyses in terms of functionalism, this perspective argues that social events and social institutions can be explained in terms of the contributions they make to the continuity and stability of a society. In other words, functionalism looks at the functions and roles different institutions perform and how these and the functions of other institutions work together to contribute towards the stability of a society.

We saw in Chapter 6 how Parsons, one of most influential functionalists, developed an explanation of the experience of acute illness based around the concept of the 'sick role'. Not only did Parsons put forward a functionalist explanation about being ill, he also developed a functionalist approach to the family (this was briefly mentioned in Chapter 1). He focused specifically on the nuclear family in western industrialized society and said that this sort of family predominates because its structure and the way it functions are optimal for meeting the needs of this type of society.

There are several stages in his argument. First of all, he said that that the nuclear family serves universal human and social needs such as the care and socialization of children, in order that they can successfully carry out their roles in society, and the provision of food and shelter. In addition, the nuclear family meets the needs of individuals for intimacy, love, security and sexual expression. Parsons then went on to argue that because the nuclear family meets such a range of needs, it therefore also meets both the instrumental and more expressive requirements of industrialized societies for a disciplined and adaptable workforce. Furthermore, nuclear families are self-contained units because they only need to perform functions for themselves as opposed to meeting the obligations to a wider network of family members that are a feature of life in extended families. As nuclear families are not tied to particular locations or extended family units they are also mobile. Such small mobile units are ideally suited to the economic needs of modern industrial economies. This was yet another reason why Parsons promulgated the value of the nuclear family in western industrialized society and concluded that it is functionally necessary to such a society.

The final strand to this explanation of the family reflects functionalism's 'consensual' representation of society. Parsons emphasized that as people broadly accept the importance of socialization, there is a consensus about such socialization and how important it is for the stability of society. Hence there is a recognition that if a family does not perform this role properly, problems and dangers arise. For instance, children are at risk of developing into deviant adults who do not perform their roles in society properly by refusing to work, turning to crime and/or not fulfilling their caring role in their families. Thus Parsons argued that the nuclear family is based on a consensus about the way it both serves the interests of, and is vital to, society (Parsons and Bales 1955; Parsons 1964).

Integral to this version of family life are traditional ideologies about the roles of men and women. Essentially, functionalism assumes an unequal sexual division of labour whereby men adopt instrumental roles and women have primary responsibility for taking care of the home and carrying out the expressive roles (see Chapter 2). Unsurprisingly, criticisms have been levied at the stereotyped picture of the family presented in Parsons' theory of the family. Moreover, this theory fails to accommodate the diversity of family arrangements that exist (Bittman and Pixley 1997; Silva and Smart 1999).

Feminism

When theorizing about the family, there is a general agreement among feminists about the inequitable sexual division of labour within family life and its likely continuation. They expand this point to argue that the family is a significant and continuing source of female oppression. The blame for this situation is laid firmly on patriarchy, because it leads to inequalities between men and women. Within patriarchy, men are given power which meant that, historically, women were subordinate to men and restricted to domesticity and motherhood, had little autonomy and power of their own and were legally and financially dependent on men, be they husbands or fathers. Despite the fact that women do have more rights and freedom today, feminists argue that women still bear the scars of their oppression in the family: within the family, the division of labour is still asymmetrical and the legacy of the sexual and financial subordination of women remains. Women are also more likely to occupy the lowest-paid jobs (see Chapter 2). Feminists are emphatic that the male domination and female subordination that occurs because of the existence of patriarchy in society are powerful ideological and social constructions that must be challenged (Jackson 1997; Giddens 2009)

However, as discussed in Chapters 1 and 2, feminists do differ in their views and these differences manifest themselves very clearly when theorizing about the family. In order to illustrate this point, the distinctive feminist perspectives on the family that have been addressed in this book are set out below.

- **Marxist feminism:** within this perspective, patriarchy is seen as serving the interests of capitalism. In addition, Marxist feminists have been highly critical of the promotion of the nuclear family under capitalism as an the 'ideal type' of family.

- **Radical feminism:** radical feminists' emphasis on how male domination is based on their biology and physical strength has led them to concentrate on physical abuse and violence in the family as the expressions of male power.

- **Liberal feminism:** this argues that the campaigning and legal changes that have occurred over the past few decades have led to some limited moves towards greater equality between men and women. Liberal feminists point to evidence of more symmetry in the household division of labour in terms of more equal sharing of domestic tasks and shifts in fatherhood, and women's increasing participation in the workforce.

Activity 10.2

As stated above, functionalism and feminism were chosen because they illustrate the differences in theoretical approaches to the family. What do you think the main differences are? Compare your ideas with those set out in the 'Activity feedback' chapter on page 233.

The role of the family in contemporary society

Despite being a complex and fluid institution and the source of theoretical dissension, the family is still a fundamental and important social institution because of the role it plays in the lives of its members and in society in general. While there are some who argue that the family fulfils certain universal functions in society, others maintain its role is shaped by political agendas. Three interlinked themes can be identified in the views on the role of the family in contemporary society. These are outlined below and include examples of further theorizing about the family.

Support and 'reproduce' the workforce

The Marxist perspective sees the family as being responsible for not just the biological reproduction of people but also for their social reproduction in terms of caring for them physically and emotionally. The latter enables children to become members of society and adults in the family to maintain their position in the social structure, such as their occupational status. The combined responsibility for this biological and social reproduction is referred to as the **reproduction of people**.

Primary responsibility for the bringing up of children

Integral to the concept of the reproduction of people is the responsibility for bringing up children. The family is one of the main agencies in the socialization of children so that they fit into society. As already established, socialization refers to the social process by which individuals are brought up and 'shaped' according to the roles, norms and values of a society. A socialized individual knows the 'appropriate' way to act in different social situations, can 'fit' into society and has taken on the values of their society.

Healthcare

Once again reproduction of people and socialization cannot be separated from attending to the healthcare needs of family members. Hence another role of the family is informal and unpaid healthcare (see Chapter 2). This has always taken place through the extensive range of tasks carried out on a daily basis by families. These include practical tasks such as shopping, cooking and cleaning as well as emotional support that naturally ensues from the mutual interdependence between family members. Although these tasks are usually taken for granted, they are essential for the maintenance of good health. There has been a greater emphasis on the family's role in health-care in recent years for several reasons. One is the expansion of public health which has meant that the family has more responsibility for the health education of its individual members. Recently, the health and well-being of children and young people specifically has 'been the subject of unprecedented attention and scrutiny' (Allen 2008: 4) within this agenda. In addition, research has repeatedly highlighted the influence that the family has on the adoption of a healthy lifestyle by children and young people. This has led to the conclusion that 'parents are the key to achieving the best physical and mental health and well-being outcomes for their children' (Department of Health 2009c: 5) and an emphasis in initiatives on the role of the family in encouraging children to eat healthily and take exercise (Sluijs *et al.* 2008; Department of Health 2009c; Velleman 2009).

Another reason is that the policy trends referred to in the Introduction to the chapter mean that the amount and level of informal healthcare now expected of families for acute and chronic conditions has also increased considerably. While this will be discussed in more detail in the next section, the following are examples of the types of healthcare tasks that families undertake as a consequence of policy developments in this area:

- physical tasks (feeding and washing), some of which can be physically demanding (lifting and hoisting);

- provision of emotional support, empathy and affection;

- administering medication;

- transporting dependants;

- organizing services for the dependant in order to manage their illness.
  (Twigg and Atkin 1994; Cancian and Oliker 1999; Seale 2000)

The different roles of the family in contemporary society and some of the changes in these roles indicate that the construction of the family can vary according to the needs of society at particular times. Implicit in such a conclusion is an acknowledgement of the politicization of the family and, indeed, such constructions vary according to political ideologies. While both the **New Right** and **New Labour** political discourses placed a strong emphasis on the value of stable family life and suggested that 'two parents are better than one', there are differences in their approaches to the family. The New Right placed more emphasis on 'traditional family life' and appropriate sexuality whereas New Labour viewed families as being essential in the transmission of moral values to, and support of, their members (Silva and Smart 1999; Powell 2000; Johnson 2000).

Nonetheless, this section has shown that the family, whatever its structure, theoretical or political construction, plays a major role in maintaining its members' 'health' in the broadest sense of the word by ensuring their welfare and providing healthcare when they are ill and/or elderly. The former includes the physical and emotional care of family members, and the bringing up of the young members in an appropriate manner not only to ensure they fit into society but also to maximize their health and well-being. The latter incorporates the informal care of dependent members of the family, such as those who are elderly and sick. The importance of the family in the provision of healthcare has been widely acknowledged within the study of the social aspects of health. Indeed, while it is recognized that the state and the private and voluntary sectors are sources of healthcare, it is the healthcare provided by the family that is the most fundamental. Furthermore, it has been argued that state-provided healthcare cannot exist without the healthcare carried out within families (Graham 1999; Allan and Crow 2001; Means *et al.* 2008).

As indicated above, the involvement of the family in informal healthcare has increased as a result of recent policy developments. A significant influence on the level of healthcare families provide has been the move to delivering healthcare in the 'community'.

'Community' and healthcare

As mentioned in the Introduction to this chapter, there has been much more emphasis on delivering healthcare in the community in recent decades. Before exploring this further let us examine the concept of 'community'.

The concept of 'community'

A satisfactory definition of 'community' has proved elusive for many years – one study showed that *94* definitions had been developed. Unsurprisingly, this has led to arguments that the concept of 'community' is socially constructed. For example, Symonds maintains that it was only in the last century that 'the phrase "community" became a public discourse. The word itself became an organising principle for polices and practice, and gained a hold on everyday commonsense' (Symonds 1998: 12).

There are many approaches to the constructed nature of the concept of 'community' in the literature and two conflicting views have been selected to demonstrate how they vary. The first constructs 'community' as an idealized way of living which is under threat. Proponents of this view tend to romanticize traditional communities, and portray them as close-knit and mutually supportive. One such proponent was Tonnies (1963). He wrote in the late nineteenth century when sociological thought was influenced by romanticism, and 'community' was regarded as essentially beneficial to human needs and social interaction. He drew a distinction between *gemeinschaft* and *gesellschaft* to illustrate the changes to communities during industrialization. He argued that the pre-industrial world was based on *gemeinschaft*, whereby community relationships were characterized by intimacy and durability, status was ascribed rather than achieved, and kin relationships took place within a shared territory and were made meaningful by a shared culture. Industrialization and urbanism led to a replacement of *gemeinschaft* by *gesellschaft*. The latter meant that relationships became impersonal, fleeting, contractual, competitive, rational and calculative rather than affective, and were often characterized by anonymity and alienation. Status was based on merit, and was therefore achieved. Tonnies placed a high value on *gemeinschaft* and was deeply pessimistic about the inevitable change from this to *gesellschaft* that industrialization entailed because of his idealized view of the merits of traditional communities and the way that relationships would be destroyed. Such romanticized views of 'community' can also be seen in post-war sociological research into urban communities which focused on working-class neighbourhoods. An example is Young and Willmott's (1957) study of family life and kinship patterns in East London in the 1950s which showed that 'community' in the traditional sense, as referred to above, had survived in Bethnal Green despite rapid social change.

In contrast, the second view of the concept of 'community' that has been chosen for the purposes of this discussion constructs communities throughout history as having far from 'dream-like' qualities. An example of this approach is that put forward by Sennett (1993), who uses the concept 'destructive *gemeinschaft*' to explain how community feelings can be psychologically destructive. Others have argued that some groups may have negative experiences of their communities. For instance, feminist writing in the 1980s emphasized how 'community' can have negative connotations for women because of their caring responsibilities (Finch and Groves 1985; Ungerson 1987).

The construction of the concept of 'community' also varies according to political ideologies. There are those who maintain that the New Right saw the 'community' as the 'first port of call for those in need' (Mohan 1995: 102). Johnson (2000) shows how New Labour adopted a different concept of 'community' which was influenced by **communitarianism**. This ideology was opposed to purely individualistic conceptions of welfare and stressed common interest and common values arising from communal bonds. Within it, communities were seen as vital units of social organization with shared moral values, and a means for ensuring social cohesion (Johnson 2000; Powell 2000). However, ambiguities in New Labour's appeal to communitarianism have been identified: Chamberlayne and King (2000) argued that there were conservative elements in New Labour's approach, thus suggesting that political constructions of the 'community' may overlap to some extent.

This brief overview demonstrates how the concept of 'community' is subject to different constructions, has different meanings for different people and varies with political ideologies. Irrespective of the 'constructed' nature of community, there has been a progressive shift towards healthcare being provided *outside* of formal healthcare organizations in a community setting.

The move to healthcare in the community

The decrease in the number of beds, the closure of smaller hospitals, the expansion of day surgery and 'hospital at home' initiatives have reduced the amount of hospital and professional care *acutely ill* people receive and increased the demand for their short-term care in the community (Baggott 2004; Means *et al.* 2008). These developments have simultaneously increased the demand for informal and unpaid healthcare within the community. While the significance of this should not be ignored, it is the move to caring for people with *long-term conditions* within the community that has had the greatest impact on those involved in providing their informal care. Among the most influential policy trends are the move to community care, the provision of care at home for people with long-term conditions and the focus on self-care. These are discussed below.

Community care

Analysis of policy documents shows that 'community care' can be traced as far back as the early 1900s when the 1904–8 Royal Commission on the Care of the Feeble Minded first signalled the shift in emphasis from institutional to 'community care' in policy initiatives. From then on, there was a growing emphasis on 'community care' in policy documents. This gathered momentum in the 1970s and 1980s, culminating in the National Health Service and Community Care Act 1990. Other subsequent pieces of legislation which have progressed community care are the Carers Recognition and Services Act 1995 and the Carers (Equal Opportunities) Act 2004.

The policy documents produced have adopted different approaches to the concept of 'community care'. For instance, different terms such as care *in* the community and care *by* the community have been used. Furthermore, the nebulous nature of the concept of community leaves it vulnerable to a variety of interpretations. This has led to the conclusion that 'community care' is yet another 'contested term used by different people in different ways at different points in time' (Means *et al.* 2008: 3). Nonetheless, there are common themes in all of the policies introduced since the 1970s. These are that dependant people will be not be cared for in long-stay hospitals and other types of large institution. Instead they will be cared for in their own homes by family members and/ or significant others within the community, or small-scale institutions. More specifically, 'community care' has come to be used to describe care for those in need which is based on support and care in their homes provided through a **mixed economy of care**. This concept refers to care that is provided both informally through the individual and collective efforts of family members and those in the community on an unpaid basis, supported formally by paid professionals employed by statutory and voluntary services (Parker 1985; Blakemore 2007; Means *et al.* 2008).

Care at home

While various reforms have been introduced to address the problems of community care, since the late 1990s the quality and the type of community care people with long-term conditions receive has been shaped by the **modernization agenda**. Among the policies that have had the most important implications for the care of people with long-term conditions living in the community are those which have led to reductions in hospital care (Means *et al.* 2008). Reducing the role of the hospital has involved a significant move away from hospital care to care in the home and the provision of a new community-based system of clinical intervention and care coordination for chronic health conditions: 'there has been a marked shift in the location of nursing care in the UK to the community and more particularly the home . . . these changes have been supported by a number of clear policy initiatives . . . which indicate that the drive towards the home is set to continue' (McGarry 2008: 83).

One of the most recent developments in the expansion of service within the community has been the introduction of community matrons. These are a group of highly experienced nurses who 'work across health and social care services and the voluntary sector, so that this group of patients receives services that are integrated and complementary' (Department of Health 2005a: 16).

Self-care

Other initiatives within the modernization agenda that have had a major impact on the delivery of healthcare in the community are those which encourage patient self-care. Indeed, self-management of chronic disorders has become a central element in the management of long-term conditions both in this country and others. Examples of such initiatives are programmes that are designed to enhance patients' self-management capacities and lead to an improved quality of life (e.g. the Expert Patients Programme – see Chapter 6). These programmes encourage people with chronic conditions to take more control over their health by developing their understanding so that they can both manage their condition and their treatment in partnership with healthcare professionals. They also aim to build local support networks so that patients can use their expertise to support each other, thereby increasing their level of self-care management further (Department of Health 2005b; Taylor and Bury 2007; Lorig *et al.* 2008).

Caring and the family

The above discussions have demonstrated the greater emphasis on healthcare being provided *outside* of formal healthcare organizations and in the home. While the developments that have taken place bring benefits, such as greater independence and empowerment for those concerned, they have nevertheless been heavily criticized (Wilson *et al.* 2007; Lorig *et al.* 2008). Many question the principles underlying the policies that have been introduced and suggest that the main driver is the motivation to reduce healthcare costs. Others have focused on the fact that the main source of the additional informal healthcare required in the community for the acutely and chronically ill is the family (Parker 1985; Watson and Doyal 1999; Means *et al.* 2008). For instance, 'care at home' and 'self-care' initiatives assume the active involvement of families (Hudson 2005; Rogers *et al.* 2008). As a consequence of community care, more and more people have had to take on the role of an unpaid carer because of the legislative enshrinement of this role and the limited sources of alternative support available to those who need care. The increasing prevalence and incidence of chronic illness, largely due to our ageing society (see Chapter 5), will result in a continuation in the rise in the number of 'carers'. Currently, there are around 6 million carers and research suggests that there will be a need for another 3.4 million informal unpaid carers over the next 35 years (Department of Health 2006; Yeandle *et al.* 2007).

These developments, in combination with those referred to in the first section of the chapter, have led to families having a greater role in healthcare than ever before. Those who have raised the issue of the steady growth in dependence on the family for healthcare have argued that locating healthcare in the family to this extent can have serious consequences for those being cared for and those providing the care. The diverse and changing nature of the family means that some families (such as one-parent families) are unable to provide the care required. Certain groups (for instance, the elderly) are more likely to suffer from inadequate care in the family than others (McGarry 2008; Swinkels and Mitchell 2009). In addition, there is a substantial body of research about the levels of violence and physical and emotional abuse that takes place in some families. This evidence also shows that certain families can actually damage the health of those they are caring for. Furthermore, physical and emotional abuse does occur in caring relationships (Brown and Wilson 2005; Aldridge 2006; Pritchard 2006).

There have been concerns about the formal and informal support available within communities to families undertaking more substantial healthcare roles; formal services have been found to be inflexible and failures of interagency working have been identified. Despite the political reinventions of 'community' as a source of unpaid support, as explained above, living in a community is not always a positive experience and can be characterized by a lack of social cohesion. It is well established that many communities are fragmented by high crime rates, high unemployment and inequalities. Therefore, the reality of community life means that those providing unpaid healthcare for family members at home often do not receive individual and collective support from others living in the same community (Crow and Maclean 2006; Means *et al.* 2008).

With reference to those providing informal care specifically, in Chapters 3 and 5 we saw that caring affects carers' physical and psychological health. They have been found to experience a wide range of problems during caring such as depression, anxiety, emotional distress, stress, feeling tired, hernias, heart problems, arthritis, asthma, giddiness, backaches and headaches (Carers National Association 1998; Hirst 1999; Yeandle *et al.* 2007). Studies have also shown that there are many other negative effects of caring. For example, it impacts on personal and sexual relationships as well as financial and social circumstances, leads to psychological distress and loss of confidence, self-esteem and sense of identity (Lewis and Meredith 1988; McLaughlin and Ritchie 1994; Hirst 2003; Gilbert *et al.* 2009; Glendinning *et al.* 2009). Some of these effects are illustrated in the case study below.

Case example: Betty's story

Betty had been caring for her husband, Les, who had rheumatoid arthritis, for 10 years. During the past two years his condition had deteriorated rapidly to the extent that he was virtually immobilized with the arthritis and in constant pain. The length of Les's illness meant that their social life had become non-existent and, apart from one or two family members, they had very few visitors. Betty was a very gregarious person and missed mixing with friends and going out for an evening.

Les obviously no longer worked, and although he had not given up work initially, he had been unable to progress in his job because of his illness. Betty had worked part-time but then found that her caring responsibilities had increased so much that she could not manage both work and caring. Hence their family finances were not in a good state and they had to live on a very low income.

Betty had developed a chronic back condition and joint problems because of having to help Les so much physically, such as helping him to stand up and support him when he walked in the house. She also had high blood pressure and had recently started to take medication for depression.

Feminist commentators have protested that the burdens of these developments fall most heavily on women as they are more likely to carry out all types of care and healthcare within families (Finch and Groves 1985; Watson and Doyal 1999). The explanations that have been put forward vary – some have argued that women are ideologically and culturally constructed as being naturally suited to caring for members of their families. Consequently, they have no choice but to provide informal care and often carry it out in addition to paid work (Ungerson 1983; Dalley 1996). Others maintain that caring (unlike paid work) is a work role that permeates women's consciousness and identity in a way that differentiates them from men. Caring therefore defines the activity of women, gives them an identity and enables them to gain entry into, and feel accepted into, both the private world of the home and the public world of the labour market. This approach has also been used to explain why women predominate in 'caring' jobs in the labour market (Graham 1983, 1993; Walker 1983).

Activity 10.3

The following are extracts from recent official publications on the move to delivering more healthcare in the community. They illustrate several of the themes in discussions about the changes that have been introduced. Can you identify these themes? See the 'Activity feedback' chapter, page 234, for a discussion of this activity.

From: *Supporting People with Long-term Conditions: An NHS and Social Care Model for Improving Care for People with Long-term Conditions* (Department of Health 2005a).

Extract 1

Supported self care – collaboratively help individuals and their carers to develop the knowledge, skills and confidence to care for themselves and their condition effectively.

- *Focus initially on the very high intensive users of secondary care services through a case management approach.*
- *Appoint community matrons to spearhead the case management drive. In total, there will be 3000 community matrons in post by March 2007.*
- *Over time, develop a system of identifying prospective very high intensity users of services.*
- *Establish multi-professional teams based in primary or community care with support of specialist advice to manage care across all settings.*
- *Develop a local strategy to support comprehensive self care.*
- *Implement the Expert Patients Programme and other self care programmes.*
- *Take a systematic approach that links health, social care, patients and carers.*
- *Use the tools and techniques already available to start to make an impact.*

(p. 6)

Extract 2

As patients develop multiple long term conditions, their care becomes disproportionately complex and can be difficult for them and the health and social care system to manage. Such patients have an intricate mix of health and social care difficulties. Because of their vulnerability, simple problems can make their condition deteriorate rapidly, putting them at high risk of unplanned hospital admissions or long term institutionalisation. This is often older people, but could also include children and patients with complex neurological conditions or mental health problems. Evidence has shown that intensive, on-going and personalised case management can improve the quality of life and outcomes for these patients, dramatically reducing emergency admissions and enabling patients who are admitted to return home more quickly.

(p. 10)

Extract 3

For this reason, the introduction of community matrons applying a case management approach will play a significant role in helping local health communities achieve the PSA [public service agreement] target for improving care for patients with long term conditions, and in reducing the use of emergency bed days by 5% by 2008. Case management is also the first step to creating an effective delivery system and implementing the wider NHS and Social Care Long Term Conditions Model.

(p. 13)

From: *Supporting Experienced Hospital Nurses to Move into Community Matron Roles* (Department of Health 2005c).

Extract 4

Many NHS hospital Trusts and primary care organisations are employing or looking to employ hospital nurses who are experienced in the care of people with long term conditions, for case management and community matron roles. These nurses are making a transition from working in a single institution with known boundaries and visible walls to the complexity of working in the community, which includes both primary care and domiciliary settings.

(p. 7)

From: *Putting People First: A Shared Vision and Commitment to the Transformation of Adult Social Care* (Department of Health 2007c).

Extract 5

Demography means an increasing number of people are living longer, but with more complex conditions such as dementia and chronic illnesses. By 2022, 20% of the English population will be over 65. By 2027, the number of over 85-year-olds will have increased by 60%. People want, and have a right to expect, services with dignity and respect at their heart. Older people, disabled people and people with mental health problems demand equality of citizenship in every aspect of their lives, from housing to employment to leisure. The vast majority of people want to live in their own homes for as long as possible. In the context of changing family structures, caring responsibilities will impact on an increasing number of citizens. Examples include an eighty-year-old woman having to cope with her husband's dementia, a young mum pursuing a career and bringing up a family while looking after her elderly parent, a business executive working overseas whose widowed mother is hospitalised overnight following a stroke and older parents seeking for the right support to ensure their adult son with a learning disability can live independently.

(p. 1)

Theoretical interpretations of the move to delivering healthcare in the community

In addition to the feminist writing referred to above, various facets of the move from formal to informal healthcare have been analysed from a postmodernism perspective. For instance, community care has been linked to the emergence of the discourse of informal care in the 1970s and 1980s. One such explanation is that put forward by Heaton (1999) who used the Foucauldian concept of the 'gaze' to contextualize the development of this discourse. The 'gaze' can be defined as 'a way of looking at or, indeed, hearing, smelling and otherwise seeing or comprehending the world' (Heaton 1999: 769) and shows how perceptions and understandings of different aspects of society change over time. There are various types of 'gaze' which are used to reflect the particular domains that become subjected to the focus and the power of the 'gaze'. One of these variants is the 'medical gaze', which refers to 'ways in which objects of medical knowledge and practices have been viewed and understood' (Heaton 1999: 769). Until the late nineteenth century the 'medical gaze' was on 'sick bodies' in hospitals and institutions, and presenting illnesses were understood in terms of anatomy and clinical disease only. As we have seen, new and broader conceptualizations of disease and its causes were developed in the twentieth century with the result that the 'medical gaze' gradually devolved and extended to patients in the community. This simultaneously increased the visibility of those caring for them, such as family members and friends in the community, and promoted a growing emphasis on their role in informal care. Heaton argues that it was the historical transformation of the 'medical gaze' in this way that led to the emergence of the discourse of informal care in the 1970s.

This perspective has also been applied to recent developments, such as the Expert Patients Programme. As opposed to being a vehicle of empowerment, this has been accused of reinforcing the medical paradigm; in Foucauldian terms, it essentially allows the further extension of the 'medical gaze' to self-care practices that were previously concealed from this gaze because they were carried out in the privacy of individuals' homes. Therefore, as a result of the Expert Patients Programme, medicine has the power to control and define self-care practices. The medicalization of self-care practices that has occurred means that medical power can now potentially seep 'into all corners of an individual's life' (Wilson *et al.* 2007: 434).

Conclusions

This chapter has explored two key concepts within the study of the social aspects of health – 'the family' and the 'community'. The diversity and fluidity of 'the family' has been clearly demonstrated. Its complex nature is reflected in a range of theoretical perspectives on the family. We have also seen that despite the variations in families and family life that exist, the family plays a vital role in meeting many of the needs of its members and, more generally, of society. One of the most important sets of needs is that based around the 'health' of family members. The demands on the family for its services in terms of 'health' has grown considerably in recent years because of policy initiatives that have moved the care of both the acutely and the chronically ill out of formal healthcare organizations. The advantages and disadvantages of these developments were considered with particular emphasis on the additional demands they place on the family and the potential adverse consequences for those providing the care and those receiving the unpaid and informal healthcare. The question of whether communities can actually be a source of the informal support required was also addressed.

As indicated on several occasions, unpaid and informal healthcare cannot be considered in isolation from the delivery of formal care. This is particularly true for any discussion about the shift to caring for acutely and chronically ill people in their communities because of the simultaneous shift to more community-based models for formal health services. Having examined the delivery of informal healthcare in detail, it is therefore appropriate to now consider the delivery of formal healthcare, which is the subject of the next chapter.

Key points

■ Developments in the delivery of healthcare have led to a greater emphasis on provision of healthcare that is carried out on an unpaid and informal basis.

■ This has led to an increased role for the family in informal healthcare.

■ Key concepts explored in relation to these developments were 'community', community care, care at home and self-care.

■ Both feminist and postmodernist perspectives have provided useful analyses of the move from formal to informal healthcare.

Discussion points

■ What are the advantages and disadvantages of belonging to a family in contemporary society?

■ How do you think postmodernism would theoretically explain 'the family'?

■ To what extent can healthcare be delivered informally in 'the community'?

Suggestions for further study

■ Steel and Kidd (2001) provide a very thorough and clear overview of a range of theories about the family. For an account of the development of community care and recent policy initiatives, see Means *et al.* (2008).

■ Recent articles on changes in the delivery of informal healthcare can be found in journals such as *Health and Social Care in the Community* and the *Journal of Epidemiology and Community Health*.

■ It is also worth looking on the websites for the Department of Health and the Social Policy Research Unit (University of York) for details of the latest research.

■ For information about carers specifically, visit the Carers UK website at www.carersuk.org.

Healthcare organizations

The NHS is in transition . . . the old structures and organisations are being dismantled and a plethora of new organisations and agencies is evolving.

(Talbot-Smith and Pollock 2006: 1)

Introduction

In the previous chapter we explored the roles of families and communities in the delivery of healthcare. The emphasis was very much on informal healthcare provided *outside* of formal healthcare organizations. This chapter will simultaneously complement the material presented in Chapter 10 and extend your knowledge of the delivery of healthcare by addressing the organization and delivery of *formal* healthcare. The quote at the beginning of this chapter highlights several of the main issues which inform debates about our formal healthcare organizations, and the chapter aims to give the reader a greater insight into these issues. It begins by establishing what we mean when we talk about 'healthcare organizations'. Examples of different theoretical approaches to healthcare organizations are then explored. These include Weber's theory of bureaucracy, structural functionalism and post-modernism. The last part of the chapter discusses and assesses the range of reforms that have been made to the organization and delivery of formal healthcare in the UK over the past three decades.

Organizations and healthcare

In order to address the subject of healthcare organizations, it is necessary to understand what is meant by the term 'organization'. Therefore this section begins by discussing organizations in general and then explains the nature of healthcare organizations.

What is an organization?

In the pre-modern world, most of our needs were provided by relatives and neighbours. Due to the complexity of modern life and our increasing interdependency, organizations are now a central feature of all societies and influence most aspects of our lives. We spend our working lives and much of our non-working lives in them. Examples include families, schools, colleges, universities, religious bodies, sports clubs, trade unions, business corporations and hospitals. An organization typically has certain objectives and is seen as being composed of large groups of individuals and sub-groups. These have prescribed roles and are all part of a defined and relatively stable set of authority relations. Together with systems of social roles, norms and shared meanings that exist in organizations, these defined lines of authority mean that interaction within organizations is regular and predictable. Several characteristics that organizations have in common have been identified (Handy 2005; Giddens 2009). These are set out below.

- **External reality:** organizations are not figments of the imagination but are based in reality. While many organizations, such as hospitals and schools, have a physical presence, they can also have a more abstract presence. For instance, the family – even though our 'family' might be geographically disparate, we are still part of it and it is a constant feature of our daily lives.

- **Coercive power:** it is the norm that members of an organization consent to the power of that organization. Taking schools as an example, while there are exceptions, the wearing of distinctive uniforms, and arrival and departure times, are usually unquestioned. Organizational sanctions are imposed, such as withdrawal of privileges and exclusion, if this power is ignored.

- **Moral authority or legitimacy:** an organization's authority is accepted as being just and rightfully given. This can be seen in the public acceptance of the right of hospitals not to discharge patients until they see fit to do so and of educational establishments to maintain academic standards when making decisions.

- **Historicity:** a basic characteristic of organizations is their enduring nature. Most have a history which extends beyond the life of the people who are part of those organizations today. Using the family and the Church of England to illustrate this point, these have been in existence for centuries and although their structures may change, they are likely to endure for a considerable time.

- **Culture:** organizations have differing sets of norms and values which are reflected in different structures and systems. These 'cultures' are affected by factors such as the people that work in the organization, its historical development, the economic climate, new technology and global changes.

Activity 11.1

Choose two 'organizations' to which you belong. Using the grid below, analyse them in terms of the characteristics of organizations presented above. Then ask yourself:

- What differences between the two organizations emerge from your analysis?

- What can the reasons for these differences be attributed to?

	ORGANIZATION 1	**ORGANIZATION 2**
External reality		
Coercive power		
Moral authority or legitimacy		
Historicity		
Culture		

Despite their ubiquity and importance in our lives, organizations are not totally beneficial to us. Their size, complex structures and tightly prescribed rules and regulations can render them inefficient, inflexible and ineffective in meeting our needs. They can also be sources of social power to the extent that they monitor and control aspects of our lives. Some of these more negative aspects are highlighted in the exploration of key theories of healthcare organizations in the next section. Before moving on to these theoretical discussions however, we need to clarify the meaning of the term 'healthcare organization'.

Healthcare organizations

The NHS is a classic example of an 'organization'. By virtue of their characteristics, there are also other healthcare organizations, both within and outside the state system of healthcare provision. Healthcare organizations within the NHS not only include hospitals (acute and long-stay) but also a whole range of organizations such as Primary Care Trusts (PCTs), NHS Direct, the National Blood Service and the Health Protection Agency, to name only a few. With reference to healthcare organizations outside the NHS, the British healthcare system has always depended on services and organizations which are privately run and financed. However, from the 1980s and into the first decade of this century, there was a marked expansion in the provision of healthcare by private and voluntary sector organizations (see Chapter 10). Together these comprise what is referred to as the 'independent sector' (Baggott 2004; Talbot-Smith and Pollock 2006).

Let us take the provision of healthcare by private healthcare organizations first. These aim to make a profit and currently provide around 20 per cent of hospital and nursing home services, 3 per cent of GP services and 40 per cent of dental services. Within the general expansion of private healthcare, during the past three decades, private hospital provision expanded the most. Simultaneously the level of private health insurance increased – around 22 per cent of the population (mainly those in professional and managerial jobs) have private health insurance.

There were other developments that shifted the balance between the public and private sectors. These included initiatives to facilitate greater collaboration between the two, such as the contracting-out of patient care by the NHS to private hospitals and using private hospitals as a way of reducing NHS waiting lists.

Many reasons have been put forward to account for this increase in the provision of healthcare by private organizations. While it is seen in part to be driven by the political emphasis on individual choice, political and economic concerns about maximizing efficiency and cost-effectiveness were also influential. In addition, some have pointed to the fact that governments may have been motivated by certain segments of the medical profession which view this move favourably as they gain financially from the expansion of the private sector. The increase in consumer demand fuelled by patients who are dissatisfied with the NHS also played a role (Mohan 1995, 2002; Baggott 2004).

With reference to the voluntary sector organizations, although they now have to operate in a more commercial environment, these are essentially not-for-profit entities. They cover a diverse range of functions, from the small-scale activities of local volunteer groups to large national charities and non-profit-making bodies. From the 1980s the advantages of the voluntary sector in providing healthcare were widely acknowledged and voluntary provision was actively encouraged. Funding to voluntary bodies increased and they became more professional in the way they were run. Another significant change was their much closer involvement in the provision of NHS care and facilities for particular groups such as children, the elderly and those with disabilities. They also now play a lead role in representing patients, service users and carers (Kendall and Knapp 1996; Talbot-Smith and Pollock 2006; Means *et al.* 2008).

Such developments led to a new mix of public, private and voluntary healthcare services which is referred to as a 'mixed economy of healthcare'. Concerns have been consistently expressed about the quality of the services available through non-state provision (Baggott 2004; Maynard 2005; Carvel 2006). In spite of these concerns, this balance in provision between the different organizations providing healthcare not only continues to be supported at national level but also at an international level. For instance, one of the regional targets of *Health for All by the Year 2000* (World Health Organization 1990) was: 'In all Member States a wide range of organisations and groups throughout the public, private and voluntary sectors should be actively contributing to the achievement of health for all' (p. 14). Nonetheless, despite the plurality of organizations providing healthcare, the 'British healthcare system is still predominantly a public service model' (Baggott 2004: 155).

Theoretical approaches to healthcare organizations

There are many theories which have been used to understand healthcare organizations and the way they function. The main ones are outlined in this section.

Healthcare organizations as bureaucracies

You will often have heard people referring negatively to our healthcare system as 'bureaucratic'. An explanation of the concept of **bureaucracy** is required in order to appreciate why such accusations are made. Although the word 'bureaucracy' has been around since the 1700s, it was the German sociologist, Max Weber (see Chapter 3) who developed it in relation to analysing organizations in his explanation of the rise of the modern organization. He argued that modern organizations were a means of coordinating the activities of human beings in industrialized society across time and space. Integral to Weber's explanation of bureaucracy is his concept of **ideal type**. This refers to the construction of a pure or ideal form of a particular aspect of the social world which does not necessarily exist anywhere in reality. Nor is an ideal type attainable or even the most desirable, but it identifies those traits which would render the aspect of the social world under scrutiny most effective (Beetham 1996; Weber 1997). For Weber, the ideal type of bureaucracy had certain key features and the closer an organization's own characteristics were to these, the more effective it would be.

Weber's ideal bureaucracy

- *A hierarchy of authority:* those with the most authority are the most senior and there is a clear line of command from the top to the bottom of the organization.

- *Specialized division of tasks:* all employees have a clear understanding of their responsibilities.

- *Rules that govern conduct:* there are procedures and guidelines that need to be adhered to at all times by employees at all levels. The rationale for decisions taken is based on these rules, not on personal responses to issues that arise.

- *A formalized system of record-keeping:* all business is conducted in writing and hence there is much emphasis on paperwork and accurate record-keeping.

- *A clear distinction between work and home life:* employees do not own any aspect of the organization for which they work and cannot use anything associated with their employment for personal gain. In addition, activities in the workplace are physically separate from those at home.

- *An employee's position in an organization reflects their knowledge, capability and expertise:* appointment to each position depends on assessment of how well an employee performs and fixed salaries are associated with each post.

According to Weber, all large-scale modern organizations are bureaucratic and, the more they increase in size, the more bureaucratic they become. He argued that the expansion of bureaucracy is inevitable in modern societies because bureaucratic authority in the only way of coping with the administrative requirements of large-scale social systems. Weber often compared bureaucracies to sophisticated machines operating on the principle of **rationalization**, whereby all procedures are precisely calculated and are systematic. However, both he and others who have followed him have recognized that bureaucracies can be dysfunctional. Among the criticisms made is that they have resulted in depersonalizing, dull, controlling jobs which stifle employees' innovation and creativity.

On another level, bureaucracies have been seen as a threat to democracy. Central databases now allow them to hold enormous amounts of information about us (e.g. income and employment details, credit ratings and criminal records). This is not only invasive in relation to our personal lives but also gives bureaucracies the power to engage in surveillance activities (Weber 1997; Giddens 2009).

Despite such criticisms, Weber's ideas are still influential today and can help explain many of the features of our healthcare system. As a large-scale organization, the NHS can be analysed in terms of its bureaucratic characteristics. Examples are as follows.

- **Hierarchical control and specialization of tasks:** ever since it was founded, the structure of the NHS has comprised several tiers with a clear line of command and delineation of tasks between and within each tier. This structure has been subjected to numerous changes.

- **Formal and well-developed record-keeping systems:** this is exemplified through various initiatives which have been introduced within the NHS such as the National Programme for Information Technology (NPfIT). Among its many functions is the creation of 'an electronic care records service providing each patient with an integrated electronic record of every health and social care event they experience . . . and a picture archiving and communication system, to make possible the display, distribution and storage of digital medical images' (Talbot-Smith and Pollock 2006: 23). Another initiative is the establishment of the Health and Social Care Information Centre (HSCIC). This is responsible for collecting and analysing data across the health and social care systems in England and disseminating the information as required.

- **Fixed salary scales:** there are many groups of staff within the NHS workforce. These include administrative and clerical staff, ancillary and maintenance staff, laboratory technicians, GPs, nurses, midwives, health visitors, consultants and hospital doctors. They are appointed using specific selection criteria and the different groups have their own pay structures and agreed conditions of service (Talbot-Smith and Pollock 2006; Walshe and Smith 2007).

Healthcare organizations as systems

The fact that employees are embedded in a complex network of other workers is implicitly acknowledged in the above discussion about healthcare organizations as bureaucracies. The systems theory of organizations has been applied to this aspect of healthcare. This theory focuses on the way different parts of organizations interact and work together. It is dominated by the **structural functionalist** approach which is a mixture of the structural perspective and the functionalist approach. As discussed in Chapter 1, structural theories maintain that social structures constrain our experiences and that individuals have very little autonomy in society. More specifically, they stress that our behaviour, values and attitudes are largely a response to rules prescribed by the organizations, processes and structures which exist in our society as well as the groups to which we belong. The functionalist approach has been referred to many times in this book and its conceptualization of society as a system made up of different, interlocking parts, each of which has its own function and role, and which together create stability and order, will be familiar to you. Structural functionalism analyses the structure of society as self-maintaining social systems in which various social institutions perform specific functions by *shaping* individual behaviour to ensure the smooth operation of society as a whole (Cuff *et al.* 2006; Boddy 2008).

The key concepts within the systems theory of organizations are sub-systems, roles and role conflict. Each of these is now discussed in relation to healthcare organizations.

Sub-systems

Systems theory maintains that organizations are made up of a set of interdependent parts or sub-systems; all contribute towards the organization's survival. Most healthcare organizations can be divided up into sub-systems by occupational groups. For instance, the sub-systems in an antenatal clinic are:

- consultants;

- junior medical staff;

- midwifery staff;

- clerical staff;

- pregnant women;

- relatives of pregnant women.

According to systems theory, all are working towards the stated goals of the antenatal clinic which are to screen the total population of pregnant women it is responsible for, to select high- and low-risk groups, and to carefully monitor high-risk groups. If an individual's commitment to these stated goals declines, the performance of other individuals in the sub-system may decline and the overall performance of the organization will be negatively affected as all sub-systems are interdependent.

However, systems theory has been criticized for ignoring the extent to which the goals and attitudes of staff working in an organization can differ from the goals of the organization itself. For instance, clerical staff may informally disagree with the administrative procedures for processing the care of pregnant women and adapt these procedures to suit the way they think is best. The development of the concept of **informal organization** to account for the coexistence of informal and formal cultures within organizations has been seen to support this criticism (Blau 1963; Boddy 2008).

Roles

Central to systems theory is the idea that individuals occupy roles within organizations. Most of us act out **multiple roles** in our lives because we adopt different roles in different settings. For instance, a female hospital doctor can also be a mother, wife, daughter, car driver, patient and taxpayer in other settings. The term **role set** is used to describe the array of roles that an individual will confront while taking a particular role. Systems theory has shown that a doctor's role set can comprise over 100 role relationships. Simplified versions of two role sets for a female doctor are shown in Figure 11.1. These illustrate the different role relationships associated with personal and professional roles, and how role sets can be used in the analysis of roles in organizations.

The use of the concepts of 'role' and 'role sets' in systems theory tends to give the impression that roles are prescribed by the rules of the organization and that people carry them out with minimum discretion. This has been challenged by other organizational theorists who argue that systems theory does not allow for the fact that individuals create and modify their roles according to their own interpretation and in relation to the way that others interpret their own roles in their role set. This has been referred to as **role-making** and has been found to occur particularly in healthcare organizations.

Figure 11.1 Role sets for a female doctor

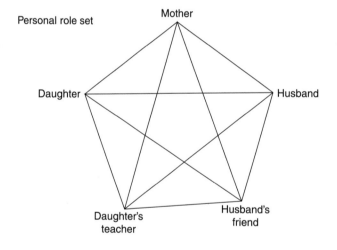

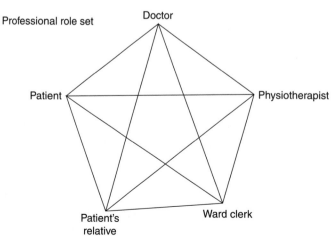

Role conflict

Role conflict is the third main concept in systems theory. It occurs when incompatible expectations are held about a role and can take two forms. One is **inter-role conflict**, which individuals experience when two roles they hold simultaneously conflict. The degree of conflict reflects the strength of attachment to the two roles. Inter-role conflict is illustrated in the case study presented in 'Susan's story' below. The second is **intra-role conflict** which occurs when we disagree with traditional beliefs about one of our roles. An example of intra-role conflict that has been cited is that of a male nurse who may have problems reconciling the role of a man with the role of a nurse, as a feminine approach has been traditionally seen as integral to this role (Parsons 1964; Walshe and Smith 2007). The following case study illustrates inter-role conflict and describes how Susan, an intensive care unit nurse and a mother, experienced such conflict when she had to work on the afternoon of her 2-year-old's birthday party.

Case example: Susan's story

Susan loved her job as an intensive care unit nurse and had undertaken a range of post-registration courses to increase her expertise and skills. As a result she was highly qualified as well as highly respected in the hospital in which she worked. Although she had delayed motherhood, when her son was born she was surprised at the intensity of her feelings for him and how much she enjoyed being a mother. When she returned to work on a part-time basis, she hated leaving him. However, she still enjoyed her job and knew that if she were to give it up to be a full-time mother, all the time and effort she had put into her successful career to date would be wasted and there would be implications for her earning potential in the future.

She managed to organize her rota to fit in with family events, but a week before her son's second birthday, she realized that she was down to work on that day and the rota could not be changed at such short notice. Both sets of grandparents had arranged to come for a 'birthday tea' and her husband had also booked annual leave for the day. She had no choice but to go ahead with the birthday party as planned even though she could not be there. On the afternoon of the party, although she tried to perform her professional role to her usual high standard, she constantly thought of the celebrations at home. She found herself constantly clock-watching and burst into tears when she telephoned her husband during her break. Each task she undertook became a hurdle that had to be overcome before she could go and fulfil the role she really wanted to on that day – being the mother of her son.

Systems theory helps us to understand the way that the different parts of a healthcare organization interact and work together so that it runs smoothly and objectives are achieved. Nonetheless, as we have seen, it is the critics of this theory who highlight some of the reasons why this smooth operation can be disrupted and hence pose questions about some of its underlying assumptions.

Healthcare organizations and surveillance

There are also postmodernist interpretations of healthcare organizations. These have been produced mainly as a result of the work of Foucault (1973), which has been used to explain why hospitals specifically can be sources of power and control. Foucault argues that every modern organization subjects those within it to surveillance. He gave this term a specialized meaning in relation to organizations in that he saw surveillance as a form of scrutiny and observation to ensure compliant behaviour. In addition, he maintained that surveillance does not necessarily depend on the physical proximity of those carrying out the surveillance to those who are being watched. Through the operation of surveillance in this way, organizations can control the behaviour of all those who enter them.

In hospitals, surveillance can take several forms. One is by virtue of their design, which features highly impersonal space with large open areas. In a Foucauldian analysis, the way hospitals are designed is not for purely utilitarian purposes, such as ensuring patients are not at risk, but so that their behaviour can be observed to see if it complies with organizational rules. The design of space in hospitals in this way simultaneously enables staff to be observed and assessments of their performance made. The design is therefore a 'power-laden process' (Evans *et al.* 2009: 717) as it creates a form of control whereby people conform to the authority and power within a hospital setting. Another form of surveillance in hospitals is the holding of personal information (referred to above) on patients and staff, whether this is in electronic or written form. Such data represents a form of control for patients as it can influence the nature and quality of their care, and for staff it can be used to monitor behaviour and promotion potential (Foucault 1973, 1979; Evans *et al.* 2009).

A strength of Foucault's analysis is that it acknowledges that despite surveillance, there is much subversion of authority and control in healthcare organizations. This is supported by others who cite Goffman's work on patients in homes for the elderly and disabled to illustrate such subversion (Goffman 1968b). This showed that although patients were subjected to continual surveillance, many did create an identity for themselves which gave them autonomy and power. For instance, some became leaders of groups of other patients within the institution.

Activity 11.2

Now test yourself on your understanding of the theoretical approaches to healthcare organizations above. Using the grid below, place the concepts listed under the correct approach. A completed version of this activity can be found in the 'Activity feedback' chapter on page 234.

Concepts

Structural functionalist; role set; specialization of tasks; power; hierarchical control; design of space; intra-role conflict; rationality; observation; multiple roles; ideal type.

Weber's theory of bureaucracy

Systems theory

Foucauldian analysis of healthcare organizations

Changes in healthcare organizations

The NHS was founded in 1948 and was based on the principle of providing free healthcare at the point of delivery to everyone. Its comprehensive and universal services were funded out of general taxation. Ever since its foundation there have been major reorganizations. Between 1948 and 1980 these involved more of an evolution of the original system and the main focus was on 'rational planning, aimed at redistributing healthcare resources and services across the country on the basis of need and ensuring efficiency through integration. The aim was to make the health service as universally available and reliable as the postal service' (Talbot-Smith and Pollock 2006: 3).

Although some of the accompanying legislation appeared far-reaching, the organizational structure of the NHS remained intact and its principles largely uncompromised. The changes introduced over the past three decades are more fundamental and effected the transition of a publically owned and publically funded system of health to a healthcare 'market'. The backdrop to these changes was the drive to reduce the cost of publically provided health care. The shift to a 'mixed economy of healthcare' which involved an increase in the provision of healthcare by independent sector organizations, as discussed in the first section, in part reflected the efforts that were been made to contain costs during this period. The rest of this section summarizes other key policy trends in the transition to a market in healthcare delivery. While the focus is on the NHS, as this has been the main target of reforms, the independent sector is referred to as appropriate.

Outsourcing

This is the 'contracting out' of non-clinical services. Initially it involved services such as hospital cleaning, catering and laundering, but more recently it has been extended to include information technology. While some of the outsourced services were turned into very competitive businesses, outsourcing has been of limited financial benefit to the NHS. There are also those who argue that any of the modest savings made have been at the expense of quality, as evidenced by concerns about the standard of hospital cleaning in recent years.

Internal markets

In the early 1990s budgets were allocated to GPs and district health authorities (DHAs) to purchase services for patients from hospitals and community units who 'would supply services and earn revenue on the basis of service contracts' (Baggott 2004: 107). In addition to creating markets within the NHS these reforms divided the NHS into 'purchasers' and 'providers'. This is referred to as the 'purchaser–provider' split. The internal market subsequently evolved and broadened. Trusts replaced fundholders and the private healthcare sector was now included. Although many different models now exist and terms such as 'commissioning', 'commissioning services' and 'service agreements' have replaced those that were originally used, it cannot be denied that the introduction of market-based delivery systems has been a significant influence on the organization of healthcare in the UK.

Public Finance Initiative

This aimed to encourage the use of private capital to build and run NHS facilities such as hospitals and intermediate care services. Under the Public Finance Initiative (PFI), private companies design, construct, finance and – with the exception of clinical services – operate facilities over a set number of years (the average is 30) for an annual fee. The advantage of this initiative is that it increases overall resources in the NHS while avoiding increasing taxes and public borrowing. It is also a way of bringing private sector managerial and commercial skills into the NHS to improve cost-effectiveness. Although the scope of PFI was extended under New Labour, it remains a controversial initiative; critics have highlighted that it has led to a reduction of spending on clinical staff and have questioned whether PFI schemes are actually value for money.

Managerialism

Since the 1980s, industrial models of management gradually replaced the administrative approach to management that previously characterized the NHS. This approach involved a consensus system of management whereby decisions were made by multidisciplinary teams comprising doctors, nurses and administrators. The move to managerialism can be traced back to the Griffiths Report in 1983 which suggested that general managers were appointed at each level to replace these consensus teams.

As a result of subsequent legislation, managerial control, performance management, target-setting and budgetary ceilings were emphasized. Professionals, and particularly doctors, within the NHS saw these initiatives as a challenge to their professional autonomy and there was considerable resistance to their implementation. Consequently, there was a plethora of initiatives to enhance management control of professionals. However, the extent of their success is much debated with many pointing to the lack of trust that now exists between management and the health professions and the way management control can repress best clinical practice. Furthermore, countervailing forces were at work. One of these was the rise of consumer power, as demonstrated below.

Consumerism

The application of consumerism to healthcare was initially criticized on the grounds that the consumption of medical care is very different from the consumption of other goods, such as food and clothing. For instance, people are not expected to pay for medical care directly, but pay indirectly through taxation, and choice is restricted. Nonetheless, consumerism was a major influence on a range of policies from the 1980s onwards. One of the justifications of the internal market was it would allow more opportunities for the views and preferences of the users to shape the culture of the NHS, as opposed to being solely determined by professionals. Other initiatives have more overtly involved patients and users in decision-making through consultation and lay representation on NHS boards. An example of the former was the establishment of Patient and Public Involvement Forums for each Primary Care or Hospital Trust in 2003. The role of these forums was to listen to people's concerns about local services, and represent their views to the relevant Trust. There were also developments, such as NHS Direct and NHS walk-in centres, which increased individual choice and were seen to demonstrate the new customer-focused approach within the NHS.

Although the rise of consumerism in the NHS certainly empowered patients in general, it had some negative consequences. There is evidence that it has contributed to the growing culture of complaints and litigation which not only undermines the morale of health professionals but has also led to a more defensive practice of medicine where the emphasis is on the safest as opposed to the best options for patients.

Quality management

Before the move to a market-based system, quality and efficiency were assured through internal regulation. Direct management and supervision were used throughout the NHS, and the clinical professions were also subject to regulation by their professional bodies. Subsequently, there was an emphasis on external regulation and extensive systems of financial incentives and penalties, audits, national standards and performance ratings were put in place. Various bodies were set up, such as the Healthcare Commission and the Care Quality Commission, to oversee the enforcement of standards in both public and private healthcare provision. As the transition to a healthcare market proceeded, the role of external regulatory systems increased (McLaughlin *et al.* 2002; Baggott 2004; Dixon-Woods 2005; Kessler *et al.* 2006; Talbot-Smith and Pollock 2006; Martin 2008; Asthana and Campbell 2009; Zigmond 2009; Cordella and Willcocks 2010).

Further changes are imminent with the extension of **personalization** from social care into healthcare. Personalization had cross-party support and is seen as being 'the cornerstone of public services' and its main objectives are that 'every person who receives support, whether it is provided by statutory services or funded by themselves, will be empowered to shape their own lives and the services they receive in all care settings' (Department of Health 2008e). Key initiatives are direct payments, individual budgets and the *in Control* programme. The strategic shift to personalization in social care has led to a transformation of the social care system (Hatton *et al.* 2008; Hiscock and Stirling 2009). This policy agenda is currently being adopted within certain areas of healthcare; personal health budgets, based on individual budgets in social care, are being piloted. The *in Control* programme was also extended into health in 2008. One of the outcomes is that 37 PCTs and their partner local authorities are exploring how the *in Control* social care model can best be adopted within the NHS (Department of Health 2008e; Hatton *et al.* 2008; Edwards and Waters 2009).

These latest developments will clearly be significant. Time will tell whether they are deemed to be a successful phase in the history of healthcare organization. Unfortunately, at the moment, despite rapid and persistent changes, costs continue to increase and our healthcare system is rarely out of the news because of its alleged failings, such as the inefficient use of resources and compromises made over the quality of care.

Activity 11.3

These are extracts from two recent newspaper articles about healthcare in the NHS and in the private healthcare sector. Read them through and then think about the questions that follow. Points relevant to each question are discussed at the 'Activity feedback' chapter on page 234.

Article 1

Paying for private medical treatment does not guarantee a safer or better quality of care than using the NHS, the Health Inspectorate said yesterday in its first analysis of the performance of the independent sector. The Healthcare Commission found only 50% of the private hospitals and clinics in England and Wales met all the required minimum standards when they were inspected in the 2005–06 period, compared with 49% of NHS trusts. About 15% of the independent providers failed on at least three tests of quality and safety. NHS trusts had to comply with more standards and their comparable failure rate was 19%. The most frequent lapses in both sectors included lack of systematic monitoring of treatment provided, poor standards of staff training and inadequate procedures to minimise risk of infection. About 14% of pregnancy termination clinics in the private and voluntary sector failed to deal with the infection issue properly.

(Carvel 2006)

Article 2

Research that ranks every general hospital in England against a range of safety measures has named 12 NHS hospital trusts judged to be 'significantly underperforming'. This is despite the fact that last month the Care Quality Commission, the health service regulator, judged overall care at eight of the trusts to be good or excellent. Today's study by Dr Foster, an NHS partner organisation that collates and analyses healthcare data, also highlights 27 trusts with unusually high death rates. Almost 5,000 more patients in their care died in the past year than was expected. Revelations of such widespread safety failings will send shockwaves through the NHS, already reeling from scandals at two trusts last week. Poor nursing care, filthy wards and hundreds of unnecessary deaths were exposed at Basildon and Thurrock University NHS Hospitals Foundation Trust, and the chair of the NHS trust in Colchester was fired. Now the new data proves that key safety failings are occurring in 11 more hospital trusts across England . . . Ministers want to know why seven in particular have had persistently high death rates over five years.

(Asthana and Campbell 2009)

(1)   Having read the articles, do you think patients are more likely to receive better care if they use private healthcare?

(2)   Which regulatory bodies are referred to the articles?

(3)   What problems seem to beset both private healthcare and the NHS despite all the recent moves to improve and monitor quality?

Conclusions

This chapter has shown that the delivery of formal healthcare is highly complex, involving a web of relationships between organizations in the public and the private sectors. Improving healthcare organization is thwarted at many different levels. As demonstrated, organizations themselves have many different features which can be interpreted in a variety of ways. In addition, they can impact negatively on those within them and others in society. Thus, the very organizations delivering healthcare defy full understanding, and their reliability is questionable when it comes to the successful implementation of policies. Moreover, initiatives which have been introduced have proved to have unintended consequences with the result that their overall outcomes have been perceived as less than positive by many. The search for innovative and creative ways of addressing the problem of healthcare organization therefore continues.

Many of the discussions in this chapter and in Chapter 10 have made implicit and explicit reference to health professionals. These people are central to the delivery of healthcare and it is on their expertise we so depend for our health and well-being. Therefore, having addressed the key issues about the delivery and organization of informal and formal healthcare in relation to the social aspects of health, we will now complete this section of the book by exploring the role that health professionals play in the delivery of healthcare in the next and penultimate chapter.

Key points

- Organizations are now a central feature of all societies and influence most aspects of our working and non-working lives.

- While the NHS is a classic example of an organization, there are also individual healthcare organizations both within and outside the NHS.

- Theoretical approaches to healthcare organizations have focused on different aspects of these as organizations. For instance, there have been theoretical analyses of healthcare organizations as bureaucracies, as systems and of the extent to which they subject those who work within them to surveillance.

- Ever since it was founded in 1948, the NHS has been subjected to major reorganizations. Since the 1980s, it has been in transition to a healthcare market. Examples of policy initiatives that have been introduced are outsourcing, internal markets, the PFI, managerialism, consumerism and quality management.

Discussion points

- What are the advantages and disadvantages of a 'mixed economy of care'?

- Which theory do you think provides the most compelling interpretation of healthcare organizations and why?

- Do you think any of the changes described in in this chapter have more significance for the future direction of healthcare organizations than others?

Suggestions for further study

- Talbot-Smith and Pollock (2006) provide a highly readable account of the organizations within the NHS and the changes to our state healthcare system.

- To keep up with very recent developments within healthcare organization and management, see the *Health Service Journal* (www.hsj.co.uk), the *British Journal of Health Care Management* (www.bjhcm.co.uk) and the Department of Health website (www.dh.gov.uk).

- Take a look at the BUPA (www.bupa.co.uk) and Nuffield Health (www.nuffieldhealth) websites if you want to get a better understanding of the types of treatment and healthcare provided by private organizations.

- For a more in-depth exploration of theoretical approaches in relation to healthcare organizations, it is worth browsing through a recently published management textbook, such as Walshe and Smith (2007) or Boddy (2008).

Health professions

Health care professions work within a complex web of power relations.
(Taylor and Hawley 2010: 150)

Introduction

The above quotation implies that the medical profession has the power to determine the organization and delivery of healthcare. However, as we saw in the previous chapter, since the 1980s there have been challenges to the medical profession's autonomy. This chapter aims to explore an issue which underpins the delivery of healthcare – the meaning and extent of professional power. This important topic within the study of the social apsects of health requires an understanding of the concept of a 'profession', the social processes involved in people becoming professionals and the recognition of certain occupations as professions. Therefore, these issues are addressed in the first part of the chapter. It then focuses on health professions themselves and examines the professionalization of medicine and other health professions, as well as the different ways that professional power has been found to operate in healthcare. Relevent theoretical perspectives, such as functionalism, symbolic interactionism and Marxist theory are incorporated into the discussions.

Professions

When asked what a **profession** is we can all think of examples such as lawyers, doctors, teachers and social workers. However, to actually define a 'profession' is more problematic because a variety of different characteristics come to mind and there are also different types of occupational group that can be regarded as professions. Indeed, professions have been analysed using different approaches since the early twentieth century, each of which has been in turn subject to major criticism. Analyses of professions in terms of their characteristics provide the most useful approach. Therefore the main characteristics of professions that have been identified in the literature are set out in the first part of this section. The extent to which some of these overlap is further evidence of the definitional problems that have been experienced. The second part briefly looks specifically at health practitioners in relation to some of the more general points made about professionals.

Professional characteristics

The extent to which an occupational group is judged as being a 'profession' or not depends on whether it has certain characteristics and meets certain criteria, as follows.

- **Possess a body of highly specialized knowledge:** professions gain their position largely from their possession of 'credentials' – degrees, diplomas and other formal qualifications – which are only awarded after prolonged and systematic training. Thus they possess a body of highly specialized knowledge. They add to this by research during the course of their professional careers.

- **Formally control the education and training of its members and the application of the relevant body of specialist knowledge:** professional occupations have control over who is trained because they are actively involved in the selection of candidates, what is taught and how that knowledge is used. In Weberian terms, this is social closure (see Chapter 3) and is seen as the way that professions preserve their prestige. Although professional training is usually provided by universities, it has traditionally taken place in institutions that may be isolated from the rest of higher education (such as medical schools and law schools). As these are controlled by the profession itself, senior members are able to mould new members into the professional image more easily.

- **Have a monopoly of their field of work:** to practise, professionals require some sort of registration (usually with a professional body – see below) and only those with such registration are allowed to be employed in their areas of work.

- **Have considerable autonomy:** this has been described as the way a profession has 'control over the determination of the substance of its own work' (Friedson 1988: xv) because its members can organize their work, define it and develop it. They also have more discretion in how they carry out some of their tasks and more freedom from external monitoring than non-professional occupations.

- **Play a positive part in society:** professional occupations have a service orientation – for example, education, healthcare and legal protection. Hence their occupational roles involve making contributions to society that are publically recognized as being positive. Several theorists have focused on other reasons why it can be argued that professions contribute positively to society. One of these was Durkheim, who argued that professions were cohesive communities based on shared values, and that systemic solidarity flows from their dense economic and non-economic relations. The social and moral integration this provides for the social system fulfils the important role of the family and traditional community which has diminished as a result of the rapid changes that have taken place in society (see Chapter 10). Therefore, professions play a vital role in supporting social structures. This theme of the ways in which the professions contribute functionally to society can also be seen in the functionalist approach. When discussing the experience of acute illness in Chapter 6 we explored Parsons' concept of the 'sick role' and how he saw the medical profession as 'policing' entry into, and exit from, that role. He also argued that illness is a form of deviance, which if left unregulated would threaten the stability of society. Therefore, according to this approach the medical profession's role in society is as an agent of social control.

- **Adhere to a code of ethics:** this prohibits the exploitation of clients and regulates intraprofessional relations.

- **Enjoy high status in society and high rewards:** professionals are in highly skilled sectors of the labour market and, as a consequence, have a prestigious position in society. They are also usually able to command more lucrative salaries than other occupations which means they can adopt more distinctive lifestyles. Moreover, professions are middle-class occupations whose members are in the top two social classes.

- **Tend to be the focus of their members' self-identity and loyalty:** for example, they may socialize together and often have a sense of vocation (Parsons 1964, 1975; Friedson 1988; Durkheim 1992; MacDonald 1995; Segre 2004; Taylor and Hawley 2010).

Even though there may be disagreement about the exact nature of these characteristics, they do ensure that professions are among the more privileged occupations in the labour market. This is because the nature of their work involves intellectual challenge and interest, and their monopoly in terms of their exclusive ownership or control of the supply of particular economic goods or services ensures a measure of job security. Their autonomy gives them relative freedom from supervision, their code of ethics gives them a feeling that they are helping others and their status provides respect and in some cases relative affluence.

Health professionals

The close alignment between its characteristics and those mentioned above has meant that the medical profession has often been used paradigmatically when theorizing about professions within the study of the social aspects of health. However, there is now a wide range of groups of people working within healthcare who are regarded as professions. These include nurses, midwives, physiotherapists, occupational therapists, radiographers, speech therapists, biomedical scientists, pharmacists, health visitors, medical social workers, chiropractors, counsellors, podiatrists, optometrists, orthoptists, osteopaths, dieticians, arts therapists and psychologists. Like the medical profession, these professions also have their own professional bodies, their own codes of professional practice and powers of self-regulation. Professional bodies include the Royal Pharmaceutical Society, the College of Optometrists, the British Association of Counselling and Psychotherapy, the General Chiropractic Council, the General Osteopathic Council, the Nursing and Midwifery Council, the Health Professions Council and the British Psychological Society. Together with that of the General Medical Council, examples of two of the codes of practice of these other healthcare professions are set out in Table 12.1. This enables you to observe the similarities between their approaches to their professional codes of conduct (Baggott 2004; Talbot-Smith and Pollock 2006).

Table 12.1 Codes of practice in the health professions

General Medical Council *Good Medical Practice: Duties of a Doctor Registered with the General Medical Council*	Patients must be able to trust doctors with their lives and health. To justify that trust you must show respect for human life and you must: 1 Make the care of your patient your first concern 2 Protect and promote the health of patients and the public 3 Provide a good standard of practice and care 4 Treat patients as individuals and respect their dignity 5 Work in partnership with patients 6 Be honest and open and act with integrity Never abuse your patients' trust in you or the public's trust in the profession (www.gmcuk.org/guidance/good_medical_practice/duties_of_a_doctor.asp)
The Royal Pharmaceutical Society of Great Britain *Code of Ethics for Pharmacists and Pharmacy Technicians*	The *Code* is founded on seven principles which express the values central to the identity of the pharmacy professions. The seven principles and their supporting explanations encapsulate what it means to be a registered pharmacist or pharmacy technician. Making these principles part of your professional life will maintain patient safety and public confidence in the professions. As a pharmacist or pharmacy technician you must: 1 Make the care of patients your first concern 2 Exercise your professional judgement in the interests of patients and the public

	3 Show respect for others
	4 Encourage patients to participate in decisions about their care
	5 Develop your professional knowledge and competence
	6 Be honest and trustworthy
	7 Take responsibility for your working practices.
	(hwww.rpsgb.org.uk)
Nursing and Midwifery Council *Standards of Conduct, Performance and Ethics for Nurses and Midwives*	The people in your care must be able to trust you with their health and well-being. To justify that trust, you must: ■ Make the care of people your first concern, treating them as individuals and respecting their dignity ■ Work with others to protect and promote the health and well-being of those in your care, their families and carers, and the wider community ■ Provide a high standard of practice and care at all times ■ Be open and honest, act with integrity and uphold the reputation of your profession As a professional, you are personally accountable for actions and omissions in your practice and must always be able to justify your decisions. You must always act lawfully, whether those laws relate to your professional practice or personal life. Failure to comply with this code may bring your fitness to practise into question and endanger your registration. (www.nmc-uk.org/aArticle.aspx?ArticleID=3056)

It is argued that the emergence of these new professions is due to a change in the power base in medicine. This is a major issue that needs exploring in this chapter but, before we can do so, we need to gain a better understanding of professionals themselves and look at two more key concepts: professional **socialization** and **professionalization**. Despite the change in approach to profession-alism in healthcare, much of the seminal work about health professionals has focused on the medical profession and this is reflected in the discussions that follow about these two concepts.

Professional socialization

Each profession has a distinctive identity and members of a profession possess a strong sense of this. The nature of the characteristics identified in the first section clearly indicates that becoming a professional involves more than the acquisition of knowledge. So how are lay people turned into 'professionals'? There has been much written in sociology about the social processes involved in acquiring a professional identity using the analogy of socialization.

Early work focused on the socialization of medical students and this influenced later work on health professionals' socialization. Although there are differences in the perspectives used in this early work, the studies carried out can be credited with distinguishing between 'formal' and 'informal' socialization of professionals. The 'formal' aspects refer to the transmission of the formal, codified and examinable knowledge and skills required. 'Informal socialization' refers to the transfer of what are considered appropriate professional attitudes and behaviour and occurs in different ways, depending on which perspective is adopted. Most perspectives agree that the rigorous selection process by senior members in professional occupations means that only those who are considered to have not only the academic ability but the appropriate values are selected in the first place. After selection, the accounts of the informal socialization process vary in their explanations.

Merton *et al.* (1957) adopted a functionalist perspective. Their study involved interviewing a range of staff in medical schools. They found that in addition to the formal curriculum, which consisted of the knowledge considered necessary to be a doctor, there was an informal curriculum. This involved the passing on of the attitudes, values, beliefs and behaviour required to fulfil the role of doctor appropriately in society. The students' performance and progress in the formal curriculum was monitored through regular examinations. While there was no formal assessment of the students' performance and progress in the informal curriculum, the extent to which they adopted professional norms and values was noted by senior staff and did influence decisions that were made about the students. For example, if they were a borderline case in end of year exams, the extent to which they had demonstrated that their attitudes and behaviour were aligned with those of the medical profession influenced decisions taken as to their progress into the next year of study.

This view, with its emphasis on the internalization of appropriate norms and values in order to perform social roles has been criticized for presenting medical students as passive recipients of medical school culture. An alternative account was put forward by Becker *et al.* (1961) using a symbolic interactionist perspective. This depicted medical students as adopting an instrumental approach to achieving their goal of successfully graduating from medical school. Part of this entailed testing out others' perceptions of their behaviour and actively managing any conflict they personally experienced between the medical profession's norms and values and student culture. Strategies that the students used to avoid their lack of adherence to professional norms being detected, such as 'making out', were identified.

Subsequent studies have developed this idea that medical students are active social actors focusing on how they define their own reality through their interpretations of medical school and the medical profession. For instance, research has been conducted into how medical students go through a process of intensive adult resocialization as they repeatedly encounter situations during their training in which they experience conflict between lay and medical norms. As a result of working through their own reactions to these experiences, they gradually come to define the latter as being superior to the former. Other research has highlighted the way that medical schools are not wholly homogenizing institutions and there are variations in the degree to which different groups of medical students (such as male and female) are socialized into the medical profession (MacDonald 1995; Turner 1995; Saks 2000).

Activity 12.1

Which of the two approaches do you find most convincing? Revisit the sections on functionalism and symbolic interactionism in Chapter 1 to help you with this activity.

Relatively little research about the socialization of other health professionals exists. There are a few studies about nursing education and these reflect the tensions between professional and lay norms referred to above. Some have argued that socialization into nursing occurs in stages, which involves a progressive internalization of the self as a professional nurse. Others have identified the ways nursing students make choices about strategies they use to cope with disjunctures in norms they encounter during their professional socialization. The influences on these choices, such as healthcare reforms and social changes, have also been addressed (Davis 1975; Melia 1987; Mackintosh 2006; Brennan and McSherry 2007).

As mentioned when discussing the characteristics of professions in the previous section, professional training has traditionally taken place in institutionally separate schools within higher education, where students were trained for one profession only. However, there have been moves recently to integrate the education of health professionals and provide more interprofessional training. The move away from mono-professional education is likely to impact on the socialization of health professionals in the future (Thomas and While 2007; Lewitt *et al.* 2010).

Now that we have explored how people are made into professionals, let us see how a profession becomes recognized as such.

Professionalization

The concept of professionalization has been used to describe the complex and often political process by which occupational groups monopolize knowledge, take over other occupations' roles, expel and exclude competitors, and achieve the personal and social privileges for their members associated with the status of a profession. The focus on the medical profession in the study of health professions was discussed above. Indeed, much work on health professions from the 1960s to the 1980s concentrated on doctors before being extended to include other professions within healthcare in the 1990s. Hence this section will address the professionalization of the medical profession first and then move on to the more recent interest in the professionalization of other health professions.

The professionalization of the medical profession

The rise of the medical profession has been relatively recent. As explained in the Introduction to this book, prior to the mid-nineteenth century health professionals did not have a consistent educational background. Nor did they have much power or status. There were only a few hospitals and healthcare took place largely within the private domain and was carried out by women. While there were a few learned physicians from the sixteenth century onward, only the rich could afford to consult them. If a condition could not be dealt with in the private domain, most people used and paid for the services of a range of health practitioners whose medical training varied considerably and could be non-existent.

This plurality of health workers enabled patients to be selective and critical in their dealings with them. Treatment was a matter of bargaining over cost and diagnosis with their chosen healers. Furthermore, the sick person was seen as the central point of reference, and source of information and inspiration for the practitioner, who in turn had to listen to them because they were paying. Therefore at this point in time patients had the power.

There were several historical developments which then changed this. A major one was the rise of biomedicine which has dominated our thinking about health and disease for the last 150 years. As also explained in the Introduction, this makes extensive use of scientific knowledge in general and emphasizes scientific method and objectivity. An understanding of anatomy and physiology is of paramount importance to biomedicine. In addition, disease and sickness are seen as deviations from normal functioning, and health is conceptualized largely in mechanical terms, as a state where all parts of the body function 'normally'. Therefore, if you are sick or have disease, you are seen as needing to be returned to the medical definition of 'normal'.

The rise of biomedicine increased medical dominance because the training and knowledge required by medical practitioners now gave them greater power in relation to patients and other health practitioners. It also conferred 'expert status' upon them and helped to consolidate their position as an 'autonomous' and learned profession. Simultaneously, the patient's role changed; instead of being active, patients now had a passive role and were just objects of medical enquiry. As the new breed of medical practitioners needed a mass of patients to observe and treat to develop biomedical knowledge, these changes were also accompanied by the establishment of more hospitals. Hence patients were subjected to medical surveillance and segregation which further encouraged their docility and powerlessness.

There were other social, economic, political and legislative changes which gave doctors more power and contributed to their professionalization. Examples are as follows.

- Doctors were increasingly viewed as valuable agents of the state in the matter of segregating and regulating 'problem groups' in society (see Chapter 8).

- In 1858, the Medical Registration Act was passed. This gave medical practitioners control of medical education and specialist services. Only those who had passed through a recognized system of training were now allowed to join the professional register and call themselves 'qualified medical practitioners'. This gave them the status of a profession.

- There was more emphasis on medical surveillance of people's lives. For instance, the advent and acceptance of germ theory meant that the underlying causes of some diseases were seen as being the entry of micro-organisms into the body, which then multiplied and disrupted normal bodily function. This led to the medical profession advising patients on personal habits as well as personal and domestic hygiene and represented the beginning of the 'medicalization of life' (see Chapter 6).

- The establishment of the NHS in 1948 consolidated their power; the principle of professional autonomy was enshrined in the 1948 Act. Doctors were given a generous package of appointments, promotions and merit awards. Hospital doctors had disproportionate influence over resources and practices and GPs were self-employed and made their own decisions about standards and service. As we will see in the next section, despite attempts during subsequent restructurings and policy initiatives to reduce the power of doctors, they have managed to retain considerable professional influence over the making and enforcement of decisions because of their pivotal role in the diagnosis and treatment of patients.

During this process of professionalization, the medical profession gained many of the characteristics of a profession that were discussed earlier, such as the possession of a body of highly specialized knowledge, the requirement for registration to practise, and employment in highly skilled sectors of the labour market with an accompanying status and salary (Larkin 1993; Busfield 2000a; Saks 2000; Porter 2002).

The professionalization of other health professions

There are now many health professions. However, because medicine is viewed as the archetypal profession within healthcare, they have failed to achieve the same professional recognition as doctors. The explanations that have been put forward for this are accurately summarized in the following quotation.

Over the years the medical profession successfully monopolised important areas of work and was able to insulate itself from external interference. Within healthcare, medical knowledge has been the dominant form of expertise with doctors enjoying superior status relative to other professional groups. The medical profession has adopted two approaches: exclusion and incorporation.

(Baggott 2004: 41)

These strategies of exclusion and incorporation can be illustrated by using the example of nursing and its attempts to achieve professional parity with the medical profession. For many years the nursing profession has sought similar professional status but has failed to meet all the criteria that would render it equal and comparable to the medical profession. Indeed, in the 1950s and 1960s, nursing was classified as a semi-profession. Central to its professionalizing strategy was the transformation of nurse education in the 1990s, when nursing qualifications were replaced by degrees and these can only be obtained in universities.

Although this in part reflected real changes in the complexity of the tasks nurses were required to undertake, the philosophy behind this move was to stress nursing's unique contribution to patient care and to develop a distinctive knowledge base. As a result of a gradual extension of nursing tasks, nurses now increasingly undertake roles that were previously performed by doctors. This in turn has led to new clinical roles such as nurse practitioners, clinical nurse specialists and community matrons, for which additional training and education are required. The nurse–doctor relationship has also developed into one of greater equality (Harvey 1995; Apesoa-Varano 2007; Taylor and Hawley 2010). Nonetheless, nursing remains subordinate to the medical profession and this has been attributed to the strategy of incorporation. Nurses are still under medical jurisdiction and control because they are only 'permitted to occupy roles which doctors allow them to perform and operate under protocols, through accreditation or under conditions controlled by the medical profession' (Baggott 2004: 42). Furthermore, as long as doctors have overall accountability for patient care, nursing will retain its subordinate position because doctors will not want to relinquish their professional oversight (Friedson 1988; Denny 2005).

The dominance of the medical profession has been heavily criticized as being exclusive and elitist. It has been argued that a more inclusive view of what it is to be a professional is required – one that encompasses all professions within healthcare, particularly those new professions which place more value on reflective practice and multidisciplinary work in the interests of adapting to the diverse needs of patients (Fish and Coles 1998; Taylor and Hawley 2010).

Professional power in healthcare

Activity 12.2

Read through this scenario of involving the mother of a critically ill baby. Think about what it is says about medical power. Make a note of your thoughts and use the material presented in the rest of this section to help you analyse them further. Some suggestions about points you could have come up with are considered in the 'Activity feedback' chapter on page 235.

Lisa Stell's daughter, Katherine, was born in May 2008 at just 24 weeks. She survived and is doing well at home. But Lisa is now frustrated that the doctors and nurses did not involve her in the critical decisions about her child's care.

Katherine was very, very tiny when she was born – just one-and-a-half pounds – and was very poorly. She was bright red and shiny and looked like a baby bird that had fallen out of its nest. The first thing that shocked me came before Katherine was born, when a neonatal care nurse warned me that, if she wasn't breathing at birth, she wouldn't be resuscitated. Over the next 15 weeks, Katherine received pretty good medical care at three different hospitals. But throughout those 15 weeks I experienced a real 'doctors know best' attitude. I found out from reading her notes that she was being treated for sepsis, a potentially lethal infection, but no one had told me that. That knocked my trust in the doctors. I felt that I was a bystander. Other parents I spoke to were frustrated, too. Neonatal care doctors do a very difficult job saving children, and often have very little time. But they should realise that it's a very emotional and worrying time for parents.

(Campbell 2009)

Medical power and healthcare

As well as contributing to knowledge about the medical profession's power in relation to other health professions, the study of the social aspects of health has provided insights into how medical power manifests itself in other areas of healthcare. From the 1960s to the 1980s there was much interest in the hegemonic nature of this power and the ways in which it was exerted. The expansion of medical jurisdiction over an increasing range of human processes and behaviours as a result of medicalization and health surveillance is seen as one example of this (see Chapters 6 and 9). Another example is the doctor–patient relationship. Research carried out into this relationship at this time highlighted its inherent inequalities (see the case study below).

Case example: A visit to the GP in the 1960s

Margaret was 16 and was plagued with acne. Despite all her attempts to improve her skin with various over-the-counter lotions and potions from the chemist, she started to feel very despondent and did not want to go out with her friends. Her mother suggested accompanying her to the doctor. She refused her mother's offer but did make an appointment to go on her own. When she went into the consultation room, the GP looked up and demanded to know where her mother was. When Margaret replied that she had wanted to come on her own, the doctor lectured her on the fact that she was only 16 and should have brought her mother. This monologue ended with him saying, 'Well I suppose I had better look at you then.' His immediate response was to warn her that she would get scarring because of the severity of the problem. Margaret could feel herself becoming tearful but managed to control her feelings for a bit longer. Her GP then said he would give her a prescription and gave her a very brief explanation about how to use the medication. When she asked a question about the correct usage, he sighed loudlly and said, 'You really should have brought your mother – she would have understood and I wouldn't have to deal with these questions.' He handed her the prescription without making eye contact or answering her question. Margaret walked home in tears.

During consultations doctors often failed to take their patients' opinions seriously because they felt they were the ones with the medical knowledge and expertise. They gathered much information from patients without explaining why they were doing so, not giving them the opportunity to ask questions, and terminated the consultation when they wanted to end it. This 'doctor-centred approach' also included using specialized language which patients could not understand to create a 'competence gap' between them and their patients. Some doctors were found to use negative typifications, such as 'anxious mothers', who were described as not having 'the sense they were born with' (Roberts 1992: 119) in one study of doctors working in an accident and emergency department. Their apparent monopoly of knowledge in turn ensured and maintained their authority and power in the doctor–patient relationship (Byrne and Long 1976). Furthermore, the quality of care for particular groups, such as those with mental illnesses and minority groups, has been found to have been compromised because of the dynamics of the doctor–patient relationship (Rogers and Pilgrim 2003; Gatrell 2008).

Those analysing these findings about the doctor–patient relationship from a Marxist perspective have argued that it reflects the dominant ideology of capitalist society. The power of the medical profession resides in the fact that it is an agent of social control for the modern capitalist state. This is because it regulates sickness and contributes towards the productivity of capitalism by treating and returning workers to the workforce. According to this perspective, the medical profession also serves the interests of capitalism by ensuring that health and illness are conceptualized in individualistic terms and that the role of industrial capitalism in the social, environmental and occupational production of health and disease is ignored (Navarro 1978; Doyal and Pennell 1979).

These early views have been criticized for politicizing the role of doctors. Furthermore, they do not acknowledge the evidence of the power of other health professions in their relationships with patients. For instance, studies found that midwives routinely labelled and classified patients. Two stereotypes commonly used on labour wards were the 'well educated, middle-class NCT type'[1] and the 'uneducated working-class woman' (Green et al. 1990: 125). Asian patients were assumed to lack 'compliance with care and abuse of the service', to 'make a fuss about nothing' and lack 'normal maternal instinct' (Bowler 1993: 157).

The decline of medical power in healthcare?

In the 1990s, research into professional power in healthcare started to focus on the decline of the autonomy of the medical profession. Several reasons that have been put forward for this, such as policy initiatives that challenge medical autonomy and the emergence of new professions in healthcare have already been mentioned in passing in this chapter and in Chapter 11. The evidence about the decline of medical autonomy over the past two decades can be most usefully analysed by categorizing the challenges into three main groups.

- **Reforms to the healthcare system:** as we saw in Chapter 11, since the 1980s the NHS has undergone some fundamental changes which have included enhanced management control of the medical professional. As a consequence, the medical profession has not only been subjected to being 'managed' by professional managers but has also faced increased internal and external regulation and monitoring through, for example, compulsory audits of their work. Research has shown that many doctors feel that they have lost a great deal of their autonomy (Taylor and Hawley 2010).

- **Patient and user empowerment:** members of the public who use healthcare services are now more likely to challenge and question the medical profession. The emphasis on disease

[1] NCT is an abbreviation used in this study for National Childbirth Trust. It used to be criticized for its middle-class membership and focus.

prevention (discussed in Chapter 6) means that patients and service users are much better informed about medical issues than ever before. Access to the internet and greater press coverage of health and health needs in general have also contributed to the increase in patients' and service users' medical knowledge. However, the quality of the information provided by these two sources cannot necessarily be guaranteed and may induce uncertainty. There is also evidence that doctors ignore internet information produced by patients. Hence the extent to which patients are truly empowered by the information available to them has been questioned. On the other hand, internet discussion forums for those with particular health problems have been found to empower patients and users. This is because they 'foster **social capital** and social support' through 'emotional support, instrumental support – both formal and informal, and community building/protection' (Drentea and Moren-Cross 2005: 920) because they facilitate the establishment of social networks and the exchange of emotional and instrumental resources. These types of discussion group can also empower people to resist medical stigma and approaches – for example, groups that resist childhood vaccinations (Hardey 1999; Drentea and Moren-Cross 2005; Hobson-West 2007; Kivits 2009). As a result of the outcomes of the introduction of consumerism into healthcare (see Chapter 11) patients and users are more actively involved in decision-making in the NHS and there are more formalized complaints systems. Such developments have encouraged the public to be more assertive in their relationships with the medical profession and have led to an increase in complaints and malpractice allegations (Lupton 1998). The numbers of incidences of violence by patients towards doctors has also risen (Elston *et al.* 2002). Nonetheless, some studies suggest that despite the influence of consumerism on the doctor–patient relationship, patients do not consistently adopt 'consumerist' behaviour during consultations and their patterns of behaviour are simultaneously or variously 'consumerist' and 'passive' depending on the context (Lupton 1997). Moreover, a move from paternalistic to more egalitarian doctor–patient relationships has been identified. These involve adoption of 'patient-centred' strategies in which there is a better balancing of power and more collaborative interaction whereby the agreed course of action is contingent on the contributions of both participants (Lupton 1997; Stevenson *et al.* 2002; Pilnick *et al.* 2009).

- **Challenges from other health professions:** the way that many other professional groups have emerged within healthcare was discussed in the second and third sections of this chapter. While it was argued that their professionalization has not led to the same professional recognition as the medical profession, changes introduced as a result of their professionalizing activities and strategies have challenged and continue to challenge that profession. An example of a change that is likely to impact on medical dominance in the future is the move to interprofessional training. Other developments that have been identified as threatening medical dominance include the significant increase in the number of alternative medical practitioners and the way that some of these, such as chiropractors, acupuncturists and homeopathists, have been incorporated into the healthcare market. The coexistence of these accepted alternatives to biomedicine within biomedical practice has been referred to as **medical pluralism**. These alternative medical practices are strenghtening their institutional bases and, should the predicted growth in their popularity be realized, they will continue to contribute to the erosion of medical dominance (Dew 2000; Saks 2000, 2003).

As indicated, some of the reasons for the decline of the autonomy of the medical profession are ambiguous. This is reflected in the lively debates that have taken place about the real extent of this decline. On the one hand there are those who argue that the status of the medical profession has diminished and it is becoming deprofessionalized (Lupton 1998; Dixon 2007). These arguments are fuelled by the way the power of the medical profession has been severely assaulted by events in recent years that have demonstrated weaknesses in its ability to self-regulate (see below). Others argue that deprofessionalization is not the issue but that it is more a question of the replacement of traditional medical professional discourses by new discourses. Although the latter may reject many of the values attributed to the more traditional discourses, they do have the potential to enable less paternalistic forms of relationships with clients. Some of those who subscribe to this view maintain that there has been a move from 'old professionalism' to 'new professionalism'. Again, this is seen as a positive development because 'new professionalism' is not only less exclusive but is also applicable across the spectrum of professions within healthcare. Furthermore, it adopts a more democratic approach to relationships between patients and health professionals (Jones and Green 2006; Taylor and Hawley 2010).

Failures of the medical profession's powers of self-regulation

- 2001: the poor quality of heart surgery for children at Bristol Royal Infirmary.

- 2005: Dr Harold Shipman found guilty of murdering dozens of his patients.

- 2010: Dr Andrew Wakefield, whose research suggesting a link between MMR vaccinations and autism, caused vaccination rates to plummet and a consequent rise in measles, found to have acted unethically.

- 2010: Dr Howard Martin admitted he had acted out of 'Christian compassion' when he gave 18 terminally ill and elderly patients what proved to be fatal doses of painkillers.

Activity 12.3

(1) Do you think the examples of failure in the medical profession outlined above are evidence of deprofessionalization?

(2) If you do not think that deprofessionalization can account for them, what other explanations can be given?

Those who oppose these sorts of arguments about deprofessionalization and new discourses of professionalism maintain that the medical monopoly still exists and that it will continue to do so because of certain features central to the practice of medicine. One of these stems from the fact that medicine adopts socially defined understandings of disease and illness. Hence it is argued that medicine is an instrument of social control. Another is the doctor–patient encounter. This will always be an 'institution of social control' (Armstrong 2008: 29) because it essentially demands that patients reveal the secrets of their minds and bodies and acquiesce to invasive medical examinations and procedures (Foucault 1973; Armstrong 2008; Bradby 2009).

Activity 12.4

Now test yourself on the knowledge that you have gained from this chapter. Help is available in the 'Activity feedback' chapter on page 235.

(1) Which one of the following statements about professions is *most* accurate?
- Require training
- Possess a body of highly specialized knowledge
- Professional knowledge is static

(2) Health professionals
- Only work in healthcare settings? T/F
- Do not have professional bodies? T/F

(3) The 'informal socialization' of professionals refers to:
- The transfer of appropriate professional attitudes and behaviour

OR

- The transmission of the knowledge and skills required to be a professional

(4) Write down two developments that contributed to the professionalization of the medical profession.

(5) Complete the following sentence:

Central to nursing's professionalizing strategy has been the transformation of nurse education in the 1990s; nursing qualifications were replaced by_____and these can only be obtained in_____ .

(6) What are the three main factors that have contributed to the decline of medical dominance over the past two decades?

Conclusions

In the exploration of what it is to be and to become a professional in this chapter, we have seen how the medical profession has professionalized and has come to be viewed as epitomizing professionalism. The ways that it has exerted its power and continues to be the dominant profession within healthcare in spite of numerous social, cultural and political challenges to this power, has also been discussed. In so doing, the emergence of new health professions and some of the implications of this were addressed.

From the arguments and material presented, it is clear that the quote at the beginning of the chapter is correct in its assertion that the power of the medical profession within healthcare is still pervasive. However, there is evidence that the medical profession is increasingly aware of this and is actively working towards addressing the negative consequences of its power in some areas, such as its relationship with patients (Campbell 2009). Nonetheless, there is still much work to be done before it can be said that changes in the way that medical power operates maximize the contribution that the medical profession can make to the effective delivery of healthcare.

Key points

■ Analyses of professions in terms of their characteristics provide the most useful approach to their definition.

■ Although the medical profession has often been used paradigmatically when theorizing about professions, there is now a wide range of groups of people working within healthcare who are regarded as professionals.

■ The concept of socialization is crucial in explanations of the social processes involved in becoming a professional.

■ The concept of professionalization has been used to describe the complex and often political process by which occupational groups monopolize knowledge, take over other occupations' roles, expel and exclude competitors and achieve the personal and social privileges for their members associated with the status of a profession.

■ While medical power has been seen as hegemonic in nature, there is much evidence there has been a decline in medical autonomy over the past two decades.

Discussion points

■ How useful is the identification of the characteristics of professions in developing an understanding of such professions?

■ To what extent do you think healthcare professions can be equal?

■ What are the positive and negative consequences of the decline in medical autonomy?

Suggestions for further study

■ For an in-depth analysis of professions in relation to the medical profession, see Friedson's work.

■ Turner (1995) provides a thorough analysis of theoretical perspectives in relation to the health profession.

■ The work by Saks (2000, 2003) on professionalization and alternative professions is useful for further exploration of changes in medical power.

■ There are many articles on healthcare professions in journals, such as *Social Science and Medicine*, the *Sociological Review* and *Sociology of Health and Illness*. Those published in the 1990s are particularly useful if you are interested in the changes that have occurred in medical power.

Afterword

I am struck by how much the events of the day both reflect, and are profoundly changing, the process of globalisation.

(Ritzer 2010: xiii)

The chapters in this book have addressed a comprehensive range of contemporary issues within the subject area of the social aspects of health. In the Introduction, the growing emphasis on global influences on our health was mentioned. Examples given included pollution, climate change and environmental degradation. The impacts of globalization have also been referred to in several of the chapters – for instance, in Chapter 5 we saw how the UK is not alone in having an 'ageing society' as ageing populations are a global phenomenon. In Chapter 10 the ways that families are subject to social and cultural practices and changes, both in our society and globally, was discussed.

The implications of global issues for our health now have a much higher profile and the author of this book felt that it was not complete without a brief introduction to this topic. Therefore, this Afterword discusses some of the key areas in the rapidly growing body of literature on the global aspects of health.

Global inequalities in health

Globalization tends to harm the poorest people in the poorest countries. Little research was carried out into health in poorer countries until recently, but some stark differences between rich and poor countries have begun to emerge:

- life expectancy in sub-Saharan Africa is 50, whereas it is 78 in high-income countries – this equates to a difference of over 20 years;

- in poorer countries, more of the lifespan is spent living with a disability – 18 per cent compared to 8 per cent in richer counties;

- the majority of maternal deaths occur in developing countries, and mainly in Africa and South Asia (World Health Organization 2008; Bywaters 2009; Graham 2009).

The effects of globalization on health

The themes in the literature on the effects of globalization on health are as follows:

- **The power of the global media has led to the rise of new health problems:** an example of a new health problem that has emerged in response to the ubiquitous western image of beauty and glamour that is projected through the global media is the growth in the use of skin-lightening products in countries where the populations are predominately non-white. The nature of these products means that their prolonged use is leading to disfigurement, increased vulnerability to skin cancer and mercury poisoning. The latter is known to cause neurological and kidney damage and may lead to psychiatric disorders. Similarly, the alarming rise of dieting and eating disorders in non-western countries has been attributed to the same cause; it is now estimated that the incidence of eating disorders in Japan is on a par with that in the USA. Rises have also been reported among Zulu women

- **Food hazards:** the increase in the food trade means that disease-producing organisms can be transported rapidly from one continent to another. In addition, global competition has led to cost-cutting in food production which can pose a risk to health.

- **Spread of non-communicable diseases:** globalization has also influenced lifestyle choices – for instance, more sedentary lives and more fast food. One of the main consequences of this is the increase in obesity rates, not just in western countries such as the USA and UK, but also countries in the less developed parts of the world. In China, where overweight people are historically uncommon, the number of people who were obese rose from 10 to 15 per cent in the early part of this century. Even in sub-Saharan Africa where under-nutrition remains a problem for many, there has been an increase in the prevalence of obesity, notably among urban women. This trend leads to increases in disease such as heart disease, diabetes and cancer.

- **Spread of communicable diseases:** as a result of globalization there is more cultural interaction and movement around the world. This can have health implications on both an individual and a wider scale. With reference to the former, air circulation systems in aeroplanes mean that bacteria are spread, making the transmission of infections a risk when flying. On a larger scale, air travel was the key means by which SARS (severe acute respiratory syndrome) was spread from southern China to 30 other countries (8,422 cases and 916 deaths) and became an epidemic. Increase in movement around the world has also led to the development of sex tourism whereby individuals from wealthy countries sexually exploit those in poorer countries. Up to 25 per cent of those attending genito-urinary clinics are reported to have contracted their infections during sex when abroad (Harris and Seid 2004; Huynen *et al.* 2005; Commission on Social Determinants of Health 2008; Ritzer 2010).

The impact of climate on health

Changing climatic patterns have been found to impact on health in many different countries. Examples are as follows.

- The rapid increase in cases of food poisoning in the UK has been linked to our warmer weather.

- Extreme weather conditions affect health. For instance, a heatwave between July and August 2003 in France led to the death of 15,000 people in a matter of weeks. Storms, floods and droughts have also claimed the lives of many. Such changes also disrupt food production systems in countries already vulnerable to malnutrition, for instance in Africa and South Asia.

- The incidence of skin cancer in the UK quadrupled in British males between 1975 and 2001, tripled in British females and is increasing in most white populations worldwide.

- The reduction in the ozone layer is seen as one of the major causes of the doubling of the number of people in the UK suffering from cataracts between 2000 and 2010 (Marmot and Wilkinson 2006; Department of Health 2008f; Schrecker *et al.* 2008; Cancer Research 2010).

However, changes in global climatic patterns are not all negative – for example, the emerging trend of warmer winters in some countries has been argued to be contributory to a reduction in seasonal mortality peaks.

Further manifestations of globalization

Further manifestations of globalization are regularly being identified. One of these is **medical tourism**. This refers to the way that people in developed countries (such as the USA, Canada and

Western Europe) are increasingly seeking medical care in Asia and Latin America because of high healthcare costs, long waiting periods or lack of access to new therapies in their own countries. The potential risk to patients is currently a matter of concern and investigation (Hopkins *et al.* 2010).

Conclusions

The above discussions show that although a considerable amount of research has been carried out into implications of global issues for our health, much more is required. As mentioned in the Introduction to this book, the increase in research into the 'social aspects of health' has led to the acknowledgement of a much greater number of social influences on health. Global influences on our health are clearly going to be highly significant in the future study of the social aspects of health. Hence this Afterword ends with a few words of advice. Keep your eye out for the latest research and information about globalization. It's all around you – not just in the academic literature but on the television and in the press, and globalization will not only affect our health – it also has the potential to remake our lives and our world in many ways. By developing your knowledge in this way, you will ensure that your understanding of the social aspects of health does not stop here but keeps apace with changes in this important subject area.

Activity feedback

Chapter 1 Studying the social aspects of health

Activity 1.1

Sociology is the study of the human social world. It is not *social work*, although social workers do study sociology, their work is about finding practical solutions to social problems, such as housing, child protection and meeting care needs. Nor is sociology the *study of individuals* as it is psychology that does this. It is inaccurate to say that sociology is the *study of society* as it does not just focus on society alone. The statement that sociology is *the study of individuals and society* is very close to the correct answer but does not capture that it not only studies individuals and society but also their relationship *with* society. Hence the right response is that sociology is the study of the human social world because this conveys how it looks at individuals operating in the social world and the two-way relationship between the individual and society.

Activity 1.2

FEMINIST THEORY	CAUSE(S) OF INEQUALITIES BETWEEN MEN AND WOMEN	SOLUTIONS	CRITICISMS
Marxist feminism	Capitalism because it leads to women's exploitation in both the private domain of the home and family, and the public sphere of work. As a result women are exploited as reproducers and producers.	Abolish capitalism.	Over-prioritization of capitalism and not enough significance attributed to patriarchy.
Radical feminism	The fundamental biological differences between men and women cause men to physically and sexually dominate women. Women's oppression by men is inherent in patriarchal societies.	Women need to wrest control of their bodies and fertility from men. New technology can help eliminate some of the obstacles to achieving this freedom.	1 Lack of recognition of the variations in the interpretation of biological differences across time and between cultures.

			2 Not all gender relationships are characterized by oppression and exploitation.
			3 Despite all the changes in women's position in society over the past 50 years, there is no evidence to suggest that a matriarchal society would be preferable.
Liberal feminism	Women do not have the same legal, social, political, and economic rights as their male counterparts.	Campaign to remove all obstacles that prevent women from having the same rights as men.	Despite all the campaigning there is evidence that women still do not have equal rights in both the public and private spheres.

Activity 1.3

Marxist theory
Alienation, bourgeoisie, capitalism, economy of a society, exploitation, means of production, proletariat.

Feminism
Education system, equality of the sexes, oppression and exclusion of women from economic power and politics, patriarchy, socialization, women's subordination to men is 'natural'.

Functionalism
Central value system, consensual representation of society, cultural and social expectations, equilibrium, social roles, social order, society is like a biological organism, sub-systems.

Symbolic interactionism
Active social actors, analysis should begin with the individual, focus on the individual rather than society, human consciousness, individuals make their own reality, understand and interpret human action.

Postmodernism
Agency, impossibility of uncovering the truth, knowledge about the social world is constantly changing, lack of objectivity, post-industrial society, social construction.

Chapter 2 Gender and health

Activity 2.1

Here are some ideas about what is 'typically' associated with being male and female in our society.

Males	Physical strength, undertaking physically demanding work such as that in the construction industry, aggressiveness, toughness, risk-taking, being emotionally unexpressive and adventurous, playing football and rugby.
Females	Beauty treatments, wearing make-up, dresses, skirts and high heels, passivity, tenderness and caring roles, being emotionally expressive.

Activity 2.2

Here are the answers in case you didn't manage to find them in the text.

Women have a lower number of inpatient hospital stays than men	F
Women are twice as likely to suffer from depression than men	T
Women live around four years longer than men	T
Heart disease and cerebrovascular disease are a major cause of death among women	F
Men tend to find their work more alienating and stressful than women	T
Smoking rates are higher for women	F
Women are more physically active in every age group	F
Men are more likely to be obese than women	F
There is a general reluctance among men to report ill health and access healthcare services	T

Activity 2.3

Some of the problems of studying gender differences in health are as follows.

- Indicators of morbidity used.
- Differing interpretations of statistics.
- Changes in the economy.
- Changes in occupations.
- Changes in family structures.
- Developments in the provision of healthcare.

These sorts of problems highlight some of the reasons why the relationship between gender and health is subject to varying interpretations, as discussed in the final section of the chapter.

Chapter 3 Social class and health

Activity 3.2

Here are some suggestions about the main similarities and differences between Marx's and Weber's theories of class.

Similarities	Both argue that: ■ society is characterized by conflicts over power and resources; ■ class influences life chances.
Differences	The two models differ in relation to the following. ■ *Means of production:* Marx argued that the ownership of the predominant means of production within an economy is the basis of class relations. In contrast, Weber argued that class is not based solely on the ownership or non-ownership of the means of production. ■ *Number of classes:* Marx said there were two (although this was increased to three in later versions of his theory) whereas Weber said there were four classes. ■ *Relationship between classes:* Marx saw this as being based on exploitation and oppression to a much greater extent than Weber. This led to a divergence in their views on the relationship between classes in that Marx's view meant that he predicted a polarization of class relations. ■ *Social mobility:* for Marx, there was a clear boundary between the classes and the social position of those within the classes was assigned and unchangeable. In Weber's model, individuals can act to change their social position and hence social mobility is possible

Activity 3.3

These are examples of similarities:

■ there is a social gradient in health with those with lower social positions experiencing the worst health and those with the higher social positions experiencing the best health;

■ the same social gradient applies to mortality rates.

This extract also adds to our understanding of the relationship between social class and health in that it provides information about the way that those in lower social positions spend more of their shorter lives in poorer health. In addition, it indicates that poverty influences the relationship between social class and health. This is one of the influences on social class differences in health that is discussed in the next section of Chapter 3.

Activity 3.4

Some ideas to help you answer the questions in this activity are as follows.

(1) The evidence in the fourth section of the chapter showed that those in the higher social classes generally have better diets and lower obesity rates than those in the lower classes. The findings from the survey by Quorn referred to in this article indicate that some professionals now have poorer and more calorific diets and are therefore at greater risk of obesity.

(2) The current economic climate and the stress of having to address its implications is presented as one cause of the change in professionals' diets. Nonetheless, more individual explanations are hinted at in terms of individuals being personally responsible for their health-related behaviour. The juxtaposition of these two explanations in one short article illustrates the inconclusive nature of theoretical debates about the causes of social class differences in health-related behaviour. The theoretical explanations of these differences are the subject of the final section of this chapter.

Chapter 4 Ethnicity and health

Activity 4.3

Here are some points that will help you think about the question posed in this activity.

Evidence of lack of 'agency' and choice	■ We saw that Pakistani, Bangladeshi and black Caribbean people report the worst health. Hence belonging to a certain minority ethnic group is closely associated with poorer health in general. Furthermore, different groups are vulnerable to particular physical and mental illnesses. For instance, the prevalence of diabetes is five times higher among African-Caribbean and Asian communities than other groups in the UK. With reference to mental illnesses, the diagnosis of psychosis is seven times higher for black Caribbean people than white British, while the Chinese have the lowest diagnosis rates.
	■ The ways in which risks to the health of those in minority ethnic groups are mediated by processes over which they have limited immediate control was demonstrated in the third section of the

chapter. Examples include the factors that lead to poverty, such as the fact that overall unemployment rates for these groups are twice those for the total working age population and, when in employment, they face earnings disadvantages in the British labour market. One of the consequences is that their income poverty rates are, on average, twice as high as white British people. Some groups, such as Bangladeshis and Pakistanis, are far more vulnerable to income poverty than others. Similarly, minority ethnic groups in general are more likely to live in the poorest housing and in the most deprived areas, and to experience reduced access to the range of healthcare available.

Evidence of 'agency' and choice	There are indications of 'agency' and choice operating in the discussions of the risks to the health of those in minority ethnic groups in the third section of the chapter. ■ One of the factors identified as contributing to the high income poverty rates among minority ethnic groups is their low uptake of some benefits. It could be argued that applying for benefits to which you are entitled is an area of our lives where we can be 'agents' and do have choice. However, studies have shown that cultural attitudes, fear of stigma and lack of knowledge are significant barriers to potential claimants in minority ethnic groups (Platt 2007). ■ Some people from minority ethnic groups may choose to live in more deprived areas so that they can have co-ethnic neighbours. However, this 'choice' may be dictated by their fear of discrimination and hostility from others in society.

It would be fair to conclude that the extent to which people from minority ethnic groups are 'agents' and have postmodernist choices in relation to their health is limited. Indeed, it seems that 'choices' are structured by a variety of constraints. These are addressed in the discussions of the relationship between ethnicity and health in the fourth section of the chapter.

Activity 4.4

These are examples of links between points made in the chapter and the quotes set out in this activity.

(1) The problems of defining ethnicity were discussed at the beginning of the chapter: its 'inherent fluidity' and the way it 'varies across situations and generations, and with time' were highlighted as well as the fact that 'systems of classification are also continually being contested and revised' and 'different terms are used in research'.

(2) Both the second and the fourth sections address the sort of ethnic inequalities that exist, variations between groups and the lack of adequate explanations for these.

(3) This quote illustrates issues that health professionals need to consider to 'reach out' to minority ethnic groups and ensure that healthcare is accessible to them. The third section outlines some of the barriers more recently identified as preventing these groups from accessing the full range of healthcare available. These also require consideration in the planning and delivery of healthcare.

Chapter 5 Ageing and health

Activity 5.2

Ideas for consideration in relation to the issues raised in this activity and the material discussed in the third section of the chapter are as follows.

(1) These are chronic illnesses; Lily suffers from two chronic physical illnesses and a chronic mental illness. As discussed, the percentages of men and women reporting both physical and mental chronic illness increases as they age. In addition, depression is one of the most common mental health problems in later life.

(2) Lily rarely leaves her home and has very few visitors. Her very restricted lifestyle and low-level non-family contact are common features of everyday life for many older people and mean that she is at risk of being socially isolated and lonely.

(3) There are several possible influences on Lily's health; the fact that she lives on her own, that her children do not live locally, that she has few social contacts and spends much of her time on her own all mean that she is socially isolated and lacks social support. This can increase vulnerability to poorer physical and mental health. Her house is old and run-down. This indicates that it is poor quality accommodation and this type of housing puts the health of older people at risk. Another influence is the way that she economizes on her heating; as explained, when older people do not keep warm enough they are vulnerable to cold-related illnesses.

(4) Although Lily's children have actively encouraged her to talk to her GP about her depression, she refuses to do so and consequently it remains undiagnosed and untreated. When compared to other groups in the population, the diagnosis and treatment rates for mental ill health are low among the elderly. This weakness in the delivery of healthcare to older people can lead to further more serious mental health problems. The confusion over the roles of, and tensions between, the health and social care professionals described resulted in Lily not receiving the healthcare in the community to which she was entitled. The fact that her children then made their own arrangements on her behalf could jeopardize the quality of the care that she receives.

Chapter 6 Experiencing illness

Activity 6.1

A summary of functionalism is set out below.

> This perspective sees society as a biological organism, such as the body, made up of different integrated parts. These parts or sub-systems have to work together as the different parts of the body do, in order for society to function properly and maintain its structure and social order. Each person has a role to fulfil in their sub-system and there are shared cultural and social expectations about the way each role should be carried out and the way others should respond. Malfunction occurs when individuals and sub-systems do not fulfil their roles and relationships as expected. Society cannot operate in the event of malfunction so it needs to be addressed effectively.

Activity 6.2

Here are possible answers to the questions in this activity.

> (1) Ruth demonstrates the different ways in which disruption can occur. One of these is how her sense of self as a 'Clooney-luvin Pollyanna' disintegrates. Despite her resolve not to 'give in', she loses the battle as the disease progresses. The euphemism she uses to convey her loss of self is 'Pollyanna commits suicide'. Her description of her family and working life at the beginning of the extract shows that she clearly had much to look forward to in the future before she became ill. However, these hopes are dashed by her illness which illustrates another of the levels on which biographical disruption can occur.
>
> (2) The extract provides some excellent examples of how 'hope and frustration alternate' as those with chronic illnesses experience the 'medical merry-go round' (Bury 1991: 457–8) associated with their condition. She talks about how the initial news that the cancer has spread to her lymph system gives her some hope 'because surgery is now futile' and at least she does not 'have to have a mastectomy and then die anyway, breastless, five years down the line'. The downside of the 'merry-go-round' is the following devastating news that the disease has spread to her major organs and the only treatment is palliative care.
>
> (3) Ruth makes many positive attempts to 'manage, mitigate, or adapt to' her illness and maintain a sense of her identity (Bury 1991: 452). Through these we see the 'coping strategies' she adopts. For instance, she shows that she is using the strategy of 'coping' in the way she pretends her hairstyle could be 'fabulously Jean Seberg' and tries to view chemotherapy as a means to losing unwanted pounds. These are some of the cognitive processes she works through in order to tolerate the effects of her illness and its treatment.

Chapter 7 Experiencing mental illness

Activity 7.1

Here are some ideas to help you with this activity.

The discussion of the range of professional representations of depression that exist provides much evidence that can be used to argue how this common form of mental illness is socially constructed. Examples of this evidence are:

- disciplines vary in their views as to what constitutes depression;

- different criteria are used to infer whether someone is depressed or not.

These examples therefore show the lack of consensus over the meaning of mental illness and the unobjective nature of its assessment

Activity 7.2

Some of the main similarities and differences between the two models in Figures 7.3 and 7.4 are as follows.

Similarities	▪ Both include social factors and processes as well as a range of other actors. ▪ Both highlight the complex interactions that take place between factors.
Differences	▪ In relation to social factors and processes *per se*, Brown and Harris's model focuses on social class and gender whereas Melzer's model focuses on different aspects of social class/position.
	▪ The causal relationships in Melzer's model are two-way. ▪ Melzer's model relates to the causes of mental disorders in general. In contrast, Brown and Harris's model is about the causes of depression.

Activity 7.3

As we saw in both Chapter 1 and Chapter 6, symbolic interactionism sees people as active social actors, who make and define their own reality through their perceptions and interpretations of the social world that arise from their face-to-face interactions with each other. It also focuses on explaining the social world from the point of view of individuals as subjective social actors.

Consequently, from a symbolic interactionist perspective, the experiences described are not so much what happens to those who live with a mental illness but the outcome of how the individuals concerned make and define their own reality in the face of their illness. For example, this perspective would argue that the fact that people with mental illnesses have fewer social and family networks than average can only be understood from the individual viewpoint of those who are mentally ill. In addition, it would see their lower than average social networks and personal relationships as the result of how they deal with the consequences and significance of their illness.

Chapter 8 Experiencing disability

Activity 8.2

① In common with Finkelstein's model, Oliver argues that the arrival of industrial society heralded the beginning of the segregation of disabled people. This was because the changes in the organization of production led to the erosion of the communities in which disabled people had a degree of integration and their gradual exclusion from paid work. In addition, these developments led to the institutionalization of disabled people and their construction as dependent.

② The emphasis on how the economy of a society determines the social relationships and divisions in that society resonates with a Marxist perspective. Changes in the mode of production during industrialization led to changes in power differentials and for disabled people also accorded with the Marxist view that social relationships change when economic relationships change within a society. Similarly, reference is made to Marxist concepts, such as dominant ideology, waged labour and proletariat.

Activity 8.3

The answer is symbolic interactionism. As explained in Chapter 1, this theory argues that people define and make their own reality because they are active social actors who develop their own interpretations of the social world. Baroness Campbell's attitude can be explained using this approach and its concepts because it is very much the outcome of the way she herself defined her own disability. She interpreted and reacted to her disability in a world where the barriers to success for disabled people are many. She was driven by her 'dreams', motivation, optimism and interpretation of what others before her had done. These factors helped her to overcome the obstacles she encountered because of her disability and make her chosen career path become her reality.

Chapter 9 Dying, death and grieving

Activity 9.1

Set out below are the sorts of factors that have been identified in this chapter as influencing the experiences of those who are dying (on the right) and those who will mourn for them (on the left). As you can see there is some overlap which explains why dying, death and bereavement are treated as one subject within the study of the social aspects of health. More importantly, these factors highlight the role of 'the social' in these life experiences.

Influences on those who will mourn	Influences on the experiences of the dying
Death is predictable; age at which death occurs	Personal and religious beliefs about death
Grieving process	Age at which death occurs

Personal and religious beliefs about death	Societal and cultural attitudes to death
Societal and cultural attitudes to death	Organization of death in society
Organization of death in society	Media
Media	Concepts of a 'good death' and a 'bad death'
Concepts of a 'good death' and a 'bad death'	Care of the dying
Care of the dying	Medical practice
The treatment and presentation of the body after death	Medical technology
Funeral ceremonies and rituals	
Norms about the expression of grief	

Chapter 10 Families, communities and healthcare

Activity 10.1

Classifying the families you listed would have been difficult for any of the following reasons.

■ They may have changed from one type to another. For example, from lone/one-parent family to a reconstituted family or from a nuclear family to a lone/one-parent family.

■ Cohabitation makes it difficult to decide whether to use the term 'family'.

■ Some may be same-sex households.

■ Some may reflect cultural differences in marriage arrangements.

■ The strength of familial bonds may vary.

These issues highlight the conclusions about the family in our society that can be drawn from the discussions in the first part of the chapter. These were that it cannot be clearly defined because it is a dynamic institution which is shaped by culture and by both national and global social changes.

Activity 10.2

	FUNCTIONALISM	FEMINISM
View of the family	Families are harmonious and meet the needs of their individual members.	Families are essentially conflict-ridden, because, for example, they are the source of female oppression.

Role of men and women	Men and women undertake traditional roles.	The sexual division of labour within family life is unequal.
Role of ideology	Ideology is not mentioned specifically but functionalism does focus on the nuclear family in western industrialized society and presents a 'consensual' representation of the family.	Patriarchy is blamed for inequalities between men and women, and for the sexual and financial subordination of women. However, its role varies according to which feminist theory is used.

Activity 10.3

Themes in these document extracts that overlap with those discussed are:

- recognition that the incidence of chronic illness will become increasingly prevalent and that this is mainly due to our ageing society;

- acknowledgement that caring responsibilities will impact on an increasing number of citizens;

- reductions in hospital care;

- provision of a new community-based system of case management and clinical intervention;

- introduction of community matrons;

- supported self-care for people with chronic health conditions;

- implementation of the Expert Patients Programme and other self-care programmes.

Chapter 11 Healthcare organizations

Activity 11.2

Weber's theory of bureaucracy: specialization of tasks, hierarchal control, rationality, ideal type.

Systems theory: structural functionalist, role-set, intra-role conflict, multiple roles.

Foucauldian analysis of healthcare organizations: power, design of space, observation.

Activity 11.3

① From the evidence and arguments presented in the articles, it would appear that patients are only marginally likely to receive better care if they use private healthcare.

② Regulatory bodies referred to in the articles are The Healthcare Commission and Care Quality Commission.

③ Examples of problems from the articles that still seem to plague both private healthcare and the NHS, despite all the recent moves to improve and monitor quality are: lack of systematic monitoring of treatment provided; poor standards of staff training; inadequate procedures to minimize risk of infection; high death rates; poor nursing care; filthy wards; and safety failings.

Chapter 12 Health professions
Activity 12.2

This case study was written in 2009. However, the experiences it describes would not seem to support the arguments presented about the decline in medical autonomy over the past two decades, and the accompanying moves to a more egalitarian doctor–patient relationship. Indeed, the medical attitudes encountered by Lisa are more representative of those identified through the research discussed as existing prior to the 1990s. Such attitudes resulted in doctors often failing to take their patients' opinions into consideration because they felt they were the ones with the medical knowledge and expertise.

Although the case study shows that the way medical power operates in neonatal care is less than satisfactory from the user's perspective, there are moves to improve the situation. New guidance is being issued by the General Medical Council about better ways of supporting parents when their children need to receive neonatal intensive care.

Activity 12.4

① Which one of the following statements about professions is *most* accurate?
- require training
- possess a body of highly specialized knowledge ✓
- professional knowledge is static

② Health professionals
- only work in healthcare settings? F
- do not have professional bodies? F

③ The 'informal socialization' of professionals refers to:
- the transfer of appropriate professional attitudes and behaviour ✓

OR

- the transmission of the knowledge and skills required to be a professional

④ Write down two developments that contributed to the professionalization of the medical profession.

Any two of the following:
- The rise of biomedicine
- Doctors were increasingly viewed as valuable agents of the state

- The 1858 Medical Registration Act
- More emphasis on medical surveillance of people's lives
- The establishment of the NHS in 1948

(5) Complete the following sentence:

Central to nursing's professionalizing strategy has been the transformation of nurse education in the 1990s; nursing qualifications were replaced by degrees and these can only be obtained in universities.

(6) What are the three main factors that have contributed to the decline of medical dominance over the past two decades?
- Reforms to the healthcare system
- Patient and user empowerment
- Challenges from other health professions

Glossary

A

absolute poverty: the lack of basic requirements to sustain a physically health existence.

acute illness: a short-term illness, such as influenza or a chest infection.

ageism: when a person is discriminated against on the grounds of age.

alienation: the experience of workers within capitalism because of their lack of control over what they produce and the production process, lack of autonomy and their separation from their fellow workers.

anti-psychiatry movement: a group of academics in the 1960s and 1970s from several different countries who criticized traditional theory and practice in psychiatry.

B

biological death: when the human body ceases to function biologically. It is also referred to as 'physical death'.

biomedicine: this rests on an assumption that all causes of disease (both mental disorders and physical disease) are understood in biological terms. It also views disease and sickness as deviations from normal functioning which medicine has the power to put right with its scientific knowledge and understanding of the human body.

body mass index (BMI): often referred to as BMI, this is is a measurement of a person's weight in kilograms divided by their height in metres squared.

bourgeoisie: one of the two social classes in Marx's theory of class. It is composed of people whose livelihood is based on the ownership of capital and on producing and trading in commodities by employing waged or salaried labour.

bureaucracy: a large-scale organization which operates on the principle of rationality and is characterized to a greater or lesser degree by hierarchical relationships, specialized division of tasks, fixed salary scales, organizational procedures, formalized system of record-keeping and a clear distinction between work and home life.

C

capitalism: a term used to characterize a society whose economy is based on the production of goods for sale using waged labour.

chronic illness: a long-term health disorder that interferes with social interaction and role performance – for example, arthritis and heart disease.

communitarianism: this ideology has strong moral and ethical elements, is opposed to pure individualism, and stresses common interests and common values arising from communal bonds. While it does emphasize the responsibilities of the state and the rights of individuals, it also emphasizes the social responsibilities of individual citizens, families and communities.

conflict theory: focuses on the fundamental conflict between groups in society because of the coercion of subordinate groups by dominant groups. As conflict theorists assume that social order can only be maintained by dominant social groups coercing subordinate groups, they argue that inequality in society is inevitable.

consensus theories: use organic analogies and argue that society survives and remains stable because of the broad acceptance by the majority of its citizens of consensual beliefs. They also assert that the natural state of society is one of dynamic equilibrium, and that balance and harmony are restored when change occurs.

culture: the values, ideas, beliefs and way of life shared within a given group. These are learned and socially transmitted through the socialization process.

D

deviance: ways of behaving that do not conform to the norms or values held by most of those in a society. Therefore, what is regarded as deviant varies from society to society.

direct racism: being subjected to verbal and/or physical abuse because of membership of an ethnic minority group.

discourse: groups of ideas or patterned ways of thinking that shape the understanding about a particular subject in society. Use of language is central to the construction of discourses. A variety of discourses can exist at any one time; some are more powerful than others and often reflect the interests of dominant and/or political groups.

discrimination: when members of a particular group in society are denied resources, rewards and opportunities that are available to and can be obtained by others in society.

dual role: refers to the way that working women tend to combine their paid work in the public sphere with their unpaid work in the private domain of the home.

E

epidemiology: the study of patterns of disease within a population over time. It involves statistical measurement to establish the risk factors of diseases as well as their social origins and transmission.

F

feminism: a body of thought and a social movement which argues for the equality of the sexes. It explains inequalities between the sexes, and focuses in particular on the historical oppression and exclusion of women and the restrictions placed on them by society.

functionalism: views society as a biological organism, such as the body, made up of different integrated parts. It argues that in order for society to function properly and maintain its structure, these parts (or sub-systems) have to fulfil their role in accordance with cultural and social expectations

G

gemeinschaft: the type of community relationships that existed in pre-industrial society. These were characterized by intimacy and durability, status was ascribed rather than achieved, kin relationships took place within a shared territory and were made meaningful by a shared culture.

gender: refers to the social (as distinct from purely biological) characteristics associated with masculinity or femininity in a particular society. These characteristics vary over time and are different in different societies and cultures.

gender differentiation: the social process whereby biological differences are given social and cultural significance and used as a basis for the social classification of males and females.

gender role: the social and behavioural characteristics that a society ascribes to masculine and feminine roles. These can form the principal categorization within social life and in some societies there are radical divisions between gender roles.

gender stereotyping: the often unwarranted generalizations made from sex differences about male and female attributes.

gesellschaft: community relationships that replaced *gemeinschaft* during and following industrialization and urbanism. These relationships were impersonal, fleeting, contractual, competitive, rational and calculative rather than affective, and were often characterized by anonymity and alienation. Status was based on merit, and was therefore achieved.

global health: refers to health issues which are determined by factors that do not respect national boundaries and are therefore beyond the control of individual countries.

globalization: the set of global processes that are widening and deepening the nature of human interaction across a broad range of social spheres. It has led to an increasing worldwide interconnectedness and a global cultural system. The uneven impact of these processes has resulted in further inequalities.

H

health surveillance: activities devised following indirect scrutiny and observation of health behaviour at both an individual and societal level which aim to prevent illness and improve the health of the population.

hegemonic masculinity: a concept used to explain how particular versions of masculinity come to be idealized and embedded in culture and in institutions in society. Characteristics of such ideals typically include stoicism and invincibility, which in turn are seen as demonstrating manliness.

I

iatrogenesis: the harmful and detrimental effects of medical intervention. Such harm does not occur in the absence of medicine and medical practice and hence is medically caused.

ideal type: the construction of a pure or ideal form of a particular feature of the social world. Ideal types do not necessarily exist anywhere in reality. Nor are they attainable or even the most desirable, but this concept identifies those traits which would render the aspect of the social world under scrutiny most effective.

identity: our distinctive sense of self which is acquired through socialization and social interaction with others. It is also both situational and contextual and hence socially produced.

illness behaviour: the actions individuals take when they experience the symptoms of ill health. These are differentially experienced by individuals, shaped by many factors, and can include not seeking medical advice and help.

indirect racism: the fear of being subjected to verbal and/or physical abuse because of membership of an ethnic minority group.

industrial society: a society in which most of the labour force live in large cities and towns and are employed in the industrial production of goods for sale. Only a small proportion work in agriculture and agricultural production itself is also highly mechanized and commercially orientated.

industrialization: the general process that originated in the early nineteenth century whereby factories, machines and large-scale production replaced agriculture and handicrafts within western economies. In its wake came the huge range of changes that created modern societies.

informal healthcare: healthcare which is unpaid and takes place outside the public sphere of paid employment. It also refers to the 'care' in a more general sense involved in 'caring' for someone who is sick or disabled.

informal organization: coexists with the formal culture within organizations and refers to ways of carrying out designated tasks and roles within an organization that depart from formally recognized procedures.

institutional racism: when a public or private body intentionally or unintentionally discriminates against people from a minority ethnic group.

inter-role conflict: when we experience conflict between two simultaneously held roles.

intra-role conflict: when we disagree with traditional beliefs about one of our roles.

L

labelling theory: focuses on the reactions of others to perceived deviance and how the deviance is maintained by their reactions.

liberalism: although the meaning of this political philosophy varies, its basic tenet is that all citizens should have equal rights and freedoms irrespective of religion and/or ethnic group. Such universal egalitarianism is achieved by eliminating discrimination. Individuals should also determine their economic position through their own efforts rather than hereditary factors.

life course perspective: there are different strands to this perspective but the predominant theme is that stages in life are not necessarily standardized, chronologically or biologically fixed, sequential or gendered, but are subject to a variety of social, historical and cultural influences.

life expectancy: provides an estimate of the average number of years a newborn baby can expect to live if patterns of mortality at the time of his or her birth were to stay the same throughout life.

M

macro: the larger, structural elements of society such as the social, economic, legal and political systems.

market situation: one of the factors identified by the German sociologist Weber as determining social class. It refers to the skills, qualifications and expertise which influence the extent to which people are 'marketable'. In turn these influence the type of work people can undertake and can therefore lead to varying earning opportunities and life chances.

Marxist theory: approaches based on this theory maintain that the way the economy of a society is run determines the social relationships, such as inequalities, in that society. Marxists blame capitalism for these inequalities; they argue that in capitalist societies there is a minority which exploits the majority and it is this exploitation that leads to inequalities.

matriarchy: a form of social organization that is female-dominated and based on public and private assumptions of female superiority.

means of production: the way goods and services are produced in a society.

medical pluralism: the coexistence of accepted alternative medical practices to biomedicine within biomedical practice.

medical tourism: people in developed countries (such as the USA, Canada and Western Europe) are increasingly seeking medical care in Asia and Latin America because of high healthcare costs, long waiting periods or lack of access to new therapies.

medicalization: the historical and social processes whereby medicine gradually defines human conditions and behaviour as medical issues or problems. As a result they are usually seen in terms of illnesses, diseases or disorders that require treatment.

micro: those elements of society which are the small-scale aspects of human behaviour such as the face-to-face interactions between individuals and between individuals and groups.

mixed economy of care: when multiple sources are involved in the provision of healthcare. These can include the state, private and voluntary organizations, as well as informal sources such as family and friends.

modernization agenda: this was introduced by New Labour across all sectors of the government. Its main themes were the promotion of parternerhips between government departments with the voluntary and private sectors, consultation with service users, target-setting, performance monitoring and greater valuing of public services.

monogamy: the practice or state of being married to one person at a time.

monopoly: the exclusive ownership or control of the supply of particular economic goods or services which enables market domination in that area.

morbidity rates: the number and patterns of physical and mental illnesses within a designated group at a given time, expressed as a rate per 100,000 of the population.

mortality rates: the number and causes of deaths within a designated group at a given time, expressed as a rate per 100,000 of the population.

multiple roles: a concept used to describe the fact that most people act out more than one role in society at any given time.

N

narratives: stories people construct to make sense of their experiences. Individuals' narratives can also shape the consequences of these experiences.

negative health: emphasizes the absence of symptoms and regards being healthy as not feeling unwell and/or having a diagnosed illness or disease.

New Labour: as well as referring to the political party, this term is also used to refer to the ideology adopted by New Labour when it came into power in 1997: opposition to individualism and a stress on common interests and common values arising from communal bonds. It emphasizes the responsibilities of the state and the rights of individuals, and the social responsibilities of individual citizens, families and communities.

New Right: the political ideology that influenced Conservative government policy in the 1980s and 1990s. It emphasized the rights of the individual and individual choice, a smaller role for the state and a greater role for markets. This was combined with strong beliefs in individual responsibility, social and moral order, 'traditional family life' and appropriate sexuality.

O

obese: a person is considered obese if they have a body mass index (BMI) of 30 or more.

organization: an organization is composed of a large group of individuals and sub-groups having particular objectives. Members have prescribed roles and are all part of a defined and relatively stable set of authority relations. Together with the systems of social roles, norms and shared meanings that exist in organizations, these defined lines of authority mean that interaction within organizations is regular and predictable. Examples of typical organizations include families, schools, colleges, universities, religious bodies, sports clubs, trade unions, business corporations and hospitals.

overweight: a person is considered overweight if they have a body mass index (BMI) of 25 or more.

P

paid work: activities that are done for money. These usually take place outside the home in the public sphere.

party: another important component of class in Weber's multiclass model because being part of a party organization, be it employment-related (such as trade unions and employers' organizations), political or religious, gives individuals access to power.

patriarchy: a social system of male dominance based on assumptions of male superiority, which is seen as being reinforced publicly and privately by social institutions such as the family, education system and the state.

personalization: the new agenda in adult social care which aims to enable service users to determine their own priorities and preferences. It is intended that there will be a strategic shift to personalization in all care settings.

polygamy: the practice or custom of having more than one wife or husband at the same time.

polyandry: the practice of a woman being married to more than one husband at any one time. This is quite rare and is usually found in impoverished societies.

polygyny: the practice of a man being married to more than one woman. This pattern of marriage is often found in tribal societies.

positive health: refers to a positive state of well-being, 'equilibrium', or fitness and energy, all of which are required to function effectively from day to day. This concept also has many distinct components which focus on both mental and physical health; it can be described as encompassing the ability to cope with stressful situations, the maintenance of a strong social support system, integration into the community, high morale and life satisfaction, psychological well-being and levels of physical fitness as well as physical health.

post-industrial society: unlike industrial societies, a post-industrial society is based primarily on the production and control of information, as opposed to the production of material goods.

private domain/sphere: the private world of the home and the family. This is also sometimes referred to as the private sphere and work done within it is usually unpaid.

profession: an occupational group which possesses a highly specialized body of knowledge, has formal control over the education and training of its members, has a monopoly of its field of work, has considerable autonomy, plays a positive role in society, adheres to a code of ethics and enjoys high status and high rewards.

professional socialization: the social processes involved in acquiring a professional identity.

professionalization: the complex and often political process by which occupational groups monopolize knowledge, take over other occupations' roles, expel and exclude competitors and achieve the personal and social privileges for their members associated with the status of a profession.

proletariat: one of the two social classes in Marx's theory of class, used to denote those people in capitalist societies who do not own capital and who are obliged to sell their labour for wages.

public health: this is concerned with improving the health of the population, rather than treating the diseases of individual patients. Public health professionals work with other professional groups to monitor the health status of the community, identify health needs, develop programmes to reduce risk and screen for early disease, control communicable disease, foster policies which promote health, plan and evaluate the provision of healthcare, and manage and implement change.

public domain/sphere: the public world outside the home where any work done is carried out within the economy and is paid.

Q

quality of life: generally refers to a range of components relating to satisfaction with life such as good general physical and mental health, satisfaction with economic and social status, sense of self-worth, social health and functional ability.

R

racism: the belief that biologically rooted racial characteristics determine social activities and abilities. The result is that those groups who believe themselves to be inherently 'superior' discriminate against those who belong to groups who are deemed to be 'inferior'. This can lead to discriminatory and aggressive behaviour towards members of minority ethnic groups.

rationalization: the process whereby modes of precise calculation and systematic organization have increasingly come to characterize and dominate modernity.

relative poverty: when people may be able to afford basic necessities but are still unable to maintain an average standard of living within their own society.

reproduction of people: refers to both the biological reproduction of people and their social reproduction in terms of helping them to be members of society and to maintain their position in the social structure – for example, their class and gender positions.

reserve army of labour: groups of workers or potential workers who are vulnerable to irregular employment, being employed on a part-time basis or laid off as the demand for labour rises and falls.

role-making: the process of creating and modifying expected behaviour in organizations.

role set: the array of roles and expectations that any individual will confront while taking a particular role.

S

serial monogamy: the practice of having a number of successive partners but only have one partner at a time.

sex: can be distinguished at birth and refers to being biologically male or female. More specifically, it relates to having male or female genitals and to the ways in which we develop anatomically in certain predictable ways.

sexual division of labour: the distribution of activities and roles between men and women both in the private sphere of the home and the public sphere of paid employment.

social capital: the resources, trust and social networks within a community which, when accessed by individuals, are beneficial as they empower them and enable them to improve their lives.

social causation: the way various social processes lead to particular social issues or problems. Those perspectives that focus on how social processes *cause* social issues/problems are referred to as social causationist explanations.

social class: groupings or classifications of the population with broadly similar occupations, levels and resources, or styles of living, perhaps with some shared perception of their collective condition. More precise meanings depend on which theory of class is adopted.

social closure: a Weberian term used to denote the way that higher social classes maintain their prestige by monopolizing resources and restricting access to their ranks.

social constructionism: the way that aspects of society or behaviour are 'constructed' in a particular way as a result of social relations and human agency rather than being 'natural' or biological in origin. Social constructions vary historically, socially and culturally and are therefore essentially contestable.

social death: the process whereby people who are dying are separated and marginalized from the rest of society. This occurs either because they are removed from society and institutionalized or because the nature of their illness (such as diseases of the mind) removes their social significance.

social determinants of health: the specific economic, political and social conditions which lead to members of different socioeconomic groups experiencing varying degrees of health and illness.

social exclusion: a contested concept that addresses the range of factors that constrain individuals' full participation in society. Examples of such factors are lack of material resources, discrimination, chronic ill health, geographical location and cultural identification.

social health: this concept goes beyond the reporting of symptoms, illness and the ability to meet the demands of everyday life. It focuses on the extent of a person's social support systems and argues that these influence mental and physical health.

social inequalities: differences in people's share of resources in society. These can involve a wide range of resources such as wealth, education, health and housing, power, status and life chances. When they are extensive and persistent, they can lead to the development of social divisions.

social integration: concerns the relationships between individuals and societal institutions, such as the family, employment, and religious, political and voluntary groups. Integration into these societal institutions helps people to cope mentally and psychologically when facing stressful life events because they provide mutual moral support and access to resources.

social model of health: acknowledges that there are a broad range of social factors that can influence health, and that health is the result of complex interactions that occur between such factors.

social networks: the patterns of individuals' social relationships and interactions with those to whom they are connected by ties such as kinship, friendship and work relationships.

social role: the behaviour, responsibilities and attributes associated with the specific social positions individuals are expected to undertake in society.

social stratification: the way that groups in society are structured into a hierarchy. Systems of social stratification usually lead to inequalities between different groups of people.

social support: this is provided by positive involvement in social networks. It has been shown to act as a buffer to stress and mental ill health, particularly if intimate and confiding relationships are involved.

socialization: the social process by which individuals are brought up and 'shaped' according to the roles, norms and values of a society. A socialized individual knows the 'appropriate' way to act in different social situations and has taken on the values of their society. The main agencies involved in socialization are the family, the education system, peer groups, the mass media, workplaces and neighbourhoods.

society: consists of social institutions and social relationships, both of which are concrete and abstract.

sociological imagination: the ability to think beyond and question our own essentially limited experiences and observations of the human social world. Such critical thinking also involves challenging what appear to be the accepted explanations of social phenomena.

status: another of the concepts developed by Weber to explain how social class is determined. Status refers to the difference in honour or prestige accorded to different social groups and is often related to 'status symbols' in terms of lifestyle.

stigma: the process by which a person is discredited and/or not fully accepted by others in particular situations.

structural functionalism: a theoretical approach that analyses the structure of society as self-maintaining social systems in which various social institutions perform specific functions by shaping individual behaviour to ensure the smooth operation of society as a whole.

structuralism: a theoretical approach which maintains that social structures determine our experiences and that individuals have very little autonomy in society.

structuration thesis: this defines structure as a duality in that it is a combination of structure and agency. It also sees structure and agency as being inextricably linked and having the potential to shape each other.

T

theory: within social science this means the set of ideas used to explain social phenomena. These explanations are systematic, consistent and supported by evidence.

U

unpaid carer: someone who cares for a dependant who cannot care for themselves and, excluding benefits, is unpaid for this work.

unpaid work: work that is necessary for a society to run and contributes to the reproduction of people and society. Unpaid work is performed in the home or private domain, does not have as much status as paid work and does not receive the public recognition of money.

References

Abbott, P. (2006) Gender, in G. Payne, (ed.) *Social Divisions*. Basingstoke: Macmillan.

Abbott, P., Wallace, C. and Tyler. M. (2005) *An Introduction to Sociology: Feminist Perspectives*, 3rd edn. London: Routledge.

Acheson, D. (1998) *Independent Inquiry into Inequalities in Health Report*. London: Stationery Office.

Action on Elder Abuse (2004) *Hidden Voices: Older People's Experience of Abuse*. London: Help the Aged.

Action on Elder Abuse (2007) *The UK Study of Abuse and Neglect of Older People*. London: King's Institute of Gerontology.

Adamson, J., Ben-Shlomo, Y., Chaturvedi, N. and Donovan, J. (2003) Ethnicity, socio-economic position and gender – do they affect reported helath-care seeking behaviour? *Social Science and Medicine*, 57(5): 895–904.

Age Concern (2008) *Undiagnosed, Untreated, At Risk. The experiences of Older People with Depression*. London: Age Concern England.

Ahlström, B.H., Skärsäter, I. and Danielson, E. (2009) Living with major depression: experiences from families' perspectives, *Scandinavian Journal of Caring Sciences*, 23(2): 309–16.

Ahmad, W. and Bradby, H. (2008) Ethnicity and health: key themes in a developing field, *Current Sociology*, 56(1): 47–56.

Aldridge, J. (2006) The experiences of children living with and caring for parents with mental illness, *Child Abuse Review*, 15(2): 79–88.

Allan, G.A. and Crow, G.P. (2001) *Families, Households and Society*. London: Palgrave.

Allen, J. (2008) *Older People and Well-being*. London: Institute for Public Policy Research.

Allender, S., Cowburn, G. and Foster, C. (2006) Understanding participation in sport and physical activity amongst children and adults: a review of qualitative studies, *Health Education Research, Theory and Practice*, 21(6): 826–35.

American Psychiatric Association (2004) *DSM-IV-TR Diagnostic and Statistical Manual of Mental Disorders*. Arlington, TX: American Psychiatric Publishing.

Anderson, P. (1974) *Passages from Antiquity to Feudalism*. London: Verso.

Annandale, E. and Hunt, K. (eds) (2000) *Gender Inequalities in Health*. Buckingham: Open University Press.

Apesoa-Varano, E.C. (2007) Educated caring: the emergence of professional identity among nurses, *Qualitative Sociology*, 30(3): 249–74.

Arber, S. and Ginn, J. (1995) *Connecting Gender and Ageing: A Sociological Approach*. Buckingham: Open University Press.

Ariès, P. (1962) *Centuries of Childhood*. London: Jonathan Cape.

Ariès, P. (1981) *The Hour of Our Death*. London: Allen Lane.

Armstrong, D. (1993) From clinical gaze to regime of total health, in A. Beattie, M. Gott, L. Jones and M. Sidell (eds) *Health and Wellbeing: A Reader*. London: Macmillan.

Armstrong, D. (1995) The rise of surveillance medicine, *Sociology of Health and Illness*, 17(3): 343–404.

Armstrong, D. (2008) The social role of medicine, in S. Earle and G. Letherby (eds) *The Sociology of Healthcare: A Reader for Health Professionals*. Basingstoke: Palgrave Macmillan.

Asthana, A. and Campbell, D. (2009) Eleven more NHS hospitals at centre of safety scandal, *The Observer*, 29 November: 16.

Astin, F. and Atkin, K. (2010) *Ethnicity and Coronary Heart Disease: Making Sense of Risk and Improving Care*. London: Race Equality Foundation.

Badger, F., Pumphrey, R., Clarke, L., Clifford, C., Gill, P., Greenfield, S. and Knight Jackson, A. (2009) The role of ethnicity in end-of-life care homes for older people in the UK: a literature review, *Diversity in Health and Care*, 6(1): 23–9.

Baggott, R. (2004) *Health and Health Care in Britain*, 3rd edn. Basingstoke: Macmillan.

Bailey, N. (2004) Does work pay? Employment, poverty and exclusion from social relations, in C. Pantazis, D. Gordon and R. Levitas (eds) *Poverty and Social Exclusion in Britain: The Millennium Survey*. Bristol: The Policy Press.

Bambra, C., Whitehead, M. and Hamilton, V. (2005) Does 'welfare-to-work' work? A systematic review of the effectiveness of the UK's welfare-to-work programmes for people with a disability or chronic illness, *Social Science and Medicine*, 60(9): 1905–18.

Bandeira, D.R., Pawlowski, J., Goncalves, T.R., Hilgert, M.C., Bozzetti, M.C. and Hugo, F.N. (2007) Psychological distress in Brazilian caregivers of relatives with dementia, *Aging and Mental Health*, 11(1): 14–19.

Barker, R. (1997) *Political Ideas in Modern Britain*. London: Routledge.

Barney, L.J., Griffiths, K.M., Christensen, H. and Jorm, A.F. (2009) Exploring the nature of stigmatising beliefs about depression and help-seeking: implications for reducing stigma, *BMC Public Health*, 9: 61.

Barry, A. and Yuill, C. (2008) *Understanding Health: A Sociological Introduction*, 2nd edn. London: Sage.

Barton, L. (2004) The disability movement: some observations, in J. Swain, S. French, C. Barnes and C. Thomas (eds) *Disabling Barriers, Enabling Environments*. London: Sage, in association with The Open University.

Becker, H.S., Geer, B., Hughes, E.C. and Strauss, A. (1961) *Boys in White: Student Culture in Medical School*. Chicago, IL: University of Chicago Press.

Beckett, C. (2009) *Human Growth and Development*, 7th edn. London: Sage.

Beetham, D. (1996) *Bureaucracy*, 2nd edn. Buckingham: Open University Press.

Bennett, W.L., Ouyang, P., Albert, W.W., Barone, B.B. and Stewart, K.J. (2008) Fatness and fitness: how do they influence health-related quality of life in type 2 diabetes mellitus? *Health and Quality of Life Outcomes*, 6: 110–31.

Berkman, L.F. (1995) The role of social relations in health promotion, *Psychosomatic Medicine*, 57: 245–54.

Berkman, L.F. and Syme, S.L (1979) Social networks, host resistance, and mortality: a nine-year follow-up of Alameda County residents, *American Journal of Epidemiology*, 109(2): 186–204.

Berkman, L.F., Glass, T., Brissette, I. and Sutman, T.E. (2000) From social integration to health: Durkheim in the new millennium, *Social Science and Medicine*, 51: 843–57.

Bhopal, R.S. (2007) *Ethnicity, Race and Health in Multicultural Societies*. Oxford: Oxford University Press.

Biggs, S. (2000) *Understanding Ageing: Images, Attitudes and Professional Practice*. Buckingham: Open University Press.

Bittman, M. and Pixley, J. (1997) *The Double Life of the Family: Myth, Hope and Experience*. Sydney: Allen & Unwin.

Black. D., Norris, J.N., Smith, C. and Townsend, P. (1980) *The Black Report*, in P. Townsend, M. Whitehead and N. Davidson (eds) (1992) *Inequalities in Health*. Harmondsworth: Penguin.

Blakemore, K. (2007) *Social Policy: An Introduction*, 3rd edn. Buckingham: Open University Press.

Blane, D., Higgs, P., Hyde, M. and Wiggins, R. (2004) Life course influences on quality of life in early old age, *Social Science and Medicine*, 58(11): 2171–9.

Blau, P. (1963) *The Dynamics of Bureaucracy*. Chicago, IL: University of Chicago Press.

Blaxter, M. (1990) *Health and Lifestyles*. London: Routledge.

Boddy, D. (2008) *Management: An Introduction*, 4th edn. Harlow: FT-Prentice Hall.

Bond, M., Clark, M. and Davies, S. (2003) The quality of life of spouse dementia caregivers: changes associated with yielding to formal care and widowhood, *Social Science and Medicine*, 57: 2385–95.

Bowler, I. (1993) 'They're not the same as us': midwives' stereotypes of South Asian descent maternity patients, *Sociology of Health & Illness*, 15(2): 157–78.

Bowling, A. (2005) *Measuring Health: A Review of Quality of Life Measurement Scales*, 3rd edn. Maidenhead: Open University Press.

Bracken, P.J. and Thomas, P. (1998) A new debate in mental health, *Open Mind*, 89(February): 17.

Bradbury, M. (2000) Contemporary representation of 'good' and 'bad' death, in D. Dickenson and M. Johnson (eds) *Death, Dying and Bereavement*. London: Sage.

Bradby, H. (2009) *Medical Sociology: An Introduction*. London: Sage.

Bradshaw, J., Hoelscher, P. and Richardson, D. (2006) *Comparing Child Well-being in OECD Countries: Concepts and Methods*. Florence: UNICEF.

Braham, P. and Janes, L. (eds) (2002) *Social Differences and Divisions*. Milton Keynes: The Open University.

Brennan, G. and McSherry, R. (2007) Exploring the transition and professional socialisation from health care assistant to student nurse, *Nurse Education in Practice*, 7(4): 206–14.

Brewer, M., Browne, J., Emmerson, C., Goodman, A., Muriel, A. and Tetlow, G. (2007) *Pensioner Poverty Over the Next Decade: What Role for Tax and Benefit Reform?* London: Institute for Fiscal Studies.

Brewer, M., Muriel, A. and Phillips, D. (2008) *Poverty and Inequality in the UK: 2008*. London: Institute for Fiscal Studies.

Briggs, A., Wild, D., Lees, M., Reaney, M., Dursun, S., Parry, D. and Mukherjee, J. (2008) Impact of schizophrenia and schizophrenia treatment related adverse events on quality of life: direct utility elicitation, *Health and Quality of Life Outcomes*, 6(105): 1–9.

Brown, G.W. and Harris, T. (1978) *The Social Origins of Depression*. London: Tavistock.

Brown, G. and Wilson, C. (2005) The family, health and caring, in E. Denny and S. Earle (eds) *Sociology for Nurses*. Cambridge: Polity Press.

Brown, M. and Stetz, K. (1999) The labor of caregiving: a theoretical model of caregiving during potentially fatal illness, *Qualitative Health Research*, 9(2): 182–97.

Bury, M. (1982) Chronic illness as biographical disruption, *Sociology of Health and Illness*, 4(2): 167–82.

Bury, M. (1991) The sociology of chronic illness: a review of research and prospects, *Sociology of Health and Illness*, 13(4): 451–68.

Bury, M. (1997) *Health and Illness in a Changing Society*. London: Routledge.

Bury, M. (2000) Health, ageing and the lifecourse, in S.J. Williams, J. Gabe and M. Calnan (eds) *Health, Medicine and Society: Key Theories, Future Agendas*. London: Routledge.

Busfield, J. (2000a) *Health and Health Care in Modern Britain*. Oxford: Oxford University Press.

Busfield, J. (2000b) Rethinking the sociology of mental health, *Sociology of Health and Illness*, 22(5): 543–58.

Bush, J., White, M., Kai, J., Rankin, J. and Bhopal, R. (2003) Understanding influences on smoking in Bangladeshi and Pakistani adults: a community based, qualitative study, *British Medical Journal*, 326: 1–6.

Byrne, P.S. and Long, B.E.L. (1976) *Doctors Talking to Patients: A Study of the Verbal Behaviours of Doctors in the Consultation*. London: HMSO.

Bywaters, P. (2009) Tackling inequalities in health: a global challenge of social work, *British Journal of Social Work*, 39(2): 353–67.

Cahill, H.A. (2001) Male appropriation and the medicalisation of childbirth: an historical analysis, *Journal of Advanced Nursing*, 33(3): 334–42.

Campbell, D. (2009) Doctors told to be more sensitive and listen to parents of very ill children, *The Observer*, 28 June: 13.

Cancer Research (2010) *Sunlight and Skin Cancer in the UK – statistics*, http://info.cancerresearchuk.org/cancerstats/causes/lifestyle/sunlight/.

Cancian, F.M. and Oliker, S.J. (1999) *Caring and Gender*. London: Sage.

Carers National Association (1998) *Facts about Carers*. London: Carers National Association.

Carvel, J. (2006) Private healthcare performance no better than NHS, *The Guardian*, 31 October.

Chamberlain, M. (1999) Brothers and sisters, uncles and aunts: a lateral perspective on Caribbean families, in E.B. Silva and C. Smart (eds) *The New Family?* London: Sage.

Chamberlayne, P. and King, A. (2000) *Cultures of Care: Biographies of Carers in Britain and the Two Germanies*. Bristol: The Policy Press.

Chun, M., Knight, B.G. and Youn, G. (2007) Differences in stress and coping models of emotional distress among Korean, Korean-American and white-American caregivers, *Aging and Mental Health*, 11(1): 20–9.

Clark, D. (2002) Between hope and acceptance: the medicalisation of dying, *British Medical Journal*, 324: 905–7.

Clark, K. and Drinkwater, S. (2007) *Ethnic Minorities in the Labour Market: Dynamics and Diversity*. Abingdon: The Policy Press.

Cohen, G. (ed.) (1987) *Social Change and the Life Course*. London: Tavistock.

Commission on Social Determinants of Health (2008) *Closing the Gap in a Generation: Health Equity Through Action on the Social Determinants of Health*. Geneva: World Health Organization.

Connell, R.W. (1995) *Masculinities*. London: Allen & Unwin.

Conrad, D. and White, A. (eds) (2010) *Promoting Men's Mental Health*. Oxford: Radcliffe Publishing.

Conrad, P. (1992) Medicalisation and social control, *Annual Review of Sociology*, 18: 209–32.

Conrad, P. (2005) The shifting engines of medicalization, *Journal of Health and Social Behavior*, 46: 3–14.

Conrad, P. and Schneider, J. (1980) Looking at levels of medicalisation: a comment on Strong's critique of the thesis of medical imperialism, *Social Science and Medicine*, 14: 75–9.

Conrad, P. and Schneider, J. (1992) *Deviance and Medicalization: From Baldness to Sickness*. St Louis, MO: Mosby.

Conway, S. (2007) The changing face of death: implications for public health, *Critical Public Health*, 17(3): 195–202.

Cordella, A. and Willcocks, L. (2010) Outsourcing, bureaucracy and public value: reappraising the notion of the 'contract state', *Government Information Quarterly*, 27(1): 82–8.

Corker, M. (2000) Disability politics, language planning and inclusive social policy, *Disability and Society*, 15(3): 445–61.

Corker, M. (2002) New disability discourse, the principle of optimisation and social change, in M. Corker and S. French (eds) *Disability Discourses*. Buckingham: Open University Press.

Corrigan, P.W. (2007) How clinical diagnosis might exacerbate the stigma of mental illness, *Social Work*, 52(1): 31–9.

Crawshaw, P. (2007) Governing the healthy male citizen: men, masculinity and popular health in *Men's Health* magazine, *Sociology of Health and Illness*, 65(8): 1606–18.

Crow, G. and Maclean, C. (2006) Community, in G. Payne (ed.) *Social Divisions*. Basingstoke: Macmillan.

Cuff, E.C., Sharrock, W.W. and Francis, D.W. (2006) *Perspectives in Sociology*, 5th edn. London: Routledge.

Culley, L. and Dyson, S. (eds) (2001) *Ethnicity and Nursing Practice*. Basingstoke: Palgrave.

Currer, C. and Stacey, M. (eds) (1986) *Concepts of Health, Illness and Disease: A Comparative Perspective*. Leamington Spa: Berg.

Currin, L.G., Jack, R.H., Linklater, K.M., Mak, V., Møller, H. and Davies, E.A. (2009) Inequalities in the incidence of cervical cancer in South East England 2001–2005: an investigation of population risk factors, *BMC Public Health*, 9: 62.

Dahrendorf, R. (1959) *Class and Class Conflict in Industrial Society*. London: Routledge.

Dalley, G. (1996) *Ideologies of Caring: Rethinking Community and Collectivism*, 2nd edn. London: Macmillan.

Darmon, N. and Drewnowski, A. (2008) Does social class predict diet quality? *American Journal of Clinical Nutrition*, 87: 1107–17.

Davar, B. (ed.) (2001) *Mental Health from a Gender Perspective*. London: Sage.

Davidson, K., Daly, T. and Arber, S. (2003) Older men, social integration and organisational activities, *Social Policy and Society*, 2(2): 81–9.

Davis, C. (1975) *Gender and the Professional Predicament in Nursing*. Buckingham: Open University Press.

Davison, T.E., McCabe, M.P., Mellor, D., Ski, C., George, K. and Moore, K.A. (2007) The prevalence and recognition of major depression among low-level aged care residents with and without cognitive impairment, *Ageing and Mental Health*, 11(1): 82–8.

de Maio, F. (2010) *Health and Social Theory*. Basingstoke: Palgrave Macmillan.

Deal, M. (2007) Aversive disablism: subtle prejudice towards disabled people, *Disability and Society*, 22(1): 93–107.

DeFranco, E.A., Lian, M., Muglia, L.A. and Schootman, M. (2008) Area level poverty and preterm birth risk: a population-based multilevel analysis, *BMC Public Health*, 8: 316.

Degnen, C. (2007) Minding the gap: the construction of old age and oldness amongst peers, *Journal of Aging Studies*, 21(1): 69–80.

Denny, E. (2005) Nursing as an occupation, in E. Denny and S. Earle (eds) *Sociology for Nurses*. Cambridge: Polity Press.

Denny, E. and Earle, S. (eds) (2005) *Sociology for Nurses*. Cambridge: Polity Press.

Department for Work and Pensions (2005) *Opportunity Age*. London: The Stationery Office.

Department for Work and Pensions (2006) *Work, Saving and Retirement Among Ethnic Minorities: A Qualitative Study*. London: The Stationery Office.

Department for Work and Pensions (2007) *In Work, Better Off*. London: The Stationery Office.

Department for Work and Pensions (2008) *Pensioners' Incomes Series 2006/07*. London: The Stationery Office.

Department of Health (1998) *Smoking Kills: A White Paper on Tobacco*. London: HMSO.

Department of Health (1999) *Saving Lives: Our Healthier Nation*. London: HMSO.

Department of Health (2001) *National Service Framework for Older People*. London: HMSO.

Department of Health (2003) *Tackling Health Inequalities: A Programme for Action*. London: HMSO.

Department of Health (2004a) *At Least Five a Day: Evidence of the Impact of Physical Activity and its Relationship to Health*. London: HMSO.

Department of Health (2004b) *Better Health in Old Age*. London: HMSO.

Department of Health (2004c) *Choosing Health: Making Healthy Choices Easier*. London: HMSO.

Department of Health (2005a) *Supporting People with Long-term Conditions: An NHS and Social Care Model for Improving Care for People with Long-term Conditions*. London: HMSO.

Department of Health (2005b) *Supporting People with Long Term Conditions: An NHS and Social Care Model to Support Local Innovation and Integration*. London: HMSO.

Department of Health (2005c) *Supporting Experienced Hospital Nurses to Move Into Community Matron Roles*. London: HMSO.

Department of Health (2006) *Government Information for Carers*. London: HMSO.

Department of Health (2007a) *The Expert Patients Programme*. London: HMSO.

Department of Health (2007b) *The Pregnancy Book 2007*. London: HMSO.

Department of Health (2007c) *Putting People First: A Shared Vision and Commitment to the Transformation of Adult Social Care*. London: HMSO.

Department of Health (2008a) *Health is Global: A UK Government Strategy 2008–13*. London: HMSO.

Department of Health (2008b) *Health Inequalities: Progress and the Next Steps*. London: HMSO.

Department of Health (2008c) *CMO Quotes: – Ethnic Minority Health*, www.dh.gov.uk/en/Aboutus/MinistersandDepartmentLeaders/ChiefMedicalOfficer/CMOPublications/QuoteUnquote/DH_4102565.

Department of Health (2008d) *National Service Framework for Older People and System Reform*. London: HMSO.

Department of Health (2008e) *An Introduction to Personalisation*, www.dh.gov.uk.

Department of Health (2008f) *Health Effects of Climate Change in the UK*. London: HMSO.

Department of Health (2009a) *Health Profiles 2009*, www.apho.org.uk/default.aspx?QN=P_HEALTH_PROFILES.

Department of Health (2009b) *Attitudes to Mental Illness: 2009 Research Report*. London: TNS UK.

Department of Health (2009c) *Healthy Lives, Brighter Futures – The Strategy for Children and Young People's Health*. London: HMSO.

Dew, K. (2000) Deviant insiders: medical acupuncturists in New Zealand, *Social Science and Medicine*, 50: 1785–95.

Diamond, I. and Quinby, L. (1988) *Feminism and Foucault: Reflections on Resistance*. Boston, MA: Northeastern University Press.

Dietze, P.M., Jolley, D.J., Chrikitzhs, T.N., Clemens, S., Catalano, P. and Stockwell, T. (2009) Income inequality and alcohol related harm in Australia, *BMC Public Health*, 9: 70–90.

Disabled People's International (1982) *Disabled People's International: Proceedings of the First World Congress*. Singapore: Disabled People's International.

Disability Rights Commission (2006) *Disability Briefing*. London: Disability Rights Commission.

Dixon, J. (2007) The politics of healthcare and the health policy process: implications for healthcare management, in K. Walshe and J. Smith (eds) *Healthcare Management*. Maidenhead: Open University Press.

Dixon-Woods, M., Kirk, D., Agarwal, S., Annandale, E., Arthur, T., Harvey, J., Hsu, R., Katbamna, S., Olsen, R., Smith, L., Riley, R. and Sutton, A. (2005) *Vulnerable Groups and Access to Health Care: A Critical Interpretive Review*. London: NCCSDO.

Doyal, L. (1995) *What Makes Women Sick? Gender and the Political Economy of Health*. Basingstoke: Macmillan.

Doyal, L. (1998) *Women and Health Services: An Agenda for Change*. Buckingham: Open University Press.

Doyal, L. and Pennell, I. (1979) *The Political Economy of Health*. London: Pluto Press.

Drentea, P. and Moren-Cross, J. (2005) Social capital and social support on the web: the case of an internet mother site, *Sociology of Health and Illness*, 27(7): 920–43.

Drieskens, S., Van Oyen, H., Demarest, S., Van der Heyden, J., Gisle, L. and Tafforeau, J. (2009) Multiple risk behaviour: increasing socio-economic gap over time?, *The European Journal of Public Health*, 11(3): 294–300.

Drummond, M. (2010) Undertanding masculinities within the context of men, body image and eating disorders, in B. Gough and S. Robertson (eds) *Men, Masculinites and Health*. Basingstoke: Palgrave Macmillan.

Dunnell, K. (2008) *Diversity and Different Experiences in the UK. National Statistician's Annual Article on Society*. London: Office for National Statistics.

Durkheim, E. (1968) *Suicide: A Study in Sociology*. London: Routledge.

Durkheim, E. (1992) *Professional Ethics and Civic Morals*. London: Routledge.

Dyson, S. (2005) *Ethnicity and Screening for Sickle Cell/Thalassaemia*. Edinburgh: Elsevier Churchill Livingstone.

Dyson, S. and Smaje, C. (2001) The health status of minority ethnic groups, in L. Culley and S. Dyson (eds) (2001) *Ethnicity and Nursing Practice*. Basingstoke: Palgrave.

Dyson, L., McCormick, F. and Renfrew, M.J. (2007) Interventions for promoting the initiation of breastfeeding, *Cochrane Database of Systematic Reviews, 2005*, 2, Art. No. CD0011688.

Earle, S. (2005) What is health?, in E. Denny and S. Earle (eds) *Sociology for Nurses*. Cambridge: Polity Press.

Earle, S. and Letherby, G. (eds) (2008) *The Sociology of Healthcare: A Reader for Health Professionals*. Basingstoke: Palgrave Macmillan.

Edwards, T. and Waters, J. (2009) *It's Your Life – Take Control. The Implementation of Self-directed Support in Hertfordshire*. Hertford: Hertfordshire County Council and In Control Partnerships.

Elias, N. (1985) *The Loneliness of Dying*. Oxford: Basil Blackwell.

Ellen, B. (2009) And you thought it was just the proles who ate all the pies, *The Observer*, 24 May: 11.

Elliot, L. and Curtis, P. (2009) UK's income gap widest since 60s, *The Guardian*, 8 May: 4.

Elston, M.A., Gabe, J., Denney, D., Lee, R. and O'Beirne, M. (2002) Violence against doctors: a medical(ised) problem?, *Sociology of Health & Illness*, 24(5): 575–98.

Engels, F. (1969) *The Condition of the Working Class in England: From Personal Observation and Authentic Sources*. St Albans: Granada.

Ermisch, J. and Francesconi, M. (2000) The increasing complexity of family relationships: lifetime experience of lone motherhood and stepfamilies in Great Britain, *European Journal of Population*, 16(3): 235–49.

Evandrou, M. and Falkingham, J. (2005) A secure retirement for all? Older people, and New Labour, in J. Hills and K. Stewart (eds) *A More Equal Society for All? New Labour, Poverty, Inequality and Exclusion*. Bristol: The Policy Press.

Evans, J., Crooks, V. and Kingsbury, P. (2009) Theoretical injections: on the therapeutic aesthetics of medical spaces, *Social Science and Medicine*, 69(5): 716–21.

Evans, O., Singleton, N., Meltzer, H., Stewart, R. and Prince, M. (2003) *The Mental Health of Older People*. London: The Stationery Office.

Fawcett, B. (2000) *Feminist Perspectives on Disability*. Harlow: Pearson Education.

Fearon, P., Kirkbride, J.B., Morgan, C., Dazzan, P., Morgan, K., Lloyd, T., Hutchinson, G., Tarrant, J., Fung, W.L.A., Holloway, J., Mallett, R., Harrison, G., Leff, J., Jones, P.B. and Murray, R.M. (2006) Incidence of schizophrenia and other psychoses in ethnic minority groups: results from the MRC AESOP study, *Psychological Medicine*, 36: 1541–50.

Field, D. and Copp, G. (1999) Communication and awareness about dying in the 1990s, *Palliative Medicine*, 13: 459–68.

Field, D. and Payne, S. (2004) Social aspects of bereavement, *Cancer Nursing Practice*, 2: 21–5.

Field, D. and Taylor, S. (1998) *Sociological Perspectives on Health, Illness and Health Care*. Oxford: Blackwell Science.

Finch, J. and Groves, D. (1985) Community care and the family, in C. Ungerson (ed.) *Women and Social Policy: A Reader*. Basingstoke: Macmillan.

Finch, N. and Searle, B. (2005) Children's lifestyles, in J. Bradshaw and E. Mayhew (eds) *The Well-being of Children in the UK*, 2nd edn. London: Save the Children Fund.

Finch, T., Latorre, M., Pollard, M. and Rutter, J. (2009) *Shall We Stay or Shall We Go? Re-migration Trends Among Britain's Immigrants*. London: Institute for Public Policy.

Finkelstein, V. (1981) Disability and the helper/helped relationship: an historical view, in A. Brechin, P. Liddiard and J. Swain (eds) *Handicap in a Social World*. London: Hodder & Stoughton.

Firestone, S. (1979) *The Dialectic of Sex: The Case for Feminist Revolution*. London: The Women's Press.

Firth, S. (2000) Approaches to death in Hindu and Sikh communities in Britain, in D. Dickenson and M. Johnson (eds) *Death, Dying and Bereavement*. London: Sage.

Fish, D. and Coles, C. (eds) (1998) *Developing Professional Judgment in Healthcare: Learning Through Critical Appreciation of Practice*. London: Butterworth Heinemann.

Floyd, B. (1997) Problems in accurate medical diagnosis of depression in female patients, *Social Science and Medicine*, 44(3): 403–12.

Foresight (2007) *Trends and Drivers of Obesity: A Literature Review for the Foresight Project on Obesity*. London: Government Office for Science.

Foster, M., Harris, J., Jackson, K., Morgan, H. and Glendinning, C. (2006) Personalised social care for adults with disabilities: a problematic concept for frontline practice, *Health and Social Care in the Community*, 14(2): 125–35.

Foucault, M. (1973) *The Birth of the Clinic: An Archaeology of Medical Perception*. London: Tavistock.

Foucault, M. (1979) *Discipline and Punish: The Birth of the Prison*. Harmondsworth: Penguin.

Frank, A.W. (2001) Can we research suffering?, *Qualitative Health Research*, 11(3): 353–62.

Freund, P. and McGuire, M. (1995) *Health, Illness and the Social Body: A Critical Sociology*. Upper Saddle River, NJ: Prentice Hall.

Friedman, H.S., Tucker, J.S., Tomlinson-Keasey, C., Schwartz, J.E., Wingard, D.L. and Criqui, M.H. (1993) Does childhood personality predict longevity? *Journal of Personality and Social Psychology*, 65: 176–85.

Friedson, E. (1988) *Profession of Medicine: A Study of the Sociology of Applied Knowledge*. London: University of Chicago Press.

Gabe, J., Bury, M. and Elston, M.A. (2004) *Key Concepts in Medical Sociology*. London: Sage.

Gallagher, E. (1976) Lines of reconstruction and extension in the Parsonian sociology of illness, *Social Science and Medicine*, 10: 207–18.

Gannon, B. and Nolan, B. (2007) The impact of disability transitions on social inclusion, *Social Science and Medicine*, 64(7): 1425–47.

Gardiner, K. and Millar, J. (2006) How low-paid employees avoid poverty: an analysis by family type and household structure, *Journal of Social Policy*, 35(3): 351–69.

Gatrell, C. (2008) *Embodying Women's Work*. Maidenhead: McGraw-Hill.

Gerhardt, U. (1989) *Ideas About Illness: An Intellectual and Political History of Medical Sociology*. London: Macmillan.

Giddens, A. (1984) *The Constitution of Society: Outline of a Theory of Structuration*. Cambridge: Polity Press.

Giddens, A. (1992) *The Consequences of Modernity*. Cambridge: Polity Press.

Giddens, A. (2009) *Sociology*, 6th edn. Cambridge: Polity Press.

Gilbert, E., Ussher, J.M. and Hawkins, Y. (2009) Accounts of disruptions to sexuality following cancer: the perspective of informal carers who are partners of a person with cancer, *Health*, 13(5): 523–41.

Glasby, J. and Littlechild, R. (2004) *The Health and Social Care Divide: The Experiences of Older People*. Bristol: Policy Press.

Glaser, B. and Strauss, A. (1965) *Awareness of Dying*. Chicago, IL: Aldine.

Glaser, B. and Strauss, A. (1968) *Time for Dying*. Chicago, IL: Aldine.

Glaser, B. and Strauss, A. (1971) *Status Passage*. London: Routledge.

Glendenning, C., Tjadens, F., Arksey, H., Moree, M., Moran, N. and Nies, H. (2009) *Care Provision Within Families and its Socio-economic Impact on Care Providers*. York: Social Policy Research Unit,

Goddard, M. (2009) Access to health care services – an English policy perspective, *Health Economics, Policy and Law*, 4: 195–208.

Goffman, E. (1968a) *Stigma: Notes on the Management of a Spoiled Identity*. Harmondsworth: Penguin.

Goffman, E. (1968b) *Asylums: Essays on the Social Situation of Mental Patients and Other Inmates*. Harmondsworth: Penguin.

Goldthorpe, J. (1980) *Social Mobility and Class Structure in Modern Britain*. Oxford: Clarendon Press.

Goodwin, A.M. and Kennedy, A. (2005) The psychosocial benefits of work for people with severe and enduring mental health problems, *Community, Work and Family*, 8(1): 23–35.

Gott, M. (2005) *Sexuality, Sexual Health and Ageing*. Maidenhead: Open University Press.

Gough, B. and Robertson, S. (2010) *Men, Masculinities and Health: Critical Perspectives*. Basingstoke: Palgrave Macmillan.

Graham, H. (1983) Caring: a labour of love, in J. Finch and D. Groves (eds) *A Labour of Love: Women, Work and Caring*. London: Routledge & Kegan Paul.

Graham, H. (1993) *Hardship and Health in Women's Lives*. London: Wheatsheaf.

Graham, H. (1999) The informal sector of welfare: a crisis in caring?, in G. Allan (ed.) *The Sociology of the Family: A Reader*. Oxford: Blackwell.

Graham, H. (ed.) (2000) *Understanding Health Inequalities*. Buckingham: Open University Press.

Graham, H. (2007) *Unequal Lives: Health and Socio-economic Inequalities*. Maidenhead: McGraw-Hill.

Graham, H. (ed.) (2009) *Understanding Health Inequalities*, 2nd edn. Maidenhead: Open University Press.

Graham, H. and Blackburn, C. (1998) The socioeconomic patterning of health and smoking behaviours among mothers with young children on income support, *Sociology of Health and Illness*, 20(2): 215–40.

Gray, L. and Leyland, A.H. (2009) Is the 'Glasgow effect' of cigarette smoking explained by socioeconomic status? A multilevel analysis, *BMC Public Health*, 9: 245.

Green, J., Kitzinger, J.V. and Coupland, V.A. (1990) Stereotypes of childbearing women: a look at some evidence, *Midwifery*, 6: 125–32.

Grue, L. and Laerum, K.T. (2002) 'Doing motherhood': some experiences of mothers with physical disabilities, *Disability and Society*, 17(6): 671–83.

Gulliford, M. (2003) Equity and access to health care, in M. Gulliford and M. Morgan (eds) *Access to Health Care*. London: Routledge.

Gulliford, M. and Morgan, M. (eds) (2003) *Access to Health Care*. London: Routledge.

Gunnarsson, E. (2009) 'I think I have had a good life': the everyday lives of older women and men from a lifecourse perspective, *Ageing and Society*, 29: 33–48.

Hall, S. (1988) Brave new world, *Marxsim Today*, October: 24–9.

Halpin, M., Philips, M. and Oliffe, J.L. (2009) Prostate cancer stories in the Canadian print media: representations of illness, disease and masculinities, *Sociology of Health and Illness*, 31(2): 155–69.

Handy, C. (2005) *Understanding Organisations*, 5th edn. London: Penguin.

Hanratty, B., Drever, F., Jacoby, A. and Whitehead, M. (2007) Retirement age caregivers and deprivation of area of residence in England and Wales, *European Journal of Ageing*, 4(1): 35–43.

Hardey, M. (1999) Doctor in the house: the internet as a source of lay health knowledge and the challenge to expertise, *Sociology of Health Illness*, 21(6): 820–35.

Hareven, T.K. (1995) Changing images of aging and the social construction of the life course, in M. Featherstone and A. Wernick (eds) *Images of Aging: Cultural Representations of Later Life*. London: Routledge.

Harman, J., Graham, H., Francis, B., Inskip, H.M. and the SWS Study Group (2006) Socioeconomic gradients in smoking among young women: a British survey, *Social Science and Medicine*, 63(11): 2791–800.

Harris, R. and Seid, M. (eds) (2004) *Globalisation and Health*. London: Brill Academic Publishers.

Harris, R., Tobias, M., Jeffreys, M., Waldegrave, K., Karlsen, S. and Nazroo, J. (2006) Racism and health: the relationship between experience of racial discrimination and health in New Zealand, *Social Science and Medicine*, 63(6): 1428–41.

Harrop, A. and Potter, C. (2009) *British Medical Association Consultation: Developing General Practice, Listening to Patients*. London: Age Concern.

Harvey, J. (1995) Up-skilling and the intensification of work: the 'extended role' in intensive care nursing and midwifery, *Sociological Review*, 43(4): 765–81.

Hatton, C., Duffy, S., Waters, J., Senker, J., Crosby, N., Poll, C., Tyson, A., Towell, D. and O'Brien, J. (2008) *An Evaluation of and Report on In Control's Work, 2005–2007*. London: In Control Publications.

Hayes, B.C. and Prior, P.M. (2003) *Gender and Health Care in the UK*. Basingstoke: Palgrave Macmillan.

Healthcare Commission (2009) *Tackling the Challenge: Promoting Race Equality in the NHS in England*. London: Commission for Healthcare Audit and Inspection.

Heaton, J. (1999) The gaze and visibility of the carer: a Foucauldian analysis of the discourse of informal care, *Sociology of Health and Illness*, 21(6): 759–77.

Heenan, D. (2002) 'It won't change the world but it turned my life around': participants' views on the Personal Advisor Scheme in the New Deal for Disabled People, *Disability and Society*, 17(4): 383–401.

Heywood, F. (2001) *Money Well Spent: The Effectiveness and Value of Housing Adaptations*. Bristol: Policy Press.

Hicks, S. and Thomas, J. (2009) *Presentation of the Gender Pay Gap*. London: Office for National Statistics.

Higgs, P. and Rees Jones, I. (2009) *Medical Sociology and Old Age: Towards a Sociology of Health in Later Life*. London: Routledge.

Hirst, M. (1999) *Informal Care-giving in the Life Course*. York: SPRU.

Hirst, M. (2003) Caring-related inequalities in psychological distress in Britain during the 1990s, *Journal of Public Health Medicine*, 25(4): 336–43.

Hiscock, D. and Stirling, S. (2009) *Prospects for More Local, More Personalised Public Services: A North East Perspective*, www.ippr.org.uk/publicationsandreports/publication.asp?id=642.

HM Government (1995) *Disability Discrimination Act 1995*. London: HMSO.

Hobson-West, P. (2007) Trusting blindly can be the biggest risk of all: organised resistance to childhood vaccination in the UK, *Sociology of Health & Illness*, 29(2): 198–215.

Hochschild, A. (1983) *The Managed Heart: Commercialisation of Human Feelings*. Berkeley, CA: University of California Press.

Hockey, J. and James, A. (2003) *Social Identities Across the Life Course*. Basingstoke: Palgrave Macmillan.

Holmes, J.D. (2007) *Liaison Psychiatry Services for Older People Project*. Leeds: NHS SDO.

Holstein, J.A. and Gubrium, J.F. (2000) *Constructing the Life Course*. New York: General Hall.

Home Office (2003) *Home Office Citizenship Survey: People, Families and Communities*. London: HMSO.

Hopkins, L., Labonte, R., Runnels, V. and Packer, C. (2010) Medical tourism today: what is the state of existing knowledge?, *Journal of Public Health Policy*, 31: 185–98.

Howarth, B. (2007) *Death and Dying. A Sociological Introduction*. Cambridge: Polity Press.

Hudson, B. (2005) Sea change or quick fix? Policy on long-term conditions in England, *Health and Social Care in the Community*, 13(4): 378–85.

Hughes, B., Russell, R. and Paterson, K. (2005) Nothing to be had 'off the peg': consumption, identity and the immobilisation of young disabled people, *Disability and Society*, 20(1): 3–17.

Hughes, G. (1998) A suitable case for treatment? Constructions of disability, in E. Saraga (ed.) *Embodying the Social: Constructions of Difference*. London: Routledge.

Humphrey, J.C. (2000) Researching disability politics, or some problems with the social model in practice, *Disability and Society*, 15(1): 63–85.

Hunt, S. (2005) *The Life Course: A Sociological Introduction*. Basingstoke: Palgrave Macmillan.

Huynen, M.M.T.E., Martens, P. and Hilderink, H.B.M. (2005) The health impacts of globalisation: a conceptual framework, *Globalization and Health*, 1: 14 (doi:10.1186/1744-8603-1-14).

Huxley, P. and Thornicroft, G. (2003) Social inclusion, social quality and mental illness, *The British Journal of Psychiatry*, 182: 289–90.

Hyde, M. (2006a) Disability, in G. Payne (ed.) *Social Divisions*, 2nd edn. Basingstoke: Macmillan.

Hyde, M. (2000b) From welfare-to-work? Social policy for disabled people of working age in the United Kingdom in the 1990s, *Disability and Society*, 15(2): 327–41.

Illich, I. (1976) *Limits to Medicine: Medical Nemesis – The Expropriation of Health*. Harmonsdworth: Penguin.

Iley, K. and Nazroo, J. (2001) Ethnic inequalities in mental health, in L. Culley and S. Dyson (eds) *Ethnicity and Nursing Practice*. Basingstoke: Palgrave.

Jackson, S. (1997) Women, marriage and family relationships, in V. Robinson and D. Richardson (eds) *Introducing Women's Studies*. Basingstoke: Macmillan.

Jamieson, A. and Victor, C. (eds) (2002) *Researching Ageing and Later Life*. Buckingham: Open University Press.

Janes, L. (2002) Understanding gender divisions, in P. Braham and L. Janes (eds) *Social Differences and Divisions*. Milton Keynes: The Open University.

Jenkins, S.P. (2008) *Marital Splits and Income Changes Over the Longer Term*. Colchester: Institute for Social and Economic Research

Johnson, N. (2000) The personal social services and community care, in M. Powell (ed.) *New Labour, New Welfare State?* Bristol: The Policy Press.

Jones, L. (1994) *The Social Context of Health and Health Work.* Basingstoke: Macmillan.

Jones, L. and Green, J. (2006) Shifting discourses of professionalism: a case study of general practitioners in the United Kingdom, *Sociology of Health and Illness*, 28(7): 927–50.

Jowsey, T., Jeon, Y.-H., Dugdale, P., Glasgow, N.J., Kljakovic, M. and Usherwood, T. (2009) Challenges for co-morbid chronic illness care and policy in Australia: a qualitative study, *Australia and New Zealand Health Policy*, 6: 22.

Judd, D. (2000) Communicating with dying children, in D. Dickenson and M. Johnson (eds) *Death, Dying and Bereavement.* London: Sage.

Karlsen, S. and Nazroo, J. (2001) Identity and structure; rethinking ethnic inequalites in health, in H. Graham (ed.) *Understanding Health Inequalities.* Buckingham: Open University Press.

Katz, J.S. (2000) Jewish perspectives on death, dying and bereavement, in D. Dickenson and M. Johnson (eds) *Death, Dying and Bereavement.* London: Sage.

Kelly, B.D. (2006) The power gap: freedom, power and mental illness, *Social Science and Medicine*, 63(8): 2118–28.

Kelly, Y.J. and Watt, R.G. (2005) Breastfeeding initiation and exclusive duration at 6 months by social class – results from the Millennium Cohort Study, *Public Health Nutrition*, 8(4): 417–21.

Kemp, L. (2002) Why are some people's needs unmet? *Disability and Society*, 17(2): 205–18.

Kendall, J. and Knapp, M. (1996) *The Voluntary Sector in the United Kingdom.* Manchester: Manchester University Press.

Kessler, D., Summerton, N. and Graham, J. (2006) Effects of the medical liability system in Australia, the UK and the USA, *Lancet*, 368: 240–6.

Kivits, J. (2009) Everyday health and the internet: a mediated health perspective on health information seeking, *Sociology of Health and Illness*, 31(5): 673–87.

Knight, M., Kurinczuk, J.J., Spark, P. and Brocklehurst, P. (2009) Inequalities in maternal health: national cohort study of ethnic variation in severe maternal morbidities, *British Medical Journal*, 338: 542.

Krieger, J. (2002) Housing and health: time again for public health action, *American Journal of Public Health*, 92(5): 758–68.

Kübler-Ross, E. (1973) *On Death and Dying.* London: Tavistock.

Kubzansky, L.D., Martin, L.T. and Buka, S.L. (2009) Early manifestatons of personality and adult health: a life course perspective, *Health Psychology*, 28(3): 364–72.

Kyle, T. and Dunn, J.R. (2008) Effects of housing circumstances on health, quality of life and healthcare use for people with severe mental illness, *Health and Social Care in the Community*, 16(1): 1–15.

Ladd, P. (2003) *Understanding Deaf Culture: In Search of Deafhood.* Bristol: Multilingual Matters.

Langani, P. (1997) Death in a Hindu family, in C. Murray Parkes, P. Langani and B. Young (eds) *Death and Bereavement Across Cultures.* London: Routledege.

Larkin, G.V. (1993) Continuity in change: medical dominance in the United Kingdom, in F.W. Hafferty and J.B. Mckinlay (eds) *The Changing Medical Profession: An International Perspective.* Oxford: Oxford University Press.

Larkin, M. (2009) *Vulnerable Groups in Health and Social Care.* London: Sage.

Larsson, K., Thorslund, M. and Kareholt, I. (2006) Are public care and services and services for older people targeted according to need? Applying the behavioural model on longitudinal data of a Swedish urban older population, *European Journal of Ageing*, 3(1): 22–33.

Law, C., Power, C., Graham, H. and Merrick, D. (2007) Obesity and health inequalities, *Obesity Reviews*, 8(1): 19–22.

Lawrence, D., Mitrou, F. and Zubrick, S.R. (2009) Smoking and mental illness: results from population surveys in Australia and the United States, *BMC Public Health*, 9: 285.

Leicester, A., O'Dea, C. and Oldfield, Z. (2008) *The Inflation Experience of Older Households*. London: Institute for Fiscal Studies.

Lester, H. and Glasby, J. (2006) *Mental Health Policy and Practice*. Basingstoke: Palgrave Macmillan.

Leutz, W. and Capitman, J. (2007) Met and unmet needs, and satisfaction among social HMO members, *Journal of Ageing and Social Policy*, 19(1): 1–19.

Levitas, R., Head, E. and Finch, N. (2006) Lone parents, poverty and social exclusion, in C. Pantazis, D. Gordon and R. Levitas (eds) *Poverty and Social Exclusion in Britain: The Millennium Survey*. Bristol: The Policy Press.

Lewis, J. and Meredith, B. (1988) *Daughters Who Care*. London: Routledge.

Lewitt, M.S., Ehrenborg, E., Scheia, M. and Brauner, A. (2010) Stereotyping at the undergraduate level revealed during interprofessional learning between future doctors and biomedical scientists, *Journal of Interprofessional Care*, 24(1): 53–62.

Link, B. and Phelan, J. (1995) Social conditions as fundamental causes of disease, *Journal of Health and Social Behaviour*, 35(extra issue): 80–94.

Littlewood, J. (1993) The denial of death and rites of passage in contemporary societies, in D. Clark (ed.) *The Sociology of Death: Theory, Culture, Practice*. Oxford: Blackwell.

Long, S.O. (2004) Cultural scripts for a good death in Japan and the United States: similarities and differences, *Social Science and Medicine*, 58(5): 913–28.

Lorig, K.R., Ritter, P.L., Dost, A., Plant, K., Laurent, D.D. and Mcneil, I. (2008) The expert patients programme online, a 1-year study of an internet-based self-management programme for people with long-term conditions, *Chronic Illness*, 4(4): 247–56.

Loudon, I. (ed.) (1997) *Western Medicine: An Illustrated History*. Oxford: Oxford University Press.

Luck, M., Bamford, M. and Williamson, P. (2000) *Men's' Health: Perspectives, Diversity and Paradox*. Oxford: Blackwell Science.

Lupton, D. (1996) *The Imperative of Health: Public Health and the Regulated Body*. London: Sage.

Lupton, D. (1997) Consumerism, reflexivity and the medical encounter, *Social Science and Medicine*, 45(3): 373–81.

Lupton, D. (1998) Doctors on the medical profession, *Sociology of Health and Illness*, 32(4): 480–97.

Lupton, D. (2008) The body, medicine and death, in S. Earle and G. Letherby (eds) *The Sociology of Healthcare: A Reader for Health Professionals*. Basingstoke: Palgrave Macmillan.

Lynch, J.W., Kaplan, G. and Salonen, J.T. (1997) Why do poor people behave poorly? Variations in adult health behaviours and psychosocial characteristics by stages of the socio-economic life course, *Social Science in Medicine*, 44(6): 809–19.

MacDonald, K.M. (1995) *The Sociology of the Professions*. London: Sage.

Mackintosh, C. (2006) Caring: the socialisation of pre-registration student nurses: a longitudinal qualitative descriptive study, *International Journal of Nursing Studies*, 43(8): 953–62.

Macleod, C. and Durrheim, K. (2002) Foucauldian feminism: the implications of governmentality, *Journal for the Theory of Social Behaviour*, 32(1): 41–60.

MacLeod, R. (2001) On reflection: doctors learning to care for people who are dying, *Social Science and Medicine*, 52(11): 1719–27.

Macpherson, W. (1999) *The Stephen Lawrence Inquiry*. London: The Stationery Office.

Markowitz, F.E. (2006) Psychiatric hospital capacity, homelessness and crime and arrest rates, *Criminology*, 44(1): 45–72.

Marmot, M. (2009) *Policy and Action for Cancer Prevention*. London: World Cancer Research Fund.

Marmot, M. (2010) *Fair Society, Healthy Lives. A Strategic Review of Health Inequalities in England Post-2010 (Marmot Review)*. London: The Marmot Review.

Marmot, M. and Wilkinson, R. (eds) (2006) *Social Determinants of Health*. Oxford: Oxford University Press.

Marmot, M., Shipley, M., Brunner, E. and Hemingway, H. (2001) Relative contribution of early life and adult socio-economic factors to adult morbidity in the Whitehall II study, *Journal of Epidemiology and Community Health*, 55(5): 301–7.

Marshall, B.L. (2006) The new virility: Viagra, male aging and sexual function, *Sexualities*, 9(3): 345–62.

Martin, G.P. (2008) Representativeness, legitimacy and power in public involvement in health-service management, *Social Science and Medicine*, 67(11): 1757–65.

Marx, K. (1867) *Das Kapital*. Moscow: Foreign Languages Publishing House.

Mason, D. (2006) Ethnicity, in G. Payne (ed.) *Social Divisions*. Basingstoke: Macmillan.

Matthewman, S., West-Newman, C.L. and Curtis, B. (eds) (2007) *Being Sociological*. Basingstoke: Palgrave Macmillan.

Maynard, A. (2005) *The Public–Private Mix for Health: Plus ça Change, Plus c'est la Même Chose?* Oxford: Radcliffe.

McCarthy, H. and Thomas, G. (2004) *Home Alone: Combating Isolation with Older Housebound People*. London: Demos.

McCrone, P., Dhanasiri, S., Patel, A., Knapp, M. and Lawton-Smith, S. (2008) *Paying the Price: The Cost of Mental Health Care in England to 2026*. London: King's Fund

McCusker, J., Cole, M., Ciampi, A., Latimer, E., Winholz, S. and Belzile, E. (2006) Does depression in older medical inpatients predict mortality?, *Journals of Gerontology*, 61(9): 975–81.

McGarry, J. (2008) Defining roles, relationships, boundaries and participation between elderly people and nurses within the home: an ethnographic study, *Health and Social Care in the Community*, 17(1): 83–91.

McLaughlin, E. and Ritchie, J. (1994) Legacies of caring: the experiences and circumstances of ex-carers, *Health and Social Care*, 2(4): 241–53.

McLaughlin, K., Osborne, S.P. and Ferlie, E. (2002) *The New Public Management: Current Trends and Future Prospects*. London: Routledge.

McNamara, B. (1994) The institutionalisation of the good death, *Social Science & Medicine*, 39(11): 1501–8.

Means, R., Richards, S. and Smith, R. (2008). *Community Care: Policy and Practice*, 4th edn. Basingstoke: Palgrave Macmillan.

Melia, K. (1987) *Learning and Working: The Occupational Socialisation of Nurses*. London: Tavistock.

Melville, C. (2005) Discrimination and health inequalities experienced by disabled people, *Medical Education*, 39(2): 124–6.

Meltzer, H., Singleton, N., Lee, A. and Bebbington, P. (2002) *The Social and Economic Circumstances of Adults with Mental Disorders*. London: Office for National Statistics.

Melzer, D., Fryers, T. and Jenkins, R. (2004) *Social Inequalities and the Distribution of the Common Mental Disorders*. Hove: Psychology Press.

Merritt, S. (2008) A new plague facing women, *The Observer*, 6 January: 26–7.

Merton, R.K., Reader, G. and Kendall, P.L. (eds) (1957) *The Student Physician: Introductory Studies in the Sociology of Medical Education*. Cambridge, MA: Harvard University Press.

Miles, A. (1991) *Women, Health and Medicine*. Buckingham: Open University Press.

Miller, A. (2003) Link no longer missing, *Community Care*, 4–10 December: 38.

Mills, C. Wright (1959) *The Sociological Imagination*. New York: Oxford University Press.

Mohan, J. (1995) *A National Health Service? The Restructuring of Health Care in Britain Since 1979*. Basingstoke: Macmillan.

Mohan, J. (2002) *Planning, Markets and Hospitals*. London: Routledge.

Molarius, A., Berglund, K., Eriksson, C., Eriksson, H.G., Lindén-Boström, M., Nordström, E., Persson, C., Sahlqvist, L., Starrin, B. and Ydreborg, B. (2009) Mental health symptoms in relation to socio-economic conditions and lifestyle factors – a population-based study in Sweden, *BMC Public Health*, 9: 302.

Montgomery, S. (1990) *Anxiety and Depression*. London: Livingstone.

Morris, P. (1969) *Put Away*. London: Routledge & Kegan Paul.

Moser, K., Patnick, J. and Beral, V. (2009) Inequalities in reported use of breast and cervical screening in Great Britain: analysis of cross sectional survey data, *British Medical Journal*, 338: b2025.

Murray-Parkes, C., Laungani, P. and Young, B. (1997) *Death and Bereavement Across Cultures*. London: Routledge.

Naidoo, J. and Wills, J. (2008) *Health Studies: An Introduction*, 2nd edn. Basingstoke: Palgrave.

National Audit Office (2007) *Improving Services and Support for People with Dementia*. London: The Stationery Office.

National Cancer Intelligence Network (2009) *Cancer Incidence and Survival by Major Ethnic Group, England, 2002–2006*. London: National Cancer Intelligence Network Co-ordinating Centre.

National Social Inclusion Programme (2007) *Third Annual Update*. London: Department of Health.

National Institute for Health and Clinical Excellence (2007) *Community Based Interventions to Reduce Substance Misuse Among Vulnerable and Disadvantaged Children and Young People*. London: National Institute for Health and Clinical Excellence.

National Statistics (2004a) *Living in Britain: No 31. Results from the 2002 General Household Survey*. London: The Stationery Office.

National Statistics (2004b) *Focus on Social Inequalities*. London: The Stationery Office.

National Statistics (2005a) *The National Statistics Socio-economic Classification User Manual*. London: The Stationery Office.

National Statistics (2005b) *Focus on Older People*. London: The Stationery Office.

National Statistics (2006a) *Population Estimates*, www.statistics.gov.uk.

National Statistics (2006b) *Focus on Ethnicity and Identity*, www.statistics.gov.uk.

National Statistics (2007) *Social Trends 37*. Basingstoke: Palgrave Macmillan.

National Statistics (2008) *Population Trends 131*. Basingstoke: Palgrave Macmillan.

Navarro, J. (1978) *Class, Struggle, the State and Medicine*. London: Martin Robertson.

Nazroo, J.Y. (1997) *The Health of Britain's Ethnic Minorities*. London: Policy Studies Institute.

Nazroo, J.Y. (2001) *Ethnicity, Class and Health*. London: Policy Studies Institute.

Nazroo, J.Y. and Williams, D.R. (2006) The social determination of ethnic/racial inequalities in health, in M. Marmot and R. Wilkinson (eds) *Social Determinants of Health*. Oxford: Oxford University Press.

Nelson, M. (2000) Childhood nutrition and poverty, *Proceedings of the Nutrition Society*, 59: 307–15.

O'Donnell, G. (2002) *Mastering Sociology*, 4th edn. Basingstoke: Palgrave.

O'Donnell, T. (2005) Social class and health, in E. Denny and S. Earle (eds) *Sociology for Nurses*. Cambridge: Polity Press.

O'Grady, A., Pleasence, P., Balmer, N.J., Buck, A. and Genn, H. (2004) Disability, social exclusion and the consequential experience of justiciable problems, *Disability and Society*, 19(4): 259–71.

O'Neill, T., Jinks, C. and Squire, A. (2006) 'Heating is more important than food': older women's perceptions of fuel poverty, *Journal of Housing for the Elderly*, 20(3): 95–108.

Oakley, A. (1972) *Sex, Gender and Society*. London: Temple Smith.

Oakley, A. (1974) *The Sociology of Housework*. London: Martin Robertson.

Oakley, A. (1980) *Women Confined: Towards a Sociology of Childbirth*. London: Martin Robertson.

Oakley, A. (1984) *The Captured Womb*. Oxford: Basil Blackwell.

Oakley, A. (1993) *Women, Medicine and Health*. Edinburgh: Edinburgh University Press.

Office for National Statistics (2001) *Psychiatric Morbidity Survey*. London: HMSO.

Office for National Statistics (2002) *National Statistics Socio-economic Classification: User Manual*. London: HMSO.

Office for National Statistics (2004) *Drinking: Adults' Behaviour and Knowledge in 2004*. London: HMSO.

Office for National Statistics (2005) *General Household Survey 2003*. London: HMSO.

Office for National Statistics (2006a) *Focus on Health*. London: HMSO.

Office for National Statistics (2006b) *General Household Survey 2004*. London: HMSO .

Office for National Statistics (2007a) *Trends in Life Expectancy by Social Class 1972–2005*, www.statistics.gov.uk/downloads/theme_population/Life_Expect_Social_ class_1972-05/life_ expect_social_class.pdf.

Office for National Statistics (2007b) *General Household Survey 2005*. London: HMSO.

Office for National Statistics (2008a) *Focus on Gender*. London: HMSO.

Office for National Statistics (2008b) *General Household Survey 2006*. London: HMSO.

Office for National Statistics (2008c) *Population Estimates*. London: HMSO.

Office for National Statistics (2009) *General Household Survey 2007*. London: HMSO.

Office of Population, Censuses and Statistics (1998) *Social Trends*. London: The Stationery Office.

Office of Population, Censuses and Statistics (2002) *Social Trends*. London: The Stationery Office.

Oliver, M. (1990) *The Politics of Disablement:* Basingstoke: Macmillan.

Oliver, M. (1996) *Understanding Disability: From Theory to Practice*. Basingstoke: Macmillan.

Oliver, M. (1998) *Disabled People and Social Policy: From Exclusion to Inclusion*. London: Longman.

Pagano, D., Freemantle, N., Bridgewater, B., Howell, N., Ray, D., Jackson, M., Fabri, B.M., Au, J., Keenan, D., Kirkup, B. and Keogh, B.E. (2009) Social deprivation and prognostic benefits of cardiac surgery: observational study of 44,902 patients from five hospitals over 10 years, *British Medical Journal*, 338: b902.

Palmer, G. and Kenway, P. (2007) *Poverty Rates Amongst Ethnic Groups in Great Britain*. York: Joseph Rowntree Foundation.

Palmer, G., MacInnes, T. and Kenway, P. (2007) *Monitoring Poverty and Social Exclusion*. York: Joseph Rowntree Trust.

Pandiani, J.A., Boyd, M.M., Banks, S.M. and Johnson, A.T. (2006) Elevated cancer incidence among adults with serious mental illness, *Psychiatric Services*, 57(7): 1032–4.

Parker, G. (1985) *With Due Care and Attention: A Review of Research on Informal Care*. London: FPSC.

Parliamentary Office of Science and Technology (2007) *Ethnicity and Health*. London: HMSO.

Parsons, T. (1964) *The Social System*. London: RKP.

Parsons, T. (1975) The sick role and the role of the physician reconsidered, *Health and Society*, 53(3): 257–78.

Parsons, T. and Bales, R. (1955) *Family, Socialization and Interaction Process*. New York: Free Press.

Patsios, D. (2006) Pensioners, poverty and social exclusion, in C. Pantazis, D. Gordon and R. Levitas (eds) *Poverty and Social Exclusion in Britain: The Millennium Survey*. Bristol: The Policy Press.

Payne, G. (ed.) (2006) *Social Divisions*. Basingstoke: Macmillan.

Payne, S. (1998) 'Hit and miss': the success and failure of psychiatric services for women, in L. Doyal (ed.) *Women and Health Services*. Buckingham: Open University Press.

Pelling, M. and Harrison, M. (2001) Pre-industrial health care, 1500–1750, in C. Webster (ed.) *Caring for Health: History and Diversity*. Buckingham: Open University Press.

Pelling, M., Harrison, M. and Weindling, P. (2001) The industrial revolution, 1750–1848, in C. Webster (ed.) *Caring for Health: History and Diversity*. Buckingham: Open University Press.

Penninx, B.W., van Tilburg, T., Deeg, D.J., Kriegsman, D.M., Boeke, A.J. and van Eijk, J.T. (1997) Direct and buffer effects of social support and personal coping resources in individuals with arthritis, *Social Science and Medicine*, 44(3): 393–402.

Perry, B.L. and Wright, E.R. (2006) The sexual partnerships of people with serious mental illness, *Journal of Sex Research*, 43: 174–81.

Petrie, K.J. and Weinman, J. (1997) *Perceptions of Health and Illness: Current Research and Applications*. Amsterdam: Harwood Academic Publishers.

Phillipson, C. (1998) *Reconstructing Old Age: New Agendas in Social Theory and Practice*. London: Sage.

Picardie, R. (1998) *Before I Say Goodbye*. London: Penguin.

Pickard, L., Wittenberg, R., Comas-Herrera, A., King, D. and Malley, J. (2007) Care by spouses, care by children: projections of informal care for older people in England to 2031, *Social Policy and Society*, 6(3): 353–66.

Pilgrim, D. (2007) *Key Concepts in Mental Health*. London: Sage.

Pilgrim, D. and Bentall, R. (1999) The medicalisation of misery: a critical realist analysis of the concept of depression, *Journal of Mental Health*, 8(3): 261–74.

Pilnick, A., Hindmarsh, J. and Teas Gill, V. (2009) Beyond 'doctor and patient' developments in the study of healthcare interactions, *Sociology of Health and Illness*, 31(6): 787–802.

Plant, M., Miller, P., Gmel, G., Kuntsche, S., Bergman, W.K., Bloomfield, K., Csmy, L., Ozenturk, T. and Vidal, A. (2010) The social consequences of binge drinking among 24 to 32-year-olds in six European countries, *Substance Use and Abuse*, 45(4): 528–42.

Platt, L. (2007) *Poverty and Ethnicity in the UK*. Bristol: The Policy Press.

Porter, R. (2002) *Blood and Guts: A Short History of Medicine*. London: Penguin.

Powell, M. (ed.) 2000) *New Labour, New Welfare State?* Bristol: The Policy Press.

Power, R. (2000) Death in Ireland: deaths, wakes and funerals in contemporary Irish society, in D. Dickenson and M. Johnson (eds) *Death, Dying and Bereavement*. London: Sage.

Pritchard, J. (2006) *Putting a Stop to the Abuse of Older People*. London: Help the Aged.

Puigpinós, R., Borrell, C., Leopoldo Ferreire Antunes, J., Azlor, E., Pasarín, M.I., Serral, G., Pons-Vigués, M., Rodríguez-Sanz, M. and Fernández, E. (2009) Trends in socioeconomic inequalities in cancer mortality in Barcelona: 1992–2003, *BMC Public Health*, 9: 35.

Ramazanoglu, C. and Holland, J. (2002) *Feminist Methodology: Challenges and Choices*. London: Sage.

Rayner, E. (1997) *Human Development. An Introduction to the Psychodynamics of Growth, Maturity and Aging*. London: Routledge.

Reinharz, S. (2001) Enough already! The pervasiveness of wanting in everyday life, in B. Davey, A. Gray and C. Seale (eds) *Health and Disease: A Reader*. Buckingham: Open University Press.

Reynolds, K. (1996) *Children's Literature in the 1890s and 1990s*. Tavistock: Northcote House and the British Council.

Riddell, M. (2007) But not everyone can grow old gracefully, *The Observer*, 10 June: 35.

Ritzer, G. (2010) *Globalisation: A Basic Text*. Oxford: Wiley-Blackwell.

Roberts, E. (2000) *Age Discrimination in Health and Social Care*. London: King's Fund.

Roberts, H. (1992) Professionals' and parents' perceptions of A & E use in a children's hospital, *Sociological Review*, 40(1): 10–31.

Robinson, C.C. and Morris, J.T. (1986) The gender-stereotyped nature of Christmas toys received by 36-, 48- and 60-month-old children: a comparison between nonrequested vs requested toys, *Sex Roles*, 15(1–2): 21–32.

Rogers, A. and Pilgrim, D. (2003) *Mental Health and Inequality*. Basingstoke: Palgrave.

Rogers, A. and Pilgrim, D. (2005) *A Sociology of Mental Health and Illness*. Maidenhead: Open University Press.

Rogers, A. and Pilgrim, D. (2010) *A Sociology of Mental Health and Illness*, 4th edn. Maidenhead: Open University Press.

Rogers, A., Hassell, K. and Nicolaas, G. (1999) *Demanding Patients? Analysing the Use of Primary Care*. Buckingham: Open University Press.

Rogers, A., Kennedy, A., Bower, P., Gardner, C., Gately, C., Lee, V., Reeves, D. and Richardson, G. (2008) The United Kingdom Expert Patients Programme: results and implications from a national evaluation, *The Medical Journal of Australia*, 189(10, supplement): S21–4.

Rose, S.M. and Hatzenbuehler, S. (2009) Embodying social class: the link between poverty, income inequality and health, *International Social Work*, 52(4): 459–71.

Rosenblatt, P.C. (1997) Grief in small-scale societies, in C. Murray Parkes, P. Laungani and B. Young (eds) *Death and Bereavement Across Cultures*. London: Routledge.

Rummery, K. (2006) Disabled citizens and social exclusion: the role of direct payments, *Policy and Politics*, 34(4): 633–50.

Saks, M. (2000) Professionalism and healthcare, in E. Davies, L. Finlay and A. Bullman (eds) *Changing Practice in Health and Social Care*. London: Sage.

Saks, M. (2003).*Orthodox and Alternative Medicine Politics: Professionalisation and Health Care*. London: Sage.

Sanders, C., Donovan, J. and Dieppe, P. (2002) The significance and consequences of having painful and disabled joints in older age: co-existing accounts of normal and disrupted biographies, *Sociology of Health & Illness*, 24(2): 227–53.

Sapey, B. (2004) Disability and social exclusion in the information society, in J. Swain, S. French, C. Barnes and C. Thomas (eds) *Disabling Barriers, Enabling Environments*. London: Sage in association with the The Open University.

Sayce, L. (2009) *Doing Seniority Differently: A Study of High Fliers Living with Ill-health, Injury or Disability*. London: RADAR.

Schneider, J., Slade, J., Secker, J., Rinaldi, M., Boyce, M., Johnson, R., Floyd, M. and Grove, B. (2009) SESAMI study of employment support for people with severe mental health problems: 12-month outcomes, *Health and Social Care in the Community*, 17(2): 151–8.

Schrecker, T., Labonte, R. and De Vogli, R. (2008) Globalisation and health: the need for a global vision, *Lancet*, 372(9650): 1607.

Scott, J. (2006) Class and stratification, in G. Payne (ed.) *Social Divisions*. Basingstoke: Macmillan.

Scull, A. (1979) *Museums of Madness: The Social Organisation of Insanity in Nineteenth Century England*. London: Allen Lane.

Seale, C. (1998) *Constructing Death: The Sociology of Dying and Bereavement*. Cambridge: Cambridge University Press.

Seale, C. (2000) Changing patterns of death and dying, *Social Science and Medicine*, 51(6): 917–30.

Seale, C. and Charteris-Black, J. (2008) The interaction of class and gender in illness narratives, *Sociology*, 42(3): 453–69.

Seale, C., Addington-Hall, J. and McCarthy, M. (1997) Awareness of dying: prevalence, causes and consequences, *Social Science and Medicine*, 45(3): 477–84.

Segre, S. (2004) A Durkheimian network theory, *Journal of Classical Sociology*, 4(2): 215–35.

Sennett, R. (1993) *The Fall of Public Man*. London: Faber & Faber.

Servin, A., Bohlin, G. and Berlin, L. (1999) Sex differences in 1-, 3-, and 5-year-olds' toy-choice in a structured play-session, *Scandinavian Journal of Psychology*, 40(1): 43–8.

Sharma, U. (1999) *Caste*. Buckingham: Open University Press.

Shaw, R. (2007) Relating: family, in S. Matthewman, C.L. West-Newman and B. Curtis (eds) *Being Sociological*. Basingstoke: Palgrave Macmillan.

Shelter (2007) *Older People and Housing*. London: Shelter.

Shilling, C. (2002) Culture, the sick role and the consumption of health, *British Journal of Sociology*, 53(4): 621–38.

Shilling, C. (2003) *The Body and Social Theory*, 2nd edn. London: Sage.

Showalter, E. (1987) *The Female Malady: Women, Madness and English Culture, 1830–1980*. London: Virago.

Shulman, G. and Hammer, J. (1988) Social characteristics, the diagnosis of mental disorders and the change from DSMII to DSMIII, *Sociology of Health and Illness*, 10(4): 543–60.

Silva, E.B. and Smart, C. (1999) The 'new' practices and politics of family life, in E.B. Silva and C. Smart (eds) *The New Family?* London: Sage.

Simonsen, M.K., Hundrup, Y.A., Gronbaek, M. and Hetimann, B.L. (2008) A prospective study of the association between weight changes and self-rated health, *BMC Women's Health*, 8: 13.

Slade, Z., Coulter, A. and Joyce, L. (2009) *Parental Experience of Services for Disabled Children: Qualitative Research*. London: Department for Children, Schools and Families.

Sluijs, E., Skidmore, P.M.L., Mwanza, K., Jones, A.P., Callaghan, A.M., Ekelund, U., Harrison, F., Harvey, I., Panter, J., Wareham, N.J., Cassidy, A. and Griffin, S.J. (2008) Physical activity and dietary behaviour in a population-based sample of British 10-year old children: the SPEEDY study (Sport, Physical activity and Eating behaviour: Environmental Determinants in Young people), *BMC Public Health*, 8: 388.

Smith, A. and Twomey, B. (2002) Labour market experiences of people with disabilities, *Labour Market Trends*, August: 415–27.

Social Exclusion Unit (2004a) *Breaking the Cycle: Taking Stock of Progress and Priorities for the Future*. London: Office of the Deputy Prime Minister.

Social Exclusion Unit (2004b) *Mental Health and Social Exclusion*. London: Office of the Deputy Prime Minister.

Social Exclusion Unit (2005) *Excluded Older People*. London: Office of the Deputy Prime Minister.

Steel, L. and Kidd, W. (2001) *The Family*. Basingstoke: Palgrave.

Steel, N., Bachmann, M., Maisey, S., Shekelle, P., Breeze, E., Marmot, M. and Melzer, D. (2008) Self-reported receipt of care consistent with 32 quality indicators: national population survey of adults aged 50 or more in England, *British Medical Journal*, 337: a957.

Steeman, E., Godderis, J., Grypdonck, M., De Bal, N. and Dierckx de Casterle, B. (2007) Living with dementia from the perspective of older people: is it a positive story?, *Aging and Mental Health*, 11(2): 119–30.

Stevens, A., Berto, D., Frick, U., Kerschl, V., McSweeney, T., Schaaf, S., Tartari, M. and Werdenich, W. (2007) The victimisation of dependent drug users: findings from a European study, UK, *European Journal of Criminology*, 4(4): 385–408.

Stevenson, F.A., Barry, C.A., Britten, N., Barber, N. and Bradley, C.P. (2002) Doctor–patient communication about drugs: the evidence for shared decision-making, *Social Science and Medicine*, 50(6): 829–40.

Stewart, I. and Vaitilingham, R. (2004) *Seven Ages of Man and Woman. A Look at Life in Britain in the Second Elizabethan Era*. Swindon: ERSC.

Sudnow, D. (1967) *Passing On: The Social Organisation of Dying*. Englewood Cliffs, NJ: Prentice Hall.

Sullivan, O. (2000) The division of domestic labour: twenty years of change?, *Sociology*, 34(3): 437–56.

Sunderland, R. (2009) The real victims of this credit crunch? Women, *The Observer*, 18 January: 32–3.

Swain, J., French, S., Barnes, C. and Thomas, C. (eds) (2004) *Disabling Barriers, Enabling Environments*. London: Sage in association with the Open University.

Sweeting, H. and Gilhooly, M. (1997) Dementia and the phenomenon of social death, *Sociology of Health & Illness*, 19(1): 93–117.

Swinkels, A. and Mitchell, T. (2009) Delayed transfer from hospital to community settings: the older person's perspective, *Health and Social Care Community*, 17(1): 45–53.

Symonds, A. (1998) Social construction and the concept of community, in A. Symonds and A. Kelly (eds) *The Social Construction of Community Care*. Basingstoke: Macmillan.

Szasz, T. (1974) *The Myth of Mental Illness: Foundations of a Theory of Personal Conduct*, 6th edn. London: Paladin.

Talbot-Smith, A. and Pollock, A. (2006) *The New NHS Guide*. London: Routledge.

Taylor, D. and Bury, M. (2007) Chronic illness, expert patients and care transition, *Sociology of Health and Illness*, 29(1): 27–45.

Taylor, G. and Hawley, H. (2010) *Key Debates in Healthcare*. Maidenhead: McGraw-Hill.

Taylor, P. and Gunn, J. (1999) Homicides by people with mental illness: myth and reality, *British Journal of Psychiatry*, 174: 9–14.

Taylor, S. and Field, D. (2007) *Sociology of Health and Healthcare*, 4th edn. Oxford: Blackwell.

Thomas, P. (2004) The experience of disabled people as customers in the owner occupation market, *Housing Studies*, 19(5): 781–94.

Thomas, P. and While, A. (2007) Should nurses be leaders of integrated health care?, *Journal of Nursing Management*, 15(6): 643–8.

Thorpe, R.D. (2009) 'Doing' chromic illness? Complementary medicine use amongst people living with HIV/AIDS in Australia, *Sociology of Health and Illness*, 31(3): 375–89.

Timmermans, S. (1994) Dying of awareness: the theory of awareness contexts revisited, *Sociology of Health & Illness*, 16(3): 322–39.

Timonen, V. (2008) *Ageing Societies*. Maidenhead: Open University Press.

Tinklin, T., Ridell, S. and Wilson, A. (2004) Policy provision for disabled students in higher education in Scotland and England: the current state of play, *Studies in Higher Education*, 29(5): 637–57.

Tomassini, C., Glaser, K., van Groenou, B. and Grundy, E. (2004) Living arrangements amongst older people: an overview of older people in Europe and the USA, *Population Trends*, 115: 24–34.

Tomlinson, M. and Walker, R. (2009) *Coping with Complexity: Child and Adult Poverty*. London: Child Poverty Action Group.

Tonnies, F. (1963) *Community and Association*. New York: Harper & Row.

Tregakis, C. (2002) Social model theory: the story so far . . ., *Disability and Society*, 17(4): 457–70.

Turner, B.S. (1995) *Medical Power and Social Knowledge*, 2nd edn. London: Sage.

Twigg, J. (2006) *The Body in Health and Social Care*. Basingstoke: Palgrave Macmillan.

Twigg, J. and Atkin, K. (1994) *Carers Perceived*. Buckingham: Open University Press.

UK Commission for Employment and Skills (2009) *Working Futures 2007–2017*. London: Department for Universities, Innovation and Skills.

Ungerson, C. (1983) Why do women care?, in J. Finch and D. Groves (eds) *A Labour of Love: Women, Work and Caring*. London: Routledge & Kegan Paul.

Ungerson, C. (1987) *Policy is Personal: Sex, Gender and Informal Care*. London: Tavistock.

Union of the Physically Impaired Against Segregation (1976) *Fundamental Principles of Disability*. London: Union of Physically Impaired Against Segregation.

Ussher, J. (1991) *Women's Madness: Misogyny or Mental Illness?* London: Harvester Wheatsheaf.

van de Ven, L., Post, M., de Witte, L. and van den Heuvel, W. (2005) It takes two to tango: the inegration of people with disabilities into society, *Disability and Society*, 20(3): 311–29.

Van Hoten, D. and Bellemakers, C. (2002) Equal citizenship for all: disability policies in the Netherlands – empowerment of marginals, *Disability and Society*, 17(2): 171–85.

van Lenthe, F.J., de Bourdeaudhuij, I., Klepp, K.I., Lien, N., Moore, L., Faggiano, F., Kunst, A.E. and Mackenbach, J.P. 2009) Preventing socioeconomic inequalities in health behaviour in adolescents in Europe: background, design and methods of project TEENAGE, *BMC Public Health*, 9: 125.

Velleman, R. (2009) *Children, Young People and Alcohol: How They Learn and How to Prevent Excessive Use*. York: Joseph Rowntree Foundation.

Vera-Sanso, P. (2006) Experiences in old age: a south Indian example of how functional age is socially structured, *Oxford Development Studies*, 34(4): 457–72.

Victor, C., Scrambler, S. and Bond, J. (2009) *Growing Older*. Maidenhead: McGraw-Hill.

Vincent, J.A. (2003) *Old Age*. London: Routledge.

Vincent, J.A. (2006) Age and old age, in G. Payne (ed.) *Social Divisions*. Basingstoke: Macmillan.

Walker, A. (1983). Caring for elderly people, in J. Finch and D. Groves (eds) *A Labour of Love: Women, Work and Caring*. London: Routledge & Kegan Paul.

Walker, A. (1992) The social construction of dependency in old age, in M. Loney, R. Bocock, J. Clarke, A. Cochrane, P. Graham and M. Wilson (eds) *The State or the Market*. London: Sage.

Walshe, K. and Smith, J. (eds) (2007) *Healthcare Management*. Maidenhead: Open University Press.

Walter, T. (1994) *The Revival of Death*. London: Routledge.

Walter, T. (1999) *On Bereavement: The Culture of Grief*. Buckingham: Open University Press.

Walter, T. (2001) From cathedral to supermarket: mourning, silence and solidarity, *Sociological Review*, 49(4): 494–511.

Walter, T. (2003) Historical and cultural variants on the good death, *British Medical Journal*, 327: 218–20.

Walter, T. (2005) Three ways to arrange a funeral: mortuary variations in the modern west, *Mortality*, 10(3): 173–92.

Walter, T. (2006) Disaster, modernity and the media, in K. Garces-Foley (ed.) *Death and Religion in a Changing World*. New York: M.E. Sharpe.

Walter, T. (2007) Postmodern grief, *International Review of Sociology*, 17(1): 123–34.

Wates, M. (2004) Righting the family picture: disability and family life, in J. Swain, S. French, C. Barnes and C. Thomas (eds) *Disabling Barriers, Enabling Environments*. London: Sage.

Watson, N. (2002) 'Well, I know this is going to sound very strange to you, but I don't see myself as a disabled person': identity and disability, *Disability and Society*, 17(5): 509–27.

Watson, S. and Doyal, L. (1999) *Engendering Social Policy*. Buckingham: Open University Press.

Wear, A. (ed.) (1992) *Medicine in Society: Historical Essays*. Cambridge: Cambridge University Press.

Weaver, N.F., Hayes, L., Unwin, N.C. and Murtagh, M.J. (2008) 'Obesity' and 'clinical obesity': men's understandings of obesity and its relation to the risk of diabetes: a qualitative study, *BMC Public Health*, 8: 311.

Weber, M. (1997) *Theory of Social and Economic Organisation*. London: Free Press.

Weeks, J. (2002) Elective families: lesbian and gay life experiments, in A. Carling, S. Duncan and R. Edwards (eds) *Analysing Families: Morality and Rationality in Policy and Practice*. London: Routledge.

Weires, M., Bermejo, J.L., Sundquist, K., Sundquist, J., and Hemminki, K. (2008) Socio-economic status and overall cause-specific mortality in Sweden, *BMC Public Health*, 8: 340.

Whelan, C. (1993) The role of social support in mediating the psychological consequences of economic stress, *Sociology of Health and Illness*, 15(1): 86–100.

White, K. (2009) *An Introduction to the Sociology of Health and Illness*, 2nd edn. London: Sage.

Whitehead, M. (1987) *The Health Divide: Inequalities in Health in the 1980s*. London: Health Education Council.

Wilkinson, D. (1999) *Poor Housing and Health: A Summary of Research Evidence*. Edinburgh: The Scottish Office.

Williams, A., Ylanne, V. and Wadleigh, P.M. (2007) Selling the 'elixir of life': images of the elderly in an *Olivio* advertising campaign, *Journal of Aging Studies*, 21(1): 1–21.

Williams, S. and Calnan, M. (1996) The 'limits' of medicalization? Modern medicine and the lay populace in 'late' modernity, *Social Science and Medicine*, 42(12): 1609–20.

Williams, S.J. (2000) Chronic illness as biographical disruption or biographical disruption as chronic illness? Reflections on a core concept, *Sociology of Health and Illness*, 22(1): 40–67.

Williams, S.J. (2003) *Medicine and the Body*. London: Sage.

Wilson, P.M., Kendall, S. and Brooks, F. (2007) The Expert Patients Programme: a paradox of patient empowerment and medical dominance, *Health and Social Care in the Community*, 15(5): 426–38.

Wolf, D.A., Mendes de Leon, C.F. and Glass, T.A. (2007) Trends in rates of onset of and recovery from disability at older ages: 1982–1994, *Journals of Gerontology, Series B, Psychological Sciences and Social Sciences*, 62(1): 3–10.

Worden, J.W. (1983) *Grief Counselling and Grief Therapy*. London: Tavistock.

World Health Organization (1946) *Preamble to the Constitution of the World Health Organization*. Geneva: World Health Organization.

World Health Organization (1986) *Ottawa Charter for Health Promotion*. Copenhagen: WHO Regional Office for Europe.

World Health Organization (1990) *Health for All by the Year 2000*. Geneva: World Health Organization.

World Health Organization (2008) *The Global Burden of Disease 2004 Update*. Geneva: World Health Organization.

World Health Organization (2009) *International Classification of Functioning, Disability and Health (ICF)*. Geneva: World Health Organization.

Wright, E.O. (1989) *The Debate on Classes*. London: Verso.

Wright, E.R., Wright, D., Perry, B.L. and Foote-Ardah, C.E. (2007) Stigma and the sexual isolation of people with serious mental disorders, *Social Problems*, 54: 73–93.

Yeandle, S., Bennett, C., Buckner, L., Fry, G. and Price, C. (2007) *Diversity in Caring: Towards Equality for Carers*. London: Carers UK.

Young, M. and Cullen, L. (1996) *A Good Death: Conversations with East Londoners*. London: Routledge.

Young, M. and Wilmott, P. (1957) *Family and Kinship in East London*. London: Routledge & Kegan Paul.

Zeka, A., Melly, S.J. and Schwartz, J. (2008) The effects of socioeconomic status and indices of physical environment on reduced birth weight and preterm birth in Eastern Massachusetts, *Environmental Health*, 7: 60.

Zigmond, D. (2009) No country for old men: the rise of managerialism and the new cultural vacuum, *Public Policy Research*, 16(2): 133–7.

Zola, I.K. (1972) Medicine as an institution of social control, *Sociological Review*, 20: 487–54.

Zola, I.K. (1973) Pathways to the doctor – from person to patient, *Social Science and Medicine*, 7: 677–87.

Index

The index entries appear in word-by-word alphabetical order.

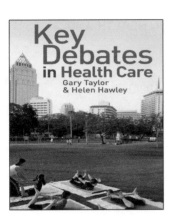

KEY DEBATES IN HEALTHCARE

Gary Taylor and Helen Hawley

9780335223947 (Paperback)
2010

eBook also available

The book examines the different models of health and healthcare delivery, and explores alternative methods of providing healthcare, using the state, the private sector or the voluntary sector. Through these debates the book will help readers explore issues such as health inequalities, health promotion and service delivery, and establish their own perspective on issues of health and society.

Key features:

- Theoretical perspectives to help understand the logic and implications of broad social and political arguments related to health
- Policy developments to show the practical application of ideas in Britain, the United States and in other parts of the world
- Healthcare scenarios to help make connections between theory, policy and practice

www.openup.co.uk

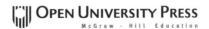 OPEN UNIVERSITY PRESS
McGraw - Hill Education

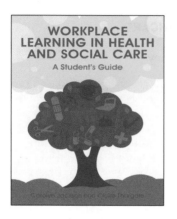

**WORKPLACE LEARNING IN HEALTH AND
SOCIAL CARE**
A Student's Guide

Carolyn Jackson and Claire Thurgate

9780335237500 (Paperback)

February 2011

eBook also available

This is a practical resource for anyone undertaking work based learning in health and social care. It introduces and explores the practicalities of learning in a healthcare setting, and is designed to help you make the most of your work based learning experience when studying for a foundation degree or other qualification.

Key features:

- Contains examples, vignettes and quotes
- Includes practical tools and worksheets to use in practice and study
- Provides practical strategies and exercises to strengthen capacity to learn at work and reflect on personal and professional development goals

www.openup.co.uk

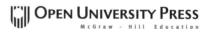

OPEN UNIVERSITY PRESS
McGraw · Hill Education